Culpeper's Complete Herbal

Culpeper's Complete Herbal

Over 400 herbs and their uses

Nicholas Culpeper

This edition published in 2023 by Arcturus Publishing Limited
26/27 Bickels Yard, 151–153 Bermondsey Street,
London SE1 3HA

AD007176UK

Printed in the US

CONTENTS

HEALTH WARNING

Some wild plants are poisonous, so please exercise caution
if you decide to experiment with the remedies in this book.
Readers should also be aware that a number of plants are
endangered and therefore protected by law, so picking
them may be forbidden. It is illegal to dig up wild plants.

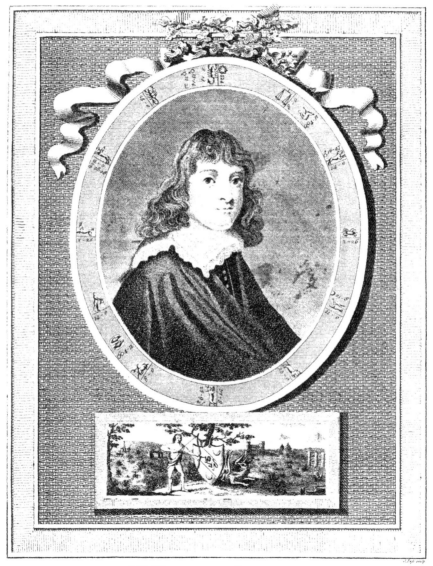

Mʳ. NICHOLAS CULPEPER.

BORN 18ᵗʰ October 11 m. PM. 1616. DEPARTED THIS LIFE 10ᵗʰ of January 1654.

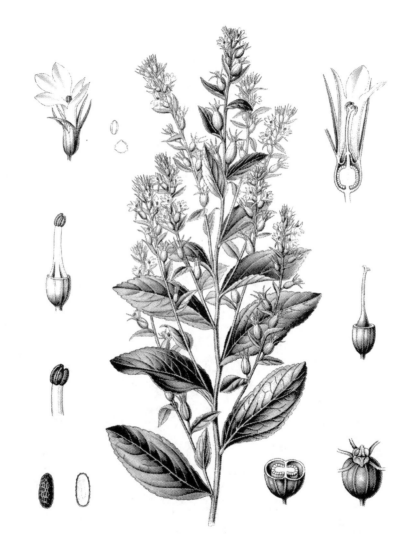

INTRODUCTION

From time to time a book is written that not only fulfils the purpose of the day but catches the imagination of generations long into the future, when the world in which it was first printed is utterly changed. Such a book is *Culpeper's Complete Herbal*, still read for what it has to tell us about the use of plants for healing as well as for its historical interest. With herbs and beauty products still bearing his name, there can be few people who haven't heard of this legendary practitioner of herbal medicine.

EARLY LIFE
Nicholas Culpeper was born on 18 October 1616 and brought up near Isfield in Sussex. His family sent him to Cambridge to study for the church, but he was far more interested in exploring anatomy and the works of the legendary Greek physicians Hippocrates and Galen, born in 460 BC and *c.*AD125 respectively. He never graduated in either discipline, however. A secret relationship with an heiress, with whom he planned to elope to the Netherlands, ended tragically when her coach was struck by lightning on route to their rendezvous. In a stroke, Culpeper had now lost not only his future wife and his place at Cambridge, but also his family's goodwill, to the extent that he was disinherited.

Determined to pursue his interest in healing the sick, Culpeper found an apprenticeship with Francis Drake, an apothecary in Threadneedle Street in London. During this period he was trained in the recognition and use of herbs by Thomas Johnson, editor of the 1633 edition of John Gerard's famous *Herbal*, first published in 1597, and studied astrology under the tutelage of William Lilly, the greatest English astrologer of the 17th century.

Equipped with these skills, Culpeper set up a practice in Red Lion Street in Spitalfields. His location in a poor area of London and his willingness to see impoverished patients without charge soon led to him taking on as many as 40 patients a day. Such people could not afford the physicians who treated the wealthy, of whom Culpeper had a very low opinion in respect to both their honesty and effectiveness.

FREEDOM TO PUBLISH
When the Civil War broke out in 1642, the Star Chamber and Court of High Commissioners were dismantled, ending the censorship of all printed material. This meant Culpeper could now disseminate knowledge previously withheld from the public. In 1649 he published an English translation of the Royal College of Physicians' *Pharmacopoeia Londinensis*; this had formerly been the preserve of doctors of medicine who understood Latin and were accustomed to writing diagnoses and prescriptions that most of their patients had no hope of comprehending. He added his own opinions on the uses of the drugs described. This assault on the Establishment caused fury at the College of Physicians.

Yet under Cromwell's Commonwealth there was nothing they could do to prevent its publication.

On 5 September 1653, Culpeper completed his masterwork, *The English Physician*, commonly known as *Culpeper's Complete Herbal*. In a letter to his wife, Alice, Culpeper predicted it would be the source of his continuing fame, and how right he was: *The English Physician* has been continuously in print since the 17th century and is the most widely disseminated secular English text ever to have existed.

Culpeper died on 10 January 1654 at the age of just 38. It is believed that tuberculosis arising from a bullet wound in the shoulder he sustained during the siege of Reading, in 1643, was the cause of his demise.

CULPEPER TODAY

Inevitably, Culpeper's view of medicine was very different from ours today. In his time, the human body was thought to be ruled by four 'humours' – black bile, yellow bile, phlegm and blood. This idea may have first arisen in Ancient Egypt or Mesopotamia but was developed in Ancient Greece, when the humours were linked with the elements fire, water, earth and air, with the seasons and with temperamental characteristics. From a medical point of view, the ideal was for the humours to be in balance in the body (a state of 'eucrasia') to give perfect health, while disease was caused by their disproportion ('dyscrasia'). The practice of bloodletting, for example, was done to remove a harmful excess of blood, linked with the liver; the gall bladder was associated with yellow bile, an overabundance of which caused a choleric or bad-tempered nature and diseases of warm and dry origin.

Although many ancient physicians disagreed with the theory of humours, it was only discredited in the mid-19th century with the discovery of cellular pathology by the German scientist Rudolf Virchow. In the *Herbal*, Culpeper's readers will find few remedies that don't discuss the role of a herb in relation to its impact on one of the four humours. More mystifying still are conditions such as 'wandering womb', referring to the belief that the womb moved around the body, sometimes rising so high up that a woman might feel as if she were being strangled, causing hysteria. Culpeper recommends rubbing the soles of the feet with burdock to persuade the womb to move downwards, which cannot but arouse scepticism in the modern reader.

Yet Culpeper's knowledge of herbs still has validity today, and modern medication is largely derived from plant material – including the ubiquitous aspirin, from the willow tree. While it's clear that one should not blithely follow Culpeper's advice, particularly for internal remedies, without further consultation, his *Herbal* combines archaic charm with a wealth of information that is much in tune with our increasing interest in the use of natural remedies to promote good health.

ACONITUM

Of this there are two sorts, the one bearing blue flowers, the other yellow; it is also called wolf's-bane, and the blue is generally known by the name of monk's-hood.

DESCRIPTION The wolf's-bane which bears the blue flower is small, but grows up to a cubit high; the leaves are split and jagged, the flowers in long rows toward the tops of the stalks, gaping like hoods; on the hoary root grows as it were a little knob, whence it spreads itself abroad, and multiplies.

PLACE The monk's-hood or blue wolf's-bane is very common in many gardens. The other is rarely found, but grows in forests and dark low woods and valleys in some parts of Germany and France.

TIME They flower in April, May, and June.

GOVERNMENT AND DANGER The plants are hot and dry in the fourth degree; if they be inwardly taken, they inflame the heart, burn the inward parts, and destroy life itself. Dodonæus reports of some men at Antwerp, who unawares did eat some of the monk's-hood in a salad, instead of some other herb, and died forthwith: this I write that people who have it in their gardens might beware of it.

ADDER'S TONGUE, OR SERPENT'S TONGUE

DESCRIPTION This small herb (*Ophioglossum*) has but one leaf, which grows with the stalk a finger's length above the ground, being fat, and of a fresh green colour; broad like the water plantain, but less so, without any middle rib in it; from the bottom of which leaf, on the inside, rises up ordinarily one, sometimes two or three, small slender stalks, the upper half whereof is somewhat bigger, and dented with small round dents of yellowish-green colour, like the tongue of an adder or serpent. The root continues all the year.

PLACE It grows in moist meadows and such-like places.

TIME It is to be found in April and May, for it quickly perishes with a little heat.

GOVERNMENT AND VIRTUES It is an herb under the dominion of the Moon in Cancer. It is temperate in respect of heat, but dry in the second degree. The said juice, given in the distilled water of oaken buds, is very good for women who have their usual menses, or discharges, slowing down too abundantly. The leaves infused or boiled in oil omphacine, or unripe olives set in the sun for certain days, or the green leaves sufficiently boiled in the said oil, make an excellent green balsam, not only for green and fresh wounds, but also for old and inveterate ulcers; especially if a little fine clear turpentine be dissolved therein.

AGRIMONY

DESCRIPTION   This has divers long leaves, some greater, some smaller, set upon a stalk, all of them dented about the edges, green above, and greyish underneath, and a little hairy withal. Among which rises up usually but one strong, round, hairy, brown stalk, two or three feet high, with smaller leaves set here and there upon it; at the top whereof grow many yellow flowers one above another in long spikes, after which come rough heads of seeds hanging downwards, which will cleave to and stick upon garments, or any thing that shall rub against them. The root is black, long, and somewhat woody, abiding many years, and shooting afresh every spring; which root, though small, has a pleasant smell.

PLACE   It grows upon banks, near the sides of hedges or rails.

TIME   It flowers in July and August, the seed being ripe shortly after.

GOVERNMENT AND VIRTUES   It is moderately hot and moist, according to the nature of Jupiter, and good for the gout, either used outwardly in an oil or ointment, or inwardly in an electuary or syrup. It has moreover been recommended in dropsies and the jaundice. Externally, it has indeed its use: I have seen very bad sore legs cured by bathing and fomenting them with a decoction of this plant. It is of a cleansing and cutting faculty, without any manifest heat, moderately drying and binding. The decoction of the herb made with wine, and drunk, helps them that have foul, troubled, or bloody water, and causes them to make water clear and speedily. A draught of the decoction, taken warm before the fit, first relieves, and in time removes, the tertian or quartan ague. The leaves and seed, taken in wine, stay the bloody-flux.

WATER-AGRIMONY

It is called in some countries water-hemp, bastard-hemp, and bastard-agrimony; also *eupatorium* and *hepatorium*, because it strengthens the liver.

DESCRIPTION   The root continues a long time, having many long slender strings; the stalks grow up about two feet high, sometimes higher; they are of a

PLATE 1

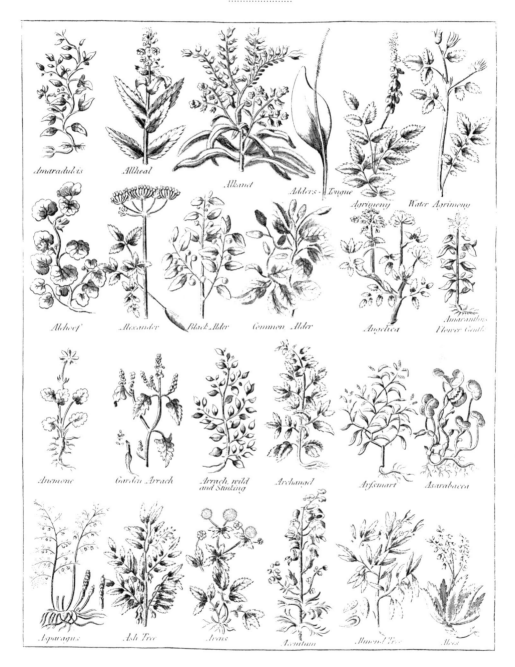

Amaradulcis   Allheal   Alkanet   Adders-Tongue   Agrimony   Water Agrimony

Alehoof   Alexander   Black Alder   Common Alder   Angelica   Amaranthus Flower Gentle

Anemone   Garden Arrach   Arrach, wild and Stinking   Archangel   Arssmart   Asarabacca

Asparagus   Ash Tree   Avens   Aconitum   Almond Tree   Moss dark purple colour; the branches are many, growing at a distance the one from the other, the one from the one side of the stalk, the other from the opposite point; the leaves are winged, and much indented at the edges; the flowers grow at the tops of the branches, of a brown-yellow colour, with black spots, having a substance within the midst of them like that of a daisy; if you rub them between your fingers, they smell like resin, or cedar when it is burnt; the seeds are long, and easily stick to any woollen thing they touch.

PLACE They delight not in heat, and therefore are not so frequently found in the southern parts of England as in the north; you may look for them in cold grounds, by ponds and ditch-sides, also by running waters; sometimes you will find them growing in the waters.

TIME They all flower in July and August, and the seed is ripe presently after.

GOVERNMENT AND VIRTUES It is a plant of Jupiter, as well as the other agrimony; only this belongs to the celestial sign Cancer. It heals and dries, cuts and cleanses thick and tough humours of the breast; and for this I hold it inferior to but few herbs that grow. It helps the dropsy and yellow jaundice. It opens obstructions of the liver, and mollifies the hardness of the spleen; being applied outwardly, it breaks abscesses; taken inwardly, it is an excellent remedy for the third-day ague. The smoke of the herb, being burnt, drives away flies, wasps, &c. and it strengthens the lungs exceedingly. Country people give it to their cattle when they are troubled with the cough, or broken winded.

BLACK ALDER-TREE

DESCRIPTION AND NAMES This grows up like a small shrub, or bush, and spreads in many branches; the wood is white, and red at the core, the bark blackish with white spots, the inner bark yellow, the leaves somewhat like the common alder; the flowers are white, and come forth at the joints with the leaves; the berries are round, first green, then red, and black when they are ripe. The Latins call it *frangula*, and *alnus nigra baccifera*; in Hampshire it is usually known by the name of dog-wood.

PLACE This tree or shrub may be found plentifully in St John's wood by Hornsey, and in the woods upon Hampstead Heath, as also at a wood called the Old Park at Barcomb in Sussex, near the brook's side.

TIME It flowers in May, and the berries are ripe in September.

GOVERNMENT AND VIRTUES It is a tree of Saturn. The inner bark thereof purges downwards both choler and phlegm, and the watery humours of such as have the dropsy, and strengthens the inward parts again by binding. The green leaves of this tree, being put into travellers' shoes, ease pain, and remove weariness. A black colour like ink is made with the bark of alder rubbed off with a rusty iron, and infused in water for some days. Some use it to dye. If the dried bark hereof be boiled with agrimony, wormwood, dodder, hops, and some fennel, with smallage, endive, and succory roots, and a reasonable draught taken every morning for some time together, it purges and strengthens the liver and spleen. It is to be understood, that these things are performed by the dried bark; for the fresh green bark, taken inwardly, provokes strong vomitings, pains in the stomach, and gripings in the belly. The outer bark contrarywise doth bind the body, and is helpful for all lasks and fluxes thereof; but this must also be dried first, whereby it will work the better. The inner bark boiled in vinegar is an approved remedy to kill lice, to cure the itch, and take away scabs by drying them up in a short time; it is singularly good to wash the teeth, to take away the pains, to fasten those that are loose, to cleanse them and keep them sound. The leaves are good fodder for kine, to make them give more milk.

COMMON ALDER-TREE

DESCRIPTION It grows to a reasonable height, and spreads much if it likes the place.

PLACE AND TIME It delights to grow in moist woods and watery places, flowering in April or May, and yielding the seed in September.

GOVERNMENT AND USE It is a tree under the dominion of Venus, and of Pisces; and therefore the decoction or distilled water of the leaves is excellent against burnings and inflammation, either with wounds or without, to bathe the place grieved with. If you cannot get the leaves, make use of the bark in the same manner. The leaves and bark of the alder-tree are cooling, drying, and binding. The fresh leaves laid upon swellings dissolves them, and stay the inflammations; the leaves, put under the bare feet galled with travelling, are a great refreshing to them.

ALE-HOOF, OR GROUND-IVY

Several countries give it several names: it is called cat's-foot, ground-ivy, gill-go-by-ground and gill-creep-by-ground, tun-hoof, hay-maids, and ale-hoof.

DESCRIPTION This well-known herb lies, spreads, and creeps, upon the ground, shooting forth roots at the corners of the tender-jointed stalks, set all along with two round leaves at every joint, somewhat hairy, crumpled, and unevenly dented about the edges, with round dents: at the joints likewise with the leaves, towards the ends of the branches, come forth hollow long flowers, of a bluish-purple colour, with small white spots upon the lips that hang down.

PLACE It is commonly found under the hedges, and on the sides of ditches, under houses, or in shadowed lanes, and other waste grounds, in almost every part of the land.

TIME It flowers somewhat early, and abides so a great while; the leaves continue green until winter, and sometimes abide, except the winter be very sharp and cold.

GOVERNMENT AND VIRTUES It is an herb of Venus. You may usually find it all the year long, except the weather be extreme frosty. It is quick, sharp, and bitter, in taste, and is thereby found to be hot and dry; a singular herb for all inward wounds, either by itself or boiled with other like herbs; and, being drunk, it in a short time eases all griping pains, windy and choleric humours in the stomach, spleen, or belly. The decoction of it in wine, drunk for some time together, procures ease unto them that are troubled with the sciatica, or hip-gout, as also the gout in the hands, knees, or feet; and, if you put to the decoction some honey, and a little burnt allum, it is excellent good to gargle any sore mouth or throat.

ALEXANDER

It is also called alisander, horse-parsley, and wild-parsley, and black pot-herb: the seed of it is usually sold in the apothecaries shops as Macedonian parsley-seed.

DESCRIPTION It is usually sown in all the gardens in Europe, and so well known that it needs no further description.

TIME They flower in June and July, and the seed is ripe in August.

GOVERNMENT AND VIRTUES It is an herb of Jupiter, and therefore friendly to nature, for it warms a cold stomach, and opens stoppings of the liver, and wonderfully helps the spleen; it is good to expel the after-birth.

ALHEAL

It is called alheal, Hercules's alheal, and Hercules's woundwort; because it is supposed that Hercules learned the virtues of this herb from Chiron, when he learned physic of him: some call it panay, and others opopanawort.

DESCRIPTION Its root is long, thick, and full of juice, of a hot and biting taste; the leaves are large, and winged almost like ash-tree leaves, but somewhat hairy, each leaf consisting of five or six pair of such wings set one against the other, upon stalks broad below, but narrow toward the end; one of the leaves is a little deeper at the bottom than the other, of a fair, fresh, yellowish-green colour; they are of a bitterish taste, being chewed. From among these rises a green stalk, round in form, great and strong in magnitude, five or six feet in altitude, with many joints and some leaves; towards the top come forth umbels of small yellow flowers, and after they are gone you may find whitish-yellow short flat seeds.

TIME It does not flower till the latter end of the summer, and sheds its seeds presently after.

GOVERNMENT AND VIRTUES It is under the dominion of Mars. It helps the gout, cramp, and seizures; and helps all joint aches; helps all cold griefs of the head, vertigo, fits, and lethargy; obstructions of the liver and spleen, stone in the kidneys and bladder. It provokes menses; it is excellent good for the grief of the sinews, itch, sores, and toothache; and purges choler very gently.

ALKANET

Besides the common name, it is called *orchanet* and *Spanish bugloss*, and by apothecaries *anchusa*.

DESCRIPTION Of the many sorts of this herb there is but one grows commonly in this nation. It has a great and thick root of a reddish colour; long, narrow, and hairy leaves, green like the leaves of bugloss, which lie very thick upon the ground; the stalks rise up compassed about thick with leaves, which are less and narrower than the former; they are tender and slender; the flowers are hollow, small, and of a reddish-purple colour; the seed is greyish.

PLACE It grows in Kent near Rochester, and in many places in the West Country, both in Devonshire and Cornwall.

TIME They flower in July and the beginning of August, and the seed is ripe soon after; but the root is in its prime, as carrots and parsnips are, before the herb runs up to stalk.

GOVERNMENT AND VIRTUES It is an herb under the dominion of Venus. It helps ulcers, hot inflammations and burnings by common fire; for these uses, your best way is to make it into an ointment. Also if you make a vinegar of it, it helps the jaundice, spleen, and gravel in the kidneys. It stays the flux of the belly, and helps fits of the womb. An ointment made of it is excellent for green wounds, pricks, or thrusts.

ALMOND-TREE

DESCRIPTION AND NAMES Of this tree there are two kinds, the one bearing sweet fruit, the other bitter. They grow bigger than any peach-tree; I have seen a bitter almond-tree in Hampshire as big as a great plum-tree. It has leaves much like peach leaves, and is called in Latin *amigdalum*; they grow plentifully in Turkey and Barbary.

NATURE AND VIRTUES The sweet almonds are hot and moist in the first degree, the bitter dry in the second. It is a plant of Jupiter. The sweet almonds nourish the body, and increase the seed; they strengthen the breath, cleanse the kidneys, and open the passages of urine. There is a fine pleasant oil drawn out of the sweet almonds, which, being taken with sugar-candy, is excellent against dry coughs and hoarseness; it is good for those that have any inward sore, and for such as are troubled with kidney stone, because it makes slippery the passages of the urine. Bitter almonds also open obstructions of the liver and spleen, expel wind, cleanse the lungs from phlegm, and provoke urine and menses; the oil of them helps pains of the womb.

ALOE, OR ALOES

NAMES By the same name of aloe or aloes is the condensed juice of this plant called in all parts of Europe; the plant is also called sea-housleek, and sea-ay-green.

DESCRIPTION This plant has very long leaves, thick, and set round about with short points or crests, standing wide one from another; the root is thick and long; all the herb is of a strong savour, and bitter taste; out of this herb is drawn a juice, which is dried, and called aloes in different parts of the world.

PLACE Aloe grows very plenteously in India, and from thence comes the best juice; it grows also in many places of Asia and Arabia, near the sea-side.

GOVERNMENT AND VIRTUES It is a martial plant, hot in the second degree, and dry in the third, of a very bitter taste; the juice, being refined and clarified, is of a clear and blackish clean brown colour; it opens the belly, and purges cold phlegmatic and choleric humours: it is the basis in almost all pills. It may be taken with cinnamon, ginger, mace, galingal, or aniseed, to assuage and drive away pains of the stomach, and to comfort and warm the same. Aloe made into powder, and strewed upon new bloody wounds, stops the blood and heals the wound. The same, boiled with wine and honey, heals rifts and outgrowings of the fundament, and stops the flux of the hæmorrhoids. Aloes mixed with oil of roses and vinegar, and laid to the forehead and temples, assuages the headache.

AMARA-DULCIS

Besides *amara-dulcis*, some call it morral, others bitter-sweet, some wood-nightshade, and others felon-wort.

DESCRIPTION   It grows up with woody stalks even to a man's height, and sometimes higher; the leaves fall off at the approach of winter, and spring out of the same stalk again at spring-time; the branch has a whitish bark, and a pith in the middle of it; the main branch spreads itself out into many small ones, with claspers, laying hold on what is next to them, as vines do; it bears many leaves, growing in no order at all. The leaves are longish, though somewhat broad and pointed at the ends; many of them have two little leaves growing at the end of their footstalk, some of them have but one, and some none; the leaves are of a pale green colour; the flowers are of a purple colour, or of a perfect blue, like to violets, and they stand many of them together in knots; the berries are green at the first, but, when they are ripe, they are very red; if you taste them, you shall find them just as the crab apples which we in Sussex call bitter-sweet, viz. sweet at first, and bitter afterwards.

PLACE   They grow commonly almost throughout England, especially in moist and shady places.

TIME   The leaves shoot out about the latter end of March; if the temperature of the air be ordinary, it flowers in July, and the seeds are ripe soon after, usually in the next month.

GOVERNMENT AND VIRTUES   It is under the planet Mercury, and a notable herb of his also, if it be rightly gathered under his influence. It is excellent good to remove witchcraft, both in men and beasts. Being tied about the neck, it is one of the most admirable remedies for the vertigo, or dizziness in the head. Country people commonly take the berries of it, and, having bruised them, they apply them to purulent infections on the fingers.

AMARANTHUS

Besides this common name, by which it is best known by the florists of our days, it is also called flower-gentle, flower-velure, floramor, and velvet-flower.

DESCRIPTION It being a garden flower, and well known to every one that keeps of it, I might forbear the description; yet notwithstanding, because some desire it, I shall give it. It runs up with a stalk three feet high, streaked, and somewhat reddish towards the root, but very smooth, divided towards the top with small branches, among which stand long broad leaves of a reddish-green colour, and slippery. The flowers are not properly flowers, but tufts, very beautiful to behold, but of no smell, of a reddish colour; if you bruise them, they yield juice of the same colour; being gathered, they keep their beauty a long time; the seed is of a shining black colour.

TIME They continue in flower from August till the frosts nip them.

GOVERNMENT AND VIRTUES It is under the dominion of Saturn, and is an excellent qualifier of the unruly actions and passions of Venus, though Mars also should join with her. The flowers, dried, and beaten into powder, stop menses in women. The flowers stop all fluxes of blood whether in man or woman, bleeding either by the nose or wound. There is also a sort of amaranthus which bears a white flower, which stops discharges in women, and is a most singular remedy for the venereal disease.

ANEMONE

Called also wind-flower, because they say the flowers never open but when the wind blows: Pliny is my author; if it be not so, blame him. The seed also, if it bears any at all, flies away with the wind.

PLACE AND TIME They are sown usually in the gardens of the curious, and flower in the spring-time.

GOVERNMENT AND VIRTUES It is under the dominion of Mars, being supposed to be a kind of crow-foot. The leaves provoke menses mightily, being boiled and the decoction drunk. The body being bathed with the decoction of them cures the leprosy. The leaves being crushed, and the juice snuffed up the nose, purges the head greatly: so does the root being chewed in the mouth, for it brings away many watery and phlegmatic humours, and is therefore excellent for lethargy. Being made into an ointment, and the eyelids anointed therewith, it helps inflammations of the eyes.

ANGELICA

That is, the angelical or angel-like herb. Angelica grows up with great hollow stalks, four or five feet high, having broad divided leaves, of a pale green colour;

at the top comes forth large umbels of white flowers, after which succeed flat seed, somewhat whitish.

PLACE AND TIME Angelica grows commonly in our gardens, and wild also in many places; it flowers about July, and the seed is ripe soon after.

GOVERNMENT AND VIRTUES It is an herb of the Sun in Leo. The water distilled out of the roots of angelica, or the powder of the same, is good against gnawing and pains of the belly occasioned by cold. It is good against all inward diseases, such as pleurisy; for the diseases of the lungs, if they come of a cold cause; and from difficulty in passing water, or of a blockage. It is good for a woman in labour. It expels wind that is in the body, and eases the pain that comes from the same. The root may be soaked in wine or water, as the nature of the illness requires. The root or the juice, put into an hollow tooth, takes away the ache. The water, the juice, or the powder of this root, sprinkled upon the diseased place, is a very good remedy against sores. The water is good to be laid on places diseased with the gout and sciatica, for it eases the pain. The seed is of like virtue with the root.

The wild angelica, that grows here in the low woods, and by the water, is not of such virtue; yet the surgeons steep the root of it in wine to heal infected wounds. The stalks or roots, candied and eaten fasting, are good preservatives in time of infection, and at other times to warm and comfort a cold stomach. A water distilled from the root simply, or steeped in wine, and distilled in glass, is much more effectual than the water of the leaves. It helps pains of the colic and the slow and painful discharge of the urine, procures women's menses, and expels the after-birth.

ARCHANGEL

To put a gloss upon their practice, the physicians call archangel the herb which country people know by the name of dead nettles.

DESCRIPTION The red archangel has divers square stalks, somewhat hairy; at the joints grow two green leaves dented about the edges, opposite each other, the lowest upon long stalks, but without any towards the tops, which are somewhat round, yet pointed, and a little crumpled and hairy: round about the upper joints, where the leaves grow thick, are sundry gaping flowers of a pale reddish colour; after which come the seeds, three or four in a husk. The root is small and thready, perishing every year; the whole plant has a strong scent.

White archangel has divers square stalks, none standing upright, but bending downward, whereon stand two leaves at a joint, larger and more pointed than the other, dented about the edges, and greener also, more like nettle-leaves, but not stinging, yet hairy: at the joints, with the leaves, stand larger and more open gaping white flowers, in husks round about the stalks, but not with such a bush of leaves and flowers set in the top as red archangel. They have small roundish black seeds. The root is white, with many strings at it, not growing downward, but lying under the upper crust of the earth, and surviving many years, spreading. This has not so strong a scent as the former plant.

Yellow archangel is like the white in the stalks and leaves, but the stalks are more straight and upright, and the joints with leaves are farther asunder, having longer leaves than the former, and the flowers a little larger and more gaping, of a fair yellow colour in most, in some paler. The roots are like the white, only they creep not so much on the ground.

PLACE They grow almost every where, unless it be in the middle of the street; the yellow most usually in the wet grounds of woods, and sometimes in the dryer, in divers counties.

TIME They flower from the beginning of the spring all the summer long.

VIRTUES AND USE The archangels are somewhat hot, and dryer than the stinging nettles, and used with better success for obstruction and hardness of the spleen, by using the decoction of the herb in wine, and afterwards applying the herb hot to the region of the spleen as a plaster, or the decoction with sponges. For women, the flowers of the white archangel are preserved to be used to stop discharges, and the flowers of the red to stop bleeding.

GARDEN ARRACH

Called also orach, and orage.

TIME It flowers and seeds from June to the end of August.

GOVERNMENT AND VIRTUES It is under the government of the Moon and in quality cold and moist like her. When eaten it softens and loosens the body of man, and encourages the expulsion of waste. The herb, whether it be bruised and applied to the throat or boiled and applied in like manner, is excellent good for swellings in the throat; the best way I suppose is to boil it, and, having drunk the decoction inwardly, apply the herb outwardly; the decoction of it besides is an excellent remedy for the yellow jaundice.

ARRACH, WILD AND STINKING

Called also *vulvaria*, from that part of the body upon which it is most used: also dog's arrach, goat's arrach, and stinking motherwort.

DESCRIPTION This has small and almost round leaves, yet a little pointed, and without dent or cut, of a dusky mealy colour, growing on the slender stalks and branches that spread on the ground, with small flowers in clusters set with the leaves, and small seeds succeeding like the rest, perishing yearly, and rising again with its own sowing. It smells like old rotten fish, or something worse.

PLACE It grows usually upon dunghills.

TIME They flower in June and July, and the seed is ripe quickly after.

GOVERNMENT AND VIRTUES It is an herb under the dominion of Venus, and under the sign Scorpio. I commend this for an universal medicine for the womb, and such a medicine as will easily, safely, and speedily, cure any disease thereof, as the fits of the mother, dislocation, or falling out thereof; it cools the womb being over-heated. It makes barren women fruitful, it cleanses the womb if it be foul, and strengthens it exceedingly; it provokes the menses if they be stopped, and stops them if they flow immoderately: you can desire no good to your womb but this herb will effect it.

ARSESMART

The hot arsesmart is called also water-pepper, and culrage; the mild arsesmart is called dead arsesmart, *persicaria*, or peach-wort, because the leaves are so like the leaves of a peach-tree; it is also called *plumbago*.

DESCRIPTION The mild arsesmart has broad leaves set at the great red joints of the stalks, with semicircular blackish marks on them usually, yet sometimes without. The flowers grow in long spikes usually, either bluish or whitish, with such-like seed following. The root is long, with many strings, perishing yearly; this has no sharp taste, as another sort has, which is quick and biting, but rather sour like sorrel.

PLACE It grows in watery places, ditches, and the like; which for the most part are dry in summer.

TIME It flowers in June, and the seed is ripe in August.

GOVERNMENT AND VIRTUES That which is hot and biting is under the dominion of Mars, but Saturn challenges the other. The water-arsesmart is of great use in the stone of the kidneys or bladder, a draught of it being taken every morning for two or three months together.

The root or seed, put into an aching hollow tooth, takes off the pain. There is scarcely any thing more effectual to drive away flies, for, whatever wounds or ulcers cattle have, if they are anointed with the juice of arsesmart, the flies will not come near. The juice thereof dropped in, or otherwise applied, consumes all cold swellings, and dissolves the congealed blood of bruises by strokes, falls, &c. The leaves bruised, and laid to the joint that has an infection thereon, takes it away. If the hot arsesmart be strewed in a chamber, it will drive away the flies, in the hottest time of summer; a good handful of the hot biting arsesmart, put under a horse's saddle, will make him travel the better, although he were half tired before: the mild arsesmart is good against abscesses and inflammations at the beginning, and to heal infected wounds.

ARTICHOKE

The latins call them *cineria*, and they are also termed *artichocus*.

GOVERNMENT AND VIRTUES They are under the dominion of Venus. They are great provocatives to lust, yet stay the involuntary course of natural seed in man; the decoction of the root boiled in wine, or the root bruised and distilled in wine, and drunk, purges the urine exceedingly.

ASARABACCA

DESCRIPTION Asarabacca has many heads rising from the roots, from whence come many smooth leaves, every one upon its own stalk, which are rounder and bigger than violet-leaves, thicker also, and of a dark green shining colour on the upper-side, and of a paler yellow-green underneath, little or nothing dented about the edges. From among them rise small, round, hollow, brown-green husks, upon short stalks about an inch long, divided at the brims into five divisions, very like the cups or heads of herbane-seed, but smaller. These are all the flowers it carries, which are somewhat sweet-smelling, and when they are ripe contain small cornered rough seeds, very like the kernels of grapes or raisins. The roots are small and whitish, spreading divers ways in the ground, and increasing into divers heads.

PLACE It grows frequently in gardens.

TIME They keep their leaves green all the winter, but shoot forth new in the spring, and with them come forth those heads or flowers which give ripe seed about midsummer, or somewhat after.

GOVERNMENT AND VIRTUES It is a plant under the dominion of Mars. Being boiled in whey, it wonderfully helps the obstructions of the liver and spleen, and is therefore profitable for the dropsy and jaundice. An oil made thereof by setting it in the Sun, with some laudanum added to it, provokes sweating, the ridge of the back being anointed therewith, and thereby drives away the shaking fits of the ague. The common use hereof, is to take the juice of five or seven leaves in a little drink to cause vomiting; the roots have also the same virtue, though they do not operate so forcibly.

I shall desire ignorant people to forbear the use of the leaves: the roots purge more gently. The truth is, I fancy purging and vomiting medicines as little as any man breathing, for they weaken nature, nor shall ever advise them to be used unless upon urgent necessity.

ASH-TREE

GOVERNMENT AND VIRTUES It is governed by the Sun. The water distilled therefrom, being taken in a small quantity every morning fasting, is a singular medicine for those that are subject to the dropsy. The decoction of the leaves, in white wine, helps to break the kidney stone and expel it, and cures the jaundice. The kernels within the husks, commonly called ashen keys, prevail against stitches and pains in the side, proceeding from wind, and void the kidney stone by provoking urine.

ASPARAGUS, SPARAGUS, OR SPERAGE

DESCRIPTION It rises up at first with divers white-green scaly heads, very brittle or easy to break while they are young, which afterwards rise up in long and slender green stalks, of the bigness of an ordinary riding-wand at the bottom of most, or bigger or lesser, as the roots are of growth; on the stalks are set divers branches of green leaves, shorter and smaller than fennel to the top; at the joints whereof come forth small mossy yellowish flowers, which turn into round berries, green at the first, and of an excellent red colour when they are ripe, looking like beads of coral, wherein are contained exceeding hard black seeds. The roots are dispersed from a spongeous head into many long, thick, and round, strings, whereby it sucks much nourishment out of the ground, and increases plentifully thereby.

PRICKLY ASPARAGUS, SPARAGUS, OR SPERAGE

DESCRIPTION It grows usually in gardens, and some of it grows wild in Appleton-meadow, in Gloucestershire, where the poor people do gather the buds, or young shoots, and sell them cheaper than our garden asparagus is sold in London.

TIME They do for the most part flower, and bear their berries, late in the year, or not at all, although they are housed in winter.

GOVERNMENT AND VIRTUES They are both under the dominion of Jupiter. The young buds or branches, boiled in ordinary broth, make the belly soluble and open, and are good against the stranguary, or difficulty of making water. It expels the gravel and stone out of the kidneys, and helps pains in the loins: if boiled in white wine or vinegar, it is prevalent for them that have their arteries loosened, or are troubled with the hip-gout, or sciatica. The decoction of the roots, being taken fasting several mornings together, stirs up bodily lust in man or woman. The garden asparagus nourishes more than the wild, yet it has the same effect in all the aforementioned diseases.

The decoction of the roots in white wine, and the back and belly bathed therewith, or kneeling or lying down in the same, or sitting therein as a bath, has been found effectual against pains of the loins and bladder, pains of the womb and colic, and generally against all pains that happen to the lower parts of the body; and is no less effectual against stiff and benumbed sinews, or those that are shrunk by cramps and convulsions; it also helps the sciatica.

AVENS, CALLED ALSO CLOVE-WORT, AND HERB BENET

DESCRIPTION The ordinary avens has many long, rough, dark green, winged leaves, rising from the root, every one made of many leaves, set on each side of the middle rib. The largest three grow at the end, and are snipped or dented round about the edges; the other being small pieces, sometimes two, and sometimes four, standing on each side of the middle rib underneath them: among which do rise up divers rough or hairy stalks, about two feet high, branching forth with leaves at every joint, not so long as those below, but almost as much cut in on the edges, some into three parts, some into more.

On the tops of the branches stand small pale yellow flowers, consisting of five leaves, like the flowers of cinquefoil, but larger. In the middle stands a large green head, which, when the flower is fallen, grows rough and round, being made of many long greenish-purple seeds, like grains, which will stick upon your clothes. The root consists of many brownish strings or fibres, smelling somewhat like cloves, especially those which grow in the higher, hotter and dryer grounds, and in the free and clear air.

PLACE They grow wild in many places under hedge-sides, and by the pathways in fields; yet they rather delight to grow in shadowy than sunny places.

TIME They flower in May and June for the most part, and their seed is ripe in July at the latest.

GOVERNMENT AND VIRTUES It is governed by Jupiter, and that gives hopes of a wholesome healthful herb. The decoction also being drunk, comforts the heart, and strengthens the stomach and a cold brain, and therefore is good in the spring-time to open obstructions of the liver, and helps the wind-colic; it also helps those that have fluxes, or have a rupture. The juice of the fresh root or powder of the dried root has the same effect as the decoction. The root in the spring-time steeped in wine doth give it a delicate savour and taste, and, being drunk fasting every morning, comforts the heart, and is a good preservative against the plague, or any other poison; it helps digestion, and warms a cold stomach, and opens obstructions of the liver and spleen.

BALSAM-TREE

Male balsam-tree

The Arabians call it *balessan*, the Greeks βαλσαμιν, and the Latins *balsamum*; the liquor they call *opobalsamum*, the berries or fruit of the tree *carpobalsamum*, and the sprigs or young branches thereof *zylobalsamum*.

Female balsam-tree

DESCRIPTION The balsam or balm-tree, in the most natural places where it grows, is never very large, seldom more than eight or nine feet high, and in some places much lower, with divers small and straight slender branches issuing from them, of a brownish-red colour, especially the younger twigs, covered with a double bark, the red first and a green one under it, which are of a very fragrant smell, and of an aromatical quick taste, somewhat astringent and gummy, cleaving to the fingers. The wood under the bark is white, and as insipid as any other wood; on these branches come forth, sparsely and without order, many stalks of winged leaves, somewhat like those of the mastic-tree, the lowest and those that first come forth consisting of but three leaves, others of five or seven leaves, but seldom more; which are set by couples, the lowest smallest, and the next bigger, and the uppermost largest of all; of a pale green colour, smelling and tasting somewhat like the bark of the branches, somewhat clammy also, and abiding on the bushes all the year. The flowers are many and small, standing by three together on small stalks at the ends of the branches, made of six small white leaves apiece, after which follow small brownish hard berries, little bigger than juniper berries, small at both ends, crested on the sides, and very like unto the berries of the turpentine-tree, of a very sharp scent, having a yellow honey-like substance in them, somewhat bitter, but aromatic in taste, and biting on the tongue like the *opobalsamum*; when they are cut there issues forth a liquor (which sometimes flows without scarifying) of a thick whitish colour at the first, but afterwards grows oily, and is somewhat thicker than oil in summer, and of so sharp a scent that it will pierce the nostrils of those that smell thereto; it is almost like oil of spike, but as it grows older so it grows thicker, and not so quick in the smell, and in colour becoming yellow like honey or brown thick turpentine as it grows old.

PLACE AND TIME The most reputed natural places where this tree has been known to grow, both in these and former days, are Arabia Felix, about Mecca and Medina, and a small village near them called Bedrumia, and the hills, valleys, and sandy grounds about them, and the country of the Sabeans adjoining them; and from thence transplanted into India and Egypt: it likewise grew on the hills of Gilead. It is reported that the Queen of Sheba brought of the balsam-trees as the richest of her presents to Solomon, who caused them to be planted in orchards in the valley of Jericho, where they flourished, and were tended and yearly pruned, until they, together with the vineyards in that country, were destroyed by the Turks. It flowers in the spring, and the fruit is ripe in autumn.

GOVERNMENT AND VIRTUES The balsam-tree is a solar plant, of temperature hot and dry in the second degree, and is sweet in smell. Taken as a scruple or two in drink, for some days together, and to sweat thereon, it opens the obstructions of the liver and spleen: it helps a cough, shortness of breath, and consumption of the lungs, warming and drying up the distillations of rheums upon them, and all other diseases of the stomach proceeding of cold or wind. It provokes the menses, expels the after-birth, and cures discharges and stopping of urine; it cleanses the loins and kidneys, and expels the stone and gravel; it is very good against the palsy, cramp, tremblings, convulsions, shrinking of the sinews, and infected wounds.

BARBERRY

GOVERNMENT AND VIRTUES Mars owns the shrub, and presents it to the use of my countrymen, to purge their bodies of choler. It is excellent for hot agues, burnings, scaldings, heat of blood, heat of the liver, and bloody diarrhoea; the berries are as good as the bark, and more pleasing; they give a man a good appetite for his victuals, by strengthening the attractive faculty, which is under Mars. Washing the hair with the lye made of the ashes of the tree, and water, will make it turn yellow, *viz.* Mars's own colour.

BARLEY

GOVERNMENT AND VIRTUES It is a notable plant of Saturn. Barley in all the parts and compositions thereof, except malt, is more cooling than wheat, and a little cleansing; and all the preparations thereof, as barley-water, and other things made thereof, do give great nourishment to persons troubled with fevers, agues, and heats in the stomach. A poultice made of barley-meal or flour, boiled in vinegar and honey, and a few dry figs put into them, dissolves all hard abscesses, and assuages inflammations, being thereto applied.

The meal of barley and fleawort boiled in water, and made into a poultice with honey and oil of lilies, applied warm, cures swellings under the ears, throat, neck, and such-like; and a plaster made thereof with tar, wax, and oil, helps the infections in the throat glands: being boiled in red wine, with pomegranate-rinds and myrtle, it stays the diarrhoea or other looseness of the belly: boiled with vinegar and a quince, it eases the pains of the gout.

GARDEN, OR SWEET BASIL

DESCRIPTION The greater ordinary basil rises up usually with one upright stalk, diversely branching forth on all sides, with two leaves at every joint, which are somewhat broad and round, yet pointed, of a pale green colour, but fresh, a little snipped about the edges, and of a strong beady scent. The flowers are small and white, standing at the tops of the branches, with two small leaves at the joints, in some places green, in others brown, after which come black seed. The root perishes at the approach of winter, and therefore must be new sown every year.

PLACE It grows in gardens only.

TIME It must be sowed late, and flowers in the heat of the summer, being a very tender plant.

GOVERNMENT AND VIRTUES With respect to the qualities of this herb most authors differ; Galen and Dioscorides hold it not fitting to be taken inwardly, as does also Crysippus; but Pliny and the Arabian physicians defend it. For mine own part I presently found that speech true; *Non nostrum inter nos tantas componere lites*, 'It is not for me to adjust such grave disputes;' and away to Dr Reason went I, who told me it was an herb of Mars, and under the Scorpion, and perhaps therefore called *basilicon*, and then no marvel if it carries a kind of virulent quality with it. Being applied to the place stung by a wasp or hornet, it speedily draws the poison to it.

BAWM

GOVERNMENT AND VIRTUES It is an herb under Jupiter, and under Cancer, and strengthens nature much in all its actions. Let a syrup made with the juice of it and sugar be kept in every gentlewoman's house, to relieve the weak stomach; as also the herb kept dry in the house, that so, with other convenient simples, you may make it into an electuary with honey, according as the disease is. It is very good to help digestion, and has such a purging quality as to expel those melancholy vapours from the spirits and blood which are in the heart and arteries, although it cannot do so in other parts of the body. Dioscorides commends the decoction thereof for women to bathe or sit in, to procure their menses; it is good to wash aching teeth therewith, and profitable for those that have the bloody diarrhoea.

The leaves also with a little saltpeter taken in drink are good against a surfeit of mushrooms, help the griping pains of the belly, and, being made into an electuary, are good for them that cannot fetch their breath with ease. Used with salt, it takes away wens, kernels or hard swellings in the flesh or throat; it cleanses soul sores, and eases pains of the gout. It is also good for the liver and spleen. A tansy or caudle made with eggs, and the juice thereof while it is young, putting to it some sugar and rose-water, is good for women in childbed, when the after-birth is not thoroughly voided, and for their faintings upon or after their sore travail. The herb bruised and boiled in a little wine and oil, and laid warm on a boil, will ripen and break it.

BAY-TREE

GOVERNMENT AND VIRTUES It is a tree of the Sun, and under the celestial sign Leo, and resists witchcraft very potently, as also all the evils old Saturn can do to the body of man; for it is said that neither witch nor devil, thunder nor lightning, will hurt a man in the place where a bay-tree is. Galen said that the leaves or bark do dry and heal very much, and the berries more than the leaves. The bark of the root is less sharp and hot, but more bitter, and has some powers of contraction withal, whereby it is effectual to break the stone, and good to open obstructions of the liver, spleen, and other inward parts, which bring the dropsy, jaundice, &c.

The berries are very effectual against the stings of wasps and bees: they likewise procure women's menses; and seven of them given to a woman in sore travail of childbirth, do cause a speedy delivery, and expel the after-birth, and therefore not to be taken but by such as have gone out their time, lest they procure abortion, or cause labour too soon: they wonderfully help all cold and rheumatic distillations from the brain to the eyes, lungs, or other parts; and being made into an electuary with honey, do help the consumption, old coughs, shortness of breath, and thin rheums: the leaves also work the like effects.

A bath of the decoction of the leaves and berries is singularly good for women to sit in who are troubled by the womb, or the diseases thereof, or the stoppings of their menses, or for the diseases of the bladder, pains in the bowels by wind, and stopping of urine. A decoction likewise of equal parts of bay-berries, cumin seed, hyssop, *origanum*, and *euphorbium*, with some honey, and the head bathed therewith, wonderfully helps watery discharge from the nose and mouth, and settles the palate of the mouth into its place.

The oil made of the berries is very comfortable in all cold griefs of the joints, nerves, arteries, stomach, belly, or womb.

BEANS

GOVERNMENT AND VIRTUES They are plants of Venus: and the distilled water of the flowers of garden-beans is good to cleanse the face and skin, and the meal or flour of them, or the small bean, does the same. The water distilled from the green husks is held to be very effectual against kidney stone.

Bean-flour is used in poultices, to assuage inflammations rising upon wounds, and the swelling of women's breasts caused by the curdling of their milk, and represses their milk. The flour of beans and fenugreek mixed with honey, and applied to infections, boils, bruises, or the abscesses of the ears, helps them all. Bean-flour boiled to a poultice with wine and vinegar, and some oil put thereto, eases both pain and swelling of the scrotum: the husks boiled in water to a consumption of a third part thereof stays diarrhoea.

The field-beans have all the aforementioned virtues as the garden-beans. Beans eaten are extreme windy meat, but if, after the Dutch fashion, when they are half-boiled, you husk them and stew them, they are more wholesome food.

FRENCH-BEANS

DESCRIPTION The French or kidney-bean arises up at first with one stalk, which afterward divides itself into many arms or branches, but all so weak, that, if they be not sustained with sticks or poles, they will lie fruitless upon the ground; at several places of these branches grow forth long stalks, with every one of them having three broad, round, and pointed, green leaves at the end of them, towards the top whereof come forth divers flowers made like unto pease-blossoms, of the same colour for the most part that the fruit will be of, that is to say, white, yellow, red, blackish, or of a deep purple, but white is the most usual; after which come long and slender flat pods, some crooked, some straight, with a string as it were running down the back thereof, wherein are contained flattish round fruit, made in the fashion of a kidney; the root is long, spreads with many strings annexed to it, and perishes every year. There is also another sort of French-bean commonly growing with us in this land, which is called the scarlet-flowered bean. This arises up with sundry branches as the other, but runs up higher to the length of hop-poles, about which they grow twining, but turning contrary to the sun; they have stalks with three leaves on each, as on the other: the flowers also are like the other in fashion, but many more set together, and of a most orient scarlet colour. The beans are larger than the ordinary kind, of a deep purple colour, turning black when they are ripe and dry: the root perishes also in winter.

GOVERNMENT AND VIRTUES These also belong to Venus, and, being dried and beaten to powder, are strengtheners of the kidneys: neither is there a better remedy than it, if taken a drachm at a time in white wine to prevent stones, or to cleanse the kidneys of gravel or blockage. The ordinary French-beans are of an easy digestion; they move the belly, provoke urine, enlarge the breast that is straitened with shortness of breath, engender sperm, and incite lust. The scarlet-coloured beans, on account of the glorious beauty of their colour, being set near a quickset hedge, will greatly adorn the same by climbing up thereon, so that they may be discerned a great way, not without admiration of the beholder at a distance.

LADY'S BED-STRAW

Besides the common name above written, it is called cheese-rennet, because it performs the same office; as also gallion, pertimugget, and maid's-hair, and, by some, wild rosemary.

DESCRIPTION This rises up with divers small, brown, square, upright stalks a yard high or more, sometimes branched forth into divers parts, full of joints, and with divers very fine small leaves at every one of them, little or nothing rough at all: at the tops of the branches there grow many long tufts or branches of yellow flowers, very thick set together, from the several joints, which consist of four leaves each, which smell somewhat strong, but not unpleasant: the seed is small and black like poppy seed, two for the most part joined together; the root is reddish with many small threads fastened unto it, which take strong hold of the ground, and creeps a little; and the branches, leaning a little down to the ground, take root at the joints thereof, whereby it is easily increased.

There is also another sort of lady's bed-straw growing frequently in England, which bears white flowers as the other does yellow.

PLACE They grow in meadows and pastures, both wet and dry, and by the sides of hedges.

TIME They flower in May for the most part, and the seed is ripe in July and August.

GOVERNMENT AND VIRTUES They are both herbs of Venus, and therefore strengthen the parts, both internal and external, which she rules. The flowers and the herb being made into an oil or into an ointment being boiled in soft animal fat or salad oil with some wax melted therein after it is strained, do help burnings with fire or scalding with water: the decoction of the herb and flower is good to bathe the feet of travellers and footmen, whose long running causes weariness and stiffness in their sinews and joints, if the decoction be used warm, and the joints afterwards anointed with the ointment; and the herb with the white flower is also very good for the sinews, arteries and joints, to comfort and strengthen them after travel, cold, and pains.

BEECH-TREE

In treating of this tree, you must understand that I mean the great mast-beech, which is, by way of distinction from that other small rough sort, called in Sussex the small beech, but in Essex, hornbeam. I suppose it needless to describe it, being already so well known to my countrymen.

PLACE It grows in woods amongst oak and other trees, and in parks, forests, and chases, to feed deer, and in other places to fatten swine.

TIME It blooms in the end of April, or beginning of May for the most part, and the fruit is ripe in September.

GOVERNMENT AND VIRTUES It is a plant of Saturn, and therefore performs his qualities and properties in these operations: the leaves of the beech-tree are cooling and binding, and therefore good to be applied to hot swellings; the nuts do much nourish such beasts as feed thereon. The water that is found within the hollow places of decaying beeches, will cure both man and beast of any scurf or scab, if they be washed therewith. You may boil the leaves into a poultice, or make an ointment of them, when the time of year serves.

BEETS

DESCRIPTION Of beets there are two sorts, which are best known generally, and whereof I shall principally treat at this time, *viz.* the white and red beets and their virtues.

The common white beet has many great leaves next the ground, somewhat large, and of a whitish-green colour; the stalk is great, strong and ribbed, bearing a great store of leaves almost to the very top of it: the flowers grow in very long tufts, small at the ends, and turning down their heads, which are small, pale, greenish-yellow burrs, giving cornered prickly seed. The root is great, long, and hard, and when it has given seed, is of no use at all.

The common red-beet differs not from the white, but only it is less, and the leaves and the roots are somewhat red: the leaves are differently red, in some only with red streaks or veins, some of a fresh red, and others of a dark red. The root is red, spongey, and is not used to be eaten.

GOVERNMENT AND VIRTUES The government of these two sorts of beet are far different, the red beet being under Saturn, and the white under Jupiter; therefore take the virtues of them apart, each by itself. The white beet is of a cleansing digesting quality: the juice of it opens obstructions both of the liver and spleen, and helps burnings. Beet is hot and dry, and loosens the belly by reason of its nitrosity. It purges the head, especially the root; for the juice of it received into the nostrils occasions sneezing; the young plants, with their roots, gently boiled and eaten with vinegar, procure an appetite, and suppress choler in the stomach. The juice of this herb is also good for all weals, blisters and sores in the skin; the herb boiled, and laid upon chilblains or kibes, helps them: the decoction thereof in water and some vinegar, heals the itch, if bathed therewith, and cleanses the head of dandruff, scurf, and is much commended against baldness and shedding of hair. The red beet is good to stay the bloody diarrhoea, women's menses, and discharges.

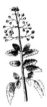

WATER-BETONY

Called also broomwort, and in Yorkshire bishop's leaves.

DESCRIPTION Winter-betony rises up with square, hard, greenish stalks, sometimes brown, set with broad dark green leaves, notched at the edges, somewhat resembling the leaves of the wood-betony, but larger, two for the most part set at a joint; the flowers are many, set at the tops of the stalks, being round-bellied, open at the brims, and divided into two parts, the uppermost being like a hood, and the lowest like a lip hanging down, of a dark red colour, They are followed by small round heads, with small points in the ends, wherein lie small brownish seeds: the root is a thick bush of strings and threads growing from the head.

PLACE It grows by ditch-sides, brooks, and other water-courses, generally through this land, and is seldom found far from the water-sides.

TIME It flowers about July, and the seed is ripe in August.

GOVERNMENT AND VIRTUES Water-betony is an herb of Jupiter in Cancer. It is of a cleansing quality; the leaves bruised and applied are effectual for ulcers; and especially if the juice of the leaves be boiled with a little honey, and then dipped therein, and the sores dressed therewith: as also for bruises or hurts, whether inward or outward. The distilled water of the leaves is used for the same purposes.

WOOD-BETONY

DESCRIPTION The common or wood-betony has many leaves rising from the root, which are somewhat broad and round at the ends, roundly dented about the edges, standing upon long stalks, from among which rise up small, square, slender, but yet upright, hairy stalks, with some leaves thereon, two apiece at the joints, smaller than the lower, whereon are set several spiked heads of flowers like lavender, but thicker and shorter for the most part, and of a reddish or purple colour, spotted with white spots both in the upper and lower part: the seeds, being contained within the husks that hold the flowers, are blackish, somewhat long and uneven. The roots are many white thready strings; the stalk perishes, but the root, with some leaves thereon, abides all the winter.

PLACE It grows frequently in woods, and delights in shady places.

TIME And it flowers in July, after which the seed is quickly ripe, yet is in its prime in May.

GOVERNMENT AND VIRTUES This herb is appropriated to the planet Jupiter, and under the sign Aries. The decoction made with mead and a little penny-royal opens obstructions both of the liver and spleen, cures stitches and pains in the back or side, the torments and griping pains of the bowels, and the wind-colic; and mixed with honey purges the belly, helps to bring down women's menses, and is of special use for those that are troubled with the falling down of the womb, and pains thereof, and causes an easy and speedy delivery of women in childbirth; it helps also to break and expel the stone either in the bladder or kidneys.

The green herb bruised, or the juice applied to any outward infected wound in the head or body, will quickly heal and close it up; as also any veins or sinews that are cut, and will draw forth any broken bone or splinter, thorn, or other thing gotten into the flesh; being applied with a little hog's-lard, it helps boils.

The root of betony is displeasing both to the taste and stomach, whereas the leaves and flowers, by virtue of their sweet and spicy taste, are comfortable both in meat and medicine.

The flowers of this herb are usually conserved.

BILBERRIES

This herb is also called by some, whorts, and whortle-berries.

DESCRIPTION Of these I shall only speak of two sorts, which are commonly known in England, *viz.* the black and red bilberries. And first of the black.

This small bush creeps along upon the ground, rising scarcely half a yard high, with divers small dark green leaves set on the green branches, not always one against another, and a little dented about the edges; at the foot of the leaves come forth small, hollow, pale, blush-coloured flowers, the brims ending in five points, with a reddish thread in the middle, which pass into small round berries, of the bigness and colour of juniper berries, but of a purple sweetish sharp taste; the juice of them gives a purplish colour to the hands and lips of those that eat and handle them, especially if they break them. The root grows aslope under ground, shooting forth in sundry places as it creeps: it loses its leaves in winter. The red bilberry or whortle-bush rises up like the former, having sundry harder leaves, like the box-tree leaves, green and round pointed, standing on the several branches; at the tops whereof only, and not from the sides as in the former, come forth divers round flowers, or a pale red colour, after which succeed round reddish sappy berries, which when ripe are of a sharp taste: the root runs in the ground as in the former, but the leaves of this abide all winter.

PLACE The first grows in forests, on the heaths, and such-like barren places; the red grows in the northern parts of this land, as Lancashire, Yorkshire, &c.

TIME They flower in March and April, and the fruit of the black bilberry bush is ripe in June and July.

GOVERNMENT AND VIRTUES They are under the dominion of Jupiter. The black bilberries are good in hot agues, and to cool the heat of the liver and stomach; they do somewhat bind the belly, and stop vomiting; the juice of the berries made into a syrup, or the pulp made into a conserve with sugar, is good for the purposes aforesaid; as also for an old cough, or an ulcer in the lungs, or other diseases therein. The red whorts are more binding, and stop women's menses.

BIRCH-TREE

DESCRIPTION This grows a goodly tall straight tree, with many boughs and branches bending downward, the old ones being covered with a discoloured chapped bark, and the younger being much browner: the leaves at first breaking out are crumpled, and afterward like beech leaves, but smaller and greener, and dented about the edges: it bears small short catkins, somewhat like those of the hasel-nut tree, which abide on the branches a long time, until grown ripe, when they fall on the ground, and their seed with them.

PLACE It usually grows in woods.

GOVERNMENT AND VIRTUES It is a tree of Venus. The juice of the leaves while young, or the distilled water of them, will break the stone in the kidneys or bladder. The leaves of the birch-tree are hot and dry, cleansing, resolving, opening, and bitter; for which reason they are of no small use in a dropsy, the itch, and the like. The bark is bituminous, and is therefore mixed with perfumes to disguise the smell. The fungus of it has an astringent quality, upon which account it stops bleeding miraculously. In the beginning of spring, before the leaves come forth, this tree when pierced yields plentifully a sweet and potable juice, which shepherds, when they are thirsty, often drink in the woods. This tree begins to yield its juice about the middle of February, and sometimes not till the beginning of March.

BIRD'S FOOT

This small herb grows not above a span high, with many branches spread upon the ground, set with many wings of small leaves; the flowers grow upon the branches, many small ones of a pale yellow colour being set at a head together, which afterwards turn into small jointed husks, well resembling the claws of small birds, whence it took its name.

Birdsfoot

There is another sort of bird's foot in all things like the former, but a little larger, the flowers of a pale whitish-red colour, and the husks distinct by joints like the other, but a little more crooked, and the roots carry many small white knots or kernels amongst the strings.

Flat-padded birdsfoot

PLACE   These grow on heaths, and in many open uncultivated places in this land.

TIME   They flower and seed in the end of summer.

GOVERNMENT AND VIRTUES   They belong to Saturn, and are of a drying binding quality, and thereby very good to be used in wound-drinks, as also to apply outwardly for the same purpose. The latter bird's foot is found to break the stones in the back or kidneys, and drive them forth, if the decoction thereof be taken.

All salts have best operation upon the stone, as ointments and plasters have upon wounds; and therefore you may make a salt of this for the stone.

BISHOP'S WEED

Besides the common name bishop's weed, it is usually known by the Greek name, *ammi* and *amios*; some call it Æthiopian cummin-seed, and other cummin royal; as also herb William, and bulwort.

DESCRIPTION   Common bishop's weed rises up with a round stalk, sometimes as high as a man, but usually three or four feet high, beset with divers small, long, and sometimes broad, leaves, cut in some places and dented about the edges, growing one against another, of a dark green colour, having sundry branches on them, and at the top small umbels of white flowers, which turn into small round brown seed, little bigger than parsley-seed, of a quick hot scent and taste. The root is white and stringy, perishing yearly after it has seeded, and usually rises again of its own sowing.

PLACE It grows wild in many places in England and Wales, as between Greenhithe and Gravesend.

GOVERNMENT AND VIRTUES It is hot and dry in the third degree, of a bitter taste, and somewhat sharp withal; it provokes women's menses, expels wind, and eases pains and gripings in the bowels.

BISTORT

It is also called snakeweed, English serpentary, dragon-wort, osterich, and passions.

DESCRIPTION This has a thick, short, knobbed root, blackish without, and somewhat reddish within, a little crooked or turned together, of an harsh astringent taste, with divers black threads hanging thereto, from whence spring up every year divers leaves, standing upon long stalks, being somewhat broad and long like a dock leaf, and a little pointed at the ends, but that it is of a bluish-green colour on the upper side, and of an ash-colour grey somewhat tinged with purple underneath, with divers veins therein; from among which rise up divers small and slender stalks, two feet high, and almost naked and without leaves, or with very few, and narrow, bearing a spiky bush of pale flesh-coloured flowers, followed by small seed, somewhat like sorrel-seed, but larger.

PLACE They grow in shadowy moist woods, and at the foot of hills, but are chiefly nourished up in gardens. The narrow-leaved bistort grows in the north: Lancashire, Yorkshire, and Cumberland.

TIME The bistorts flower about the end of May, and the seed is ripe about the beginning of July.

GOVERNMENT AND VIRTUES It belongs to Saturn, and is in operation cold and dry. The leaves, seed, or roots, are all very good in decoctions, drinks, or lotions, for inward or outward wounds or other sores; and the powder, strewed upon any cut or wound in a vein, stays the immoderate bleeding thereof. It is good also to fasten the gums, and to take away the heat and inflammations that happen in the jaws, glands of the throat, or mouth, if the decoction of the leaves, roots, or seeds bruised, or the juice of them, be applied; but the roots are most effectual to the purposes aforesaid.

BLACK BINDWEED

It is also called with-wind.

DESCRIPTION Black bindweed has smooth red branches, very small, like threads, wherewith it wraps and winds itself about trees, hedges, stakes, and everything it can lay hold upon; the leaves are like ivy, but smaller and more tender; the flowers are white and very small; the seed is black, triangular or three-square, growing thick together; every seed is closed and covered with a thin skin; the root is small and tender as a thread.

PLACE It grows in borders of fields and gardens, about hedges and ditches, and among herbs.

TIME It delivers its seed in August and September, and afterwards perishes.

GOVERNMENT AND VIRTUES Bindweed is a plant of Mercury, of a hot nature, and of subtle parts, having power to dissolve; the juice of the leaves, being drunk, do loosen and open the belly; and being pounded, and laid to the grieved place, dissolves, wastes, and consumes hard swellings.

BLACK-THORN, OR SLOE-BUSH

PLACE It grows in every country, in the hedges and borders of fields.

TIME It flowers in April, and sometimes in March, but ripens after all other plums, and is not fit to be eaten until the autumn frost have mellowed it.

GOVERNMENT AND VIRTUES All the parts of the sloe-bush are binding, cooling, and drying, and effectual to stay the bleeding at the nose and mouth, or any other place; to stay the bloody diarrhoea, and to ease the pains in the sides or bowels, by drinking the decoction of the bark of the roots, or more usually the decoction of the berries either fresh or dried. The conserve is also of very much use to the purposes aforesaid. The leaves also are good to make lotions to gargle and wash the mouth and throat. The simple distilled water of the flowers is very effectual for the said purposes. The distilled water of the green berries is used also for the same purposes.

BLIGHTS

DESCRIPTION Of these there are two sorts commonly known, *viz.* white and red. The white has leaves somewhat like beets, but smaller, rounder, and of a whitish-green colour, upon a small stalk which rises up two or three feet high; the flowers grow at the top in long round tufts, where are contained small round seed; the root is very full of strings. The red blight is in all things like the white, but that its leaves and tufted heads are exceeding red at the first, and afterwards turn more purple. There are other kinds of blights which grow wild, differing from the two former sorts but little, only the wild are smaller in every part.

PLACE They grow in gardens, and wild in many places of this land.

TIME They seed in August and September.

GOVERNMENT AND VIRTUES They are all of them cooling, drying, and binding, serving to restrain the fluxes of blood in either man or woman, especially the red, which also stays the overflowing of women's menses, as the white blight stays discharges in women. They are all under the dominion of Venus.

BLUE-BOTTLE

It is also called *syanus*, I suppose from the colour of it; hurt-sickle, because it damages the edge of the sickles that reap the corn; blue-blow and corn-flower.

DESCRIPTION I shall only describe that which is most common, and in my opinion most useful: its leaves spread upon the ground, being of a whitish-green colour, somewhat cut on the edges like those of corn-scabious, among which rises up a stalk divided into divers branches, beset with long leaves of a greenish colour, either but very little indented or not at all; the flowers are of a blue colour, from whence it took its name, consisting of an innumerable company of small flowers, set in a scaly head, not much unlike those of knapweed; the seed is smooth, bright, and shining, wrapped up in a woolly mantle: the root perishes every year.

PLACE They grow in corn-fields, amongst all sorts of corn, peas, and beans, but not in tares; if you please to take them up from thence, and transplant them in your garden, especially towards the full of the Moon, they will grow more double than they are.

TIME They flower from the beginning of May to the end of harvest.

GOVERNMENT AND VIRTUES As they are naturally cold, dry, and binding, so are they under the dominion of Saturn. The powder or dried leaves of the blue-bottle or corn-flower is given with good success to those that are bruised by a fall, or have broken a vein inwardly. The juice put into fresh wounds quickly closes the lips of them together, and is very effectual to heal ulcers and sores in the mouth.

BORAGE AND BUGLOSS

These plants are so well known to be inhabitants of every garden, that I hold it needless to give them a description here. To these I may add a third sort, which is not so common, nor yet so well known, and therefore I shall give you its name and its description.

NAME It is called *langue-de-boeuf*: but why they should call one herb by the name of *bugloss*, and another by the name of *langue-de-boeuf*, is to me a question, seeing one signifies ox-tongue in Greek, and the other signifies the same in French.

DESCRIPTION The leaves thereof are smaller than those of bugloss, but much rougher, the stalk rising up about a foot and a half high, and is most commonly of a red colour: the flowers stand in scaly rough heads, being composed of many small yellow flowers, not much unlike those of the dandelion, and the seed flies away in thistledown in the same way: you may easily know the flowers by the taste, for they are very bitter.

PLACE It grows wild in many places of the land, and may be plentifully found near London, between Rotherhithe and Deptford, by the ditch sides; its virtues are held to be the same with borage and bugloss, only this is something hotter.

TIME They flower in June and July, and the seed is ripe shortly after.

GOVERNMENT AND VIRTUES They are all three herbs of Jupiter, and under Leo, all great cordials and strengtheners of nature. The seed and leaves are good to increase milk in women's breasts: the leaves, flowers, and seed, all or any of them, are good to expel pensiveness and melancholy, to clarify the blood, and to mitigate heat in fevers. The juice made into a syrup prevails much to all the purposes aforesaid. The flowers candied, or made into a conserve, are chiefly used as a cordial, and are good for those that are weak with long sickness; the distilled water is no less effectual; the dried herb is never used, but the green; yet the ashes thereof boiled in mead, or honey-water, are available against inflammations and ulcers in the mouth or throat, to wash and gargle it therewith.

BRAMBLE

GOVERNMENT AND VIRTUES It is a plant of Venus in Aries. The buds, leaves, and branches, while they are green, are of good use in the ulcers and sores of the mouth and throat, and for the quinsey; and likewise to heal other fresh wounds and sores. Either the decoction or powder of the root, being taken, is good to break or drive forth gravel and the stone in the kidneys. The leaves and brambles, as well green as dry, are excellent lotions for sores; the decoction of them and of the dried branches does much bind the belly, and is good for too much flowing of women's menses. The distilled water of the branches, leaves, flowers, or fruit, is very pleasant in taste, and very effectual in fevers and hot distempers of the body, head, eyes, and other parts.

BRANK-URSINE

Besides the common name brank-ursine, it IS also called bear's breech, and *acanthus*, though I think our English names more proper, for the Greek word *acanthus* signifies any thistle whatsoever.

DESCRIPTION This thistle shoots forth many large, thick, smooth green leaves upon the ground, with a thick, juicy middle rib; the leaves have deep gashes on the edge; they remain a long time before any stalk appears; afterwards rises up a stalk three or four feet high, finely decked with flowers from the middle upwards, for on the lower part there is neither branch nor leaf; the flowers are hooded and gaping, white in colour, and stand in brownish husks, with a small, long, undivided, leaf under each leaf; they seldom seed in our country; its roots are many and thick, blackish without and whitish within, full of clammy sap; if you set a piece of them in a garden, defending it from the first winter's cold, it will grow and flourish.

PLACE They are only nursed up in gardens in England, where they will grow very well.

TIME It flowers in June and July.

GOVERNMENT AND VIRTUES An excellent plant under the dominion of the Moon, its leaves being boiled, and used in enemas, are exceeding good to mollify the belly; the decoction, drunk, is excellent good for the bloody diarrhoea; the leaves being bruised, or rather boiled, and applied like a poultice, are exceeding good to strengthen joints that have been put out; there is scarcely a better remedy to be applied to such places as are burnt with fire than this is; for it fetcheth out the fire, and heals it without a scar; either taken inwardly or applied to the place, it helps the cramp and the gout.

BRIONY

It is called wild-vine, wood-vine, *tamus*, and our lady's seal; the white is called white-vine by some, and the black black-vine.

DESCRIPTION   The common white briony grows creeping upon the hedges, sending forth many long, rough, very tender, branches at the beginning, with many very rough broad leaves thereon, cut for the most part into five partitions, in form very like a vine-leaf, but smaller, rougher, and of a whitish or hoary-green colour, spreading very far; and twining with its small claspers, that come forth at the joints with the leaves, very fast on whatsoever standeth next to it; at the several joints also, especially towards the tops of branches, comes forth a long stalk bearing many whitish flowers, together in a long tuft, consisting of small branches each, laid open like a star; after which come the berries, separated one from another more than a cluster of grapes, green at the first, and very red when they are thoroughly ripe; of no good scent, and of a most loathsome taste, provoking vomit: the root grows very large, with many long branches growing from it, of a pale whitish colour on the outside, and more white within, and of a sharp, bitter, loathsome taste.

PLACE   It grows on banks, or under hedges, through this land, and the roots lie very deep.

TIME   It flowers in July and August, some earlier and some later than others.

GOVERNMENT AND VIRTUES   The roots of briony purge the belly with great violence, troubling the stomach, and burning the liver, and are therefore not rashly to be taken, but, used correctly, are very profitable for the diseases of the head, as also the joints and sinews; and for palsies, convulsions, cramps and stitches in the side, and the dropsy; they cleanse the kidneys from gravel and stone by opening the obstructions of the spleen, and consuming the hardness and swellings thereof.

If the juice be tempered with the vetches or fenugreek, or boiled in oil till it be consumed, it is a plant profitable for tanners to thicken their leather hides with. A drachm of the root in powder taken in white wine, brings on the menses; an electuary, made of the roots and honey, mightily cleanses the chest of rotten phlegm and wonderfully helps an old strong cough and those that are troubled with shortness of breath; it is very good for them that are bruised inwardly, to help to expel the clotted or congealed blood.

BROOKLIME

It is also called water-pimpernel.

DESCRIPTION   It rises from a creeping root, that shoots forth strings at every joint as it runs; it has divers and sundry green stalks, round and sappy, with some branches on them, and somewhat broad, round, deep, green, and thick, leaves set by couples thereon; from these shoot forth long stalks, with

PLATE 2

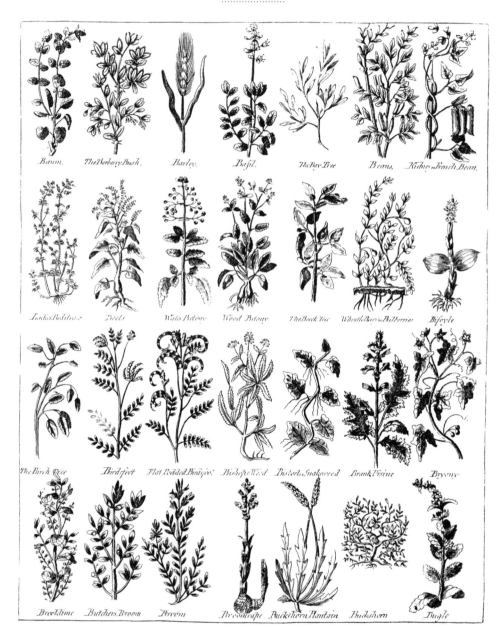

Balm.   The Berbary Bush.   Barley.   Basil.   The Bay Tree   Beans.   Kidney or French Bean.

Ladies Bedstraw   Beets   Water Betony   Wood Betony   The Beech Tree   Wheatle Berry or Billberries   Bifoyle

The Birch Tree   Birdsfoot   Flat Podded Birdsfoot   Bishops Weed   Bistort or Snakeweed   Brank Ursine   Bryony

Brooklime   Butchers Broom   Broom   Broomrape   Buckthorn Plantain   Buckshorn   Bugle sundry small blue flowers on them, that consist of five small round-pointed leaves each. There is another sort differing from the former only in that it is larger, and the flowers are of a paler blue colour.

PLACE They sometimes grow in small standing waters, but generally near water-cresses, and are sometimes sold for them in the markets.

TIME They flower in June and July, giving seed the month after.

GOVERNMENT AND VIRTUES It is a hot and biting martial plant: brooklime and water-cresses are generally used to purge the blood and body, and are helpful for the scurvy: they also provoke urine, and help to break the stone and pass it away. Being fried with butter and vinegar, and applied warm, it helps all manner of tumours, swellings, and inflammations.

BROOM AND **BROOM-RAPE**

Broom

The broom-rape springs up on many places from the roots of the broom, but more often in fields, or by hedge-sides, and on heaths. The stalk is of the size of a finger or thumb, above two feet high, having a show of leaves on them, and many flowers at the top, of a deadish-yellow colour.

Broom-rape

PLACE They grow in many places of this land commonly, and as commonly spoil all the land they grow in.

TIME They flower in summer months, and give their seed before winter.

GOVERNMENT AND VIRTUES The juice or decoction of the young branches or seed, or the powder of the seed taken in drink, purges downwards and draws phlegmatic and watery humours from the joints, whereby it helps the dropsy, gout, sciatica, and pains in the hips and joints: it also provokes strong vomiting, and helps the pains of the sides, and swellings of the spleen; cleanses also the kidneys and bladder of the stone, provokes urine abundantly, and hinders the growing again of the stone in the body. The continual use of the powder of the leaves and seed cures the black-jaundice: the distilled water of the flowers is profitable for all the same purposes; it also alters the fits of agues. The oil or water that is drawn from the ends of the green sticks heated in the fire helps the toothache.

The broom-rape also is not without its virtues. The decoction in wine is thought to be as effectual to avoid the stone in the kidneys and bladder, and to provoke urine, as the broom itself. The juice thereof is a singular good help to cure infected wounds and malignant ulcers. As for the broom and broom-rape, Mars owns them; and it is exceeding prejudicial to the liver, I suppose by reason of the antipathy between Jupiter and Mars: therefore, if the liver be disaffected, administer none of it.

BUCKSHORN

It is also called hartshorn, herbastella and *herbastellaria*, *sanguinaria*, herb-eve, herb-ivy, wort-cresses, and swine-cresses.

DESCRIPTION It has many small and weak straggling branches trailing here and there upon the ground; the leaves are many, small, and jagged, and are not much unlike those of the buckshorn plantain, but much smaller, and not so hairy: the flowers grow among the leaves in small, rough, whitish, clusters; the seeds are smaller and brownish, and of a bitter taste.

PLACE They grow in dry, barren, and sandy, grounds.

TIME They flower and seed with the other plantains.

GOVERNMENT AND VIRTUES This is under the dominion of Saturn: the virtues are held to be the same as buckshorn plantain, the leaves being bruised, and applied to warts, will make them waste away in a short time.

BUCKSHORN PLANTAIN

DESCRIPTION This being sown of seed, rises up at the first with small, long, narrow, hairy, dark green leaves, like grass, without any division or gash in them; but those that follow are gashed in on both sides into three or four gashes, and pointed at the ends, resembling a buck's horn, whereof it took its name; and being well grown round about the root upon the ground, they resemble the form of a star, from among which rise up divers hairy stalks, about a hand-breadth high, bearing every one a small, long, spiky head, like those of the common plantain, having similar flowers and seed after them: the root is single, long, small, and stringy.

PLACE They grow in dry sandy ground, as in Tothill-fields, Westminster, and many other places in this kingdom.

TIME They flower and seed in May, June, and July; and their leaves, in a manner, abide green all the winter.

GOVERNMENT AND VIRTUES It is under the dominion of Saturn, and is of a drying and binding quality: this boiled in wine and drunk, helps those that are troubled with the stone in the kidneys, by cooling the heat of the parts afflicted, and strengthening them; it stays bloody diarrhoea, and stops looseness of the belly and bowels: the leaves hereof bruised, and laid to the sides of a person with an ague, suddenly ease the fit; and the leaves and roots beaten with some bay-salt, and applied to the wrists, work the same effects.

BUCK-WHEAT

NAMES   In most counties of England this grain goes by the general name of French wheat, as in Hampshire, Surrey, Berkshire, Wiltshire, and Buckinghamshire, and especially in those barren parts of the counties where it is most usually sown and delights to grow; it is also in many parts of England called buckwheat: some take it to be the *erysinum* of Theophrastus, and the *ireo* of Pliny, and it is called *frumentum sarasenicum* by Mathiolus; the Dutch names are *bockweyd* and *buckenweydt*.

DESCRIPTION   Buck-wheat rises up with divers round hollow reddish stalks, set with many leaves, each by itself on a stalk, which is broad and round, and lies forked at the bottom, small and pointed at the end; they somewhat resemble an ivy-leaf in appearance, but are softer to handle; at the top of the stalks come forth clusters of small white flowers, which turn into small three-cornered blackish seed, with a white pulp therein; the root is small and thready.

PLACE AND TIME   It is said to have its original birth-place in Arabia, whereby it had the Latin name *frumentum sarasenicum*, and was transplanted from thence into Italy, but now is very commonly sown in most of our northern counties, where for the use and profit made of it, many fields are sown therewith; it is not usually sown before April, and sometimes not until May, for at its first springing up a frosty night kills it all, and so it will do the flowers when it blossoms; it is ripe at the latter end of August, or the beginning of September, and will grow in a dry hungry ground, for which it is held as good as manure.

GOVERNMENT AND VIRTUES   This grain is attributed to Venus: it nourishes less than wheat, rye, or barley, but more than millet, and the bread or cakes made of the meal are easily digested, and soon pass out of the stomach; it gives small nourishment, though not bad, and is withal a little flatulent or windy, yet country-people in divers parts of Germany and Italy eat it as almost their only bread-corn, and are strong and lusty persons; the bread or cakes made of it are pleasant, but do lie somewhat heavy on the stomach. I never knew any bread or cakes made of it for people to eat in this country, but it is generally used to fatten hogs and poultry of all sorts, which it does very quickly.

The medicinal uses of it are these: it increases milk, and loosens the belly.

BUGLE

Besides the name bugle, it is called middle-confound, and middle-comfrey, brown-bugle, and by some sicklewort and herb-carpenter, though in Sussex they call another herb by that name.

DESCRIPTION This has larger leaves than those of the self-heal, but else of the same fashion, or rather a little longer; in some green on the upper side, and in others rather brownish, dented about the edges, somewhat hairy, as the square stalk is also, which rises up to be half a yard high sometimes, with the leaves set in pairs; from the middle upwards stand the flowers together, with many smaller and browner leaves than the rest on the stalk below, set at distances, and the stalk bare between them; among which flowers are also small ones, of a bluish, and sometimes of an ash, colour, fashioned like the flowers of the ground-ivy, after which come small, round, blackish, seed: the root is composed of many strings, and spreads upon the ground.

The white bugle differs neither in form or size from the former, save that the leaves and stalks are always green, and the flowers are white.

PLACE It grows in woods, coppices, and fields, generally throughout England, but the white-flowered bugle is not so plentiful as the other.

TIME They flower from May till July, and in the mean time perfect their seed; the root, and the leaves next the ground, abide all the winter.

GOVERNMENT AND VIRTUES This herb belongs to Venus. It is wonderful in curing all manner of ulcers and sores, whether new and fresh or old and inveterate, and even gangrenes and fistulas, if the leaves are bruised and applied, or the juice used to wash and bathe the places; and the same, made into a lotion with some honey and alum, cures all sores of the mouth or gums.

BURDOCK

Also called *personata*, *bardona*, *lappa major*, great burdock, and clotbur.

PLACE It grows plentifully by ditches and water-sides, and by the highways, almost everywhere throughout this land.

GOVERNMENT AND VIRTUES Venus challenges this herb for her own; and, by its seed or leaf, you may draw the womb which way you please, either upward by applying it to the crown of the head, in case it falls out, or downward by applying it to the soles of the feet; or, if you would stay in its place, apply it to the navel, and that is likewise a good way to stay the child in it: the burleaves are cooling, moderately drying, and good for old ulcers and sores. The leaves applied to places troubled with the shrinking of the sinews or arteries, give much ease. The juice of the leaves, taken with honey, provokes urine, and remedies the pain of the bladder: the seed being drunk in wine forty days together, wonderfully helps the sciatica: the leaves bruised with the white of an egg, and applied to any place burnt with fire, take out the heat, give sudden ease, and heal it up afterwards. Its roots may be preserved with sugar, and taken fasting, or at other times, for the said purposes.

BURNET

It is also called *sanguisorba*, *pimpinella*, *bipenula*, *solbegrella*, &c. Common garden burnet is so well known that it needs no description; but there is another sort which is wild, the description whereof take as follows.

DESCRIPTION   The great wild burnet has winged leaves arising from the roots like the garden burnet, but not so many; yet each of these leaves are at least twice as large as the other, and nicked in the same manner about the edges, of a greyish colour on the underside; the stalks are larger and rise higher, with many such-like leaves set thereon, and greater heads at the tops, of a brownish-green colour; and out of them come small, dark, purple, flowers, like the former, but larger: the root is black and long like the other, but also greater; it has almost neither scent nor taste like the garden kind.

PLACE   The first grows frequently in gardens; the wild kind grows in divers counties of this kingdom, especially in Huntingdon and Northamptonshire; also near London by Pancras church, and by a causeway side in the middle of a field by Paddington.

TIME   They flower about the end of June and beginning of July; their seed is ripe in August.

GOVERNMENT AND VIRTUES   It is an herb the Sun challenges dominion over; the continual use of it preserves the body in health, and the spirits in vigour. The smaller is the most effectual, because quicker and more aromatical; it is a friend to the heart, liver, and other principal parts of a man's body: two or three of the stalks with leaves put into a cup of wine are known to quicken the spirits, refresh and cheer the heart. They have also a drying and an astringent quality, whereby they are available in all manner of fluxes of blood or humours. It is a singularly good herb for all sorts of wounds: to be used either by the juice or the decoction, by the powder of the herb or root, or by ointment.

BUTCHER'S BROOM

It is called *ruscus* and *bruscus*, knee-holm, knee-holly, knee hulver, and pettigree.

DESCRIPTION The first shoots that sprout from the root of butcher's broom are thick, whitish, and short, somewhat like those of asparagus, but greater; they, rising up to be a foot and a half high, are spread into divers branches, green, and somewhat crested with a roundness, tough and flexible, whereon are set somewhat broad and almost round hard leaves, and prickly pointed at the ends, of a dark green colour, two for the most part set at a place, very close or near together; about the middle of the leaf, on the back and lower side from the middle rib, breaks forth a small whitish-green flower, consisting of four small round-pointed leaves, standing upon little or no stalk, and in the place whereof comes a small round berry, green at the first, and red when it is ripe, wherein are two or three white, hard, round, seeds, contained; the root is thick, white, and great at the head, and from thence sends forth divers thick, white, long, tough strings.

PLACE It grows in coppices, and on heaths and waste-grounds, and under or near holly-bushes.

TIME It shoots forth its young buds in the spring, and the berries are ripe in or about September: the branches or leaves abiding green all the winter.

GOVERNMENT AND VIRTUES It is a plant of Mars, being of a gallant cleansing and opening quality; the decoction of the root drunk, and a poultice made of the berries and leaves being applied, are effectual in knitting and consolidating broken bones, or parts out of joint.

BUTTER-BUR

This herb is called *petasitis*.

DESCRIPTION It rises up in February, with a thick stalk about a foot high, whereon are set a few small leaves, or rather pieces, and at the tops a long spiked head of flowers, of a blush or deep red colour, according to the soil wherein it grows; and, before the stalk with the flowers have been a month above ground, they will be withered and gone, and blown away with the wind, and the leaves will begin to spring, which being full blown are very large and broad, being somewhat thin and almost round, whose thick red footstalks, about a foot long, stand towards the middle of the leaves; the lower part being divided into two round parts, close almost one to another, of a pale green colour, and hoary underneath: the root is long and spreading under the ground, being in some

PLATE 3

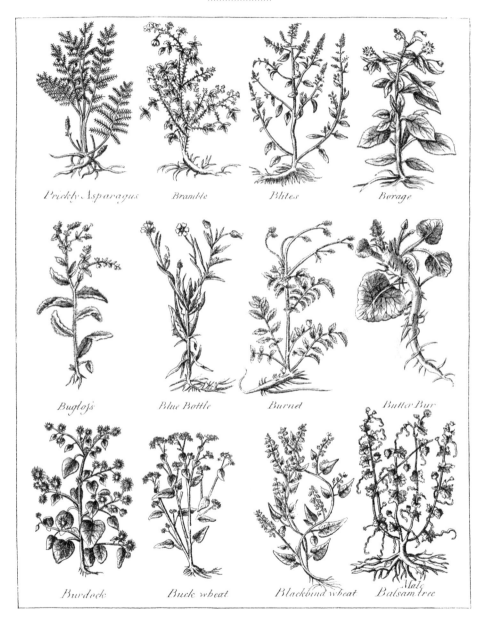

Prickly Asparagus   Bramble   Blites   Borage

Buglofs   Blue Bottle   Burnet   Butter Bur

Burdock   Buck wheat   Blackbind wheat   Male Balsam Tree

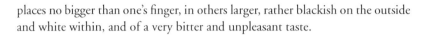

places no bigger than one's finger, in others larger, rather blackish on the outside and white within, and of a very bitter and unpleasant taste.

PLACE AND TIME They grow in low and wet grounds by rivers and watersides; their flowers (as is said) rising and decaying in February and March, before the leaves, which appear in April.

GOVERNMENT AND VIRTUES It is under the dominion of the Sun, and therefore a great strengthener of the heart, and cheers the vital spirits. Its roots are found to be very available against fevers, by provoking sweat; the root taken with the zedoary and angelica helps the rising of the womb.

BYFOIL, OR TWAYBLADE

DESCRIPTION This small herb, from a root somewhat sweet, shooting downwards many long stripes, rises up a round green stalk, bare or naked next the ground for an inch, two, or three, to the middle thereof, as it is in age or growth, as also from the middle upwards to the flowers, having only two broad plantain-like leaves, but whiter, set at the middle of the stalk, one against another, and compasses it round at the bottom of them.

PLACE It is an usual inhabitant in woods, coppices, and in many other places in this land. There is another sort grows in wet grounds and marshes, which is somewhat differing from the former: it is a smaller plant, and greener, having sometimes three leaves; the spike of flowers is less than the former, and the roots of this do run or creep in the ground.

GOVERNMENT AND VIRTUES They are much and often used by many to good purposes, for wounds both green and old, and to consolidate or knit ruptures, being a plant of Saturn.

CABBAGES AND COLEWORTS

TIME Their flowering time is towards the middle or end of July, and the seed is ripe in August.

Cabbage

GOVERNMENT AND VIRTUES The cabbages or coleworts boiled gently in broth, and eaten, open the body. They are much commended being eaten before meat to keep one from surfeiting. The decoction of coleworts takes away the pains and aches, and allays the swellings of gouty legs and knees, the place being bathed therewith warm. Cabbages are extreme windy, whether

Colewort you take them as meat or as medicine; but colewort-flowers are something more tolerable, and the wholesomer food of the two. The Moon challenges the dominion of the herb.

SEA-COLEWORT

DESCRIPTION this has divers somewhat long, broad, large, thick, wrinkled, leaves, crumpled upon the edges, growing each upon a several thick, footstalk, very brittle, of a greyish-green colour; from among which rises up a strong thick stalk, two feet high, or more, with some leaves thereon to the top, where it branches forth much, and on every branch stands a large bush of pale-whitish flowers, consisting of four leaves each: the root is somewhat large, and shoots forth many branches under ground, keeping green leaves all the winter.

PLACE They grow in many places upon the sea-coasts, as well on the Kentish as Essex shores; as, at Lid in Kent, Colchester in Essex, and divers other places, and in other counties, of this land.

TIME They flower and seed about the time the other kinds do.

GOVERNMENT AND VIRTUES The Moon claims the dominion of these also. The broth or first decoction, of the sea-colewort, does, by the sharp, nitrous, and bitter, qualities therein, open the belly and purge the body; it cleanses and digests more powerfully than the other kind.

CALAMINT

It is called also mountain mint.

DESCRIPTION It is a small herb, seldom rising above a foot high, with square, hairy, and woody, stalks, and two small hoary leaves set at a joint, about the bigness of marjoram, or not much bigger, a little dented about the edges, and of a very fierce or quick scent, as the whole herb is; the flowers stand at several spaces of the stalks, from the middle almost upwards, which are small and gaping like the common mint, and of a pale-bluish colour; after which follow small, round, blackish, seeds; the root is small and woody, with divers small sprigs spreading within the ground: it abides many years.

PLACE It grows on heaths, and upland dry grounds, in many counties of this kingdom.

TIME They flower in July, and their seed is ripe quickly after.

GOVERNMENT AND VIRTUES It is an herb of Mercury, and a strong one too, therefore excellent good in all afflictions of the brain; the decoction of the herb, being drunk, brings down women's menses; it is profitable for those that are troubled with convulsions or cramps. It helps such as have the leprosy, either taken inwardly, drinking whey after it, or the green herb outwardly applied; it hinders conception in women, being either burned or strewed in the chamber. Being applied to the hipbone, by continuance of time it spends the humours which cause the pains of the sciatica. The decoction hereof, with some sugar put thereto, is very profitable for those that have an old cough, and that are scarce able to breathe by shortness of their wind. Let no women use too much of it, for it works very violently upon the female subject.

WATER-CALTROPS

They are called also, *tribulus aquaticus*, *tribulus lacustris*, *tribulus marinus*, caltrops, faligot, water-nuts, and water-chestnuts.

DESCRIPTION As for the greater sort, or water-caltrop, it is but very rarely found here: two other sorts there are, which I shall here describe.

The first has a long, creeping, and jointed root, sending forth tufts at each joint, from which joints arise, long, flat, slender, knotted, stalks, even to the top of the water, divided towards the top into many branches, each carrying two leaves on both sides, being about two inches long and half an inch broad, thin and almost transparent; they look as though they were torn; the flowers are long, thick, and whitish, set together almost like a bunch of grapes, which being gone, there succeed, for the most part, four sharp-pointed grains all together, containing a small white kernel in them.

The second differs not much from this, except that it delights in more clear water; its stalks are not flat, but round; its leaves are not so long, but more pointed. As for the place, we need not determine, for their name shews they grow in the water.

GOVERNMENT AND VIRTUES It is under the dominion of the Moon, and, being made into a poultice, is excellent good for hot inflammations and swellings, cankers, sore throats and mouths, being washed with the decoction; it cleanses and strengthens the neck and throat much.

CAMOMILE

GOVERNMENT AND VIRTUES A decoction made of camomile, and drunk, takes away all pains and stitches in the sides. It is profitable for all sorts of agues that come either from phlegm or melancholy, or from an inflammation of the bowels; the bathing with a decoction of camomile takes away weariness, eases pains to what part of the body soever it be applied; it comforts the sinews that are overstrained; mollifies all swellings; it moderately comforts all parts that have need of warmth; digests and dissolves whatsoever has need thereof by a wonderful and speedy property. It eases all the pains of the cholic and stone, and all pains and torments of the belly, and gently provokes urine: the flowers boiled in posset-drink, provoke sweat, and help to expel colds, aches, and pains wheresoever, and are an excellent help to bring down women's menses; a syrup made of the juice of camomile with the flowers and white wine, is a remedy against the jaundice and dropsy; the oil, made of the flowers of camomile is much used against all hard swellings, pains, or aches.

WILD CAMPIONS

DESCRIPTION The wild white campion has many long and somewhat broad dark green leaves lying upon the ground, with divers roots therein, somewhat like plantain, but rather hairy, broader, and not so long; the hairy stalks rise up in the middle of them three or four feet high, and sometimes more, with divers great white joints at several places thereon, and two such-like leaves thereat up to the top, sending forth branches at several joints also, all which bear, on several footstalks, white flowers at the tops of them, consisting of five broad pointed leaves, every one cut in on the end unto the middle, making them seem to be two apiece, smelling somewhat sweet, and each of them standing in large, green, striped, hairy, husks, large and round below next to the stalk; the seed is small and greyish in the hard heads that come up afterwards; the root is white, long, and spreading.

The red wild campion grows in the same manner as the white, but its leaves are not so plainly ribbed, being somewhat shorter, rounder, and more woolly in handling: the flowers are of the same size and form, but some are of a pale and others of a bright red colour, cut in at the ends more finely, which makes the leaves seem more in number than the other: the seed and the roots are alike, the roots of both sorts abiding many years.

There are forty-five sorts of campions more: those of them which are of physical uses have the like virtues with these above described.

PLACE They grow commonly throughout this kingdom in fields, and by hedge-sides and ditches.

TIME They flower in summer, some earlier than others, and some abiding longer than others.

GOVERNMENT AND VIRTUES They belong to Saturn; the decoction of the herb, either of the white or red, being drunk, does stay inward bleedings, and applied outwardly it does the like; also, being drunk, it helps to expel urine, being stopped, and gravel or stone in the kidneys.

CARDUUS BENEDICTUS

It is called *carduus benedictus*, or blessed thistle, or holy thistle; which name was doubtless given to it on account of its excellent qualities.

PLACE It grows plentifully in gardens.

TIME They flower in August, and seed soon after.

GOVERNMENT AND VIRTUES It is an herb of Mars, and under the sign Aries. It helps swimmings and giddiness of the head, or the disease called vertigo. It is an excellent remedy against the yellow jaundice, and other infirmities of the gall, because Mars governs choler. Tis herb being eaten, or the powder or juice drunk, keeps a person from the headache and megrim. The decoction helps a weak stomach, and causes appetite to meat. The powder thereof, eaten with honey, or drunk in wine, does ripen and digest cold phlegm, purges and brings up that which is in the breast, and causes to breathe more easily. The juice, drunk with wine, is good against shortness of breath, and the diseases of the lungs. The leaves bruised or pounded, and laid to, are good against burnings, hot swellings, carbuncles, and sores that are hard to be cured. Finally, the down coming off the flowers thereof, when the seed is ripe, does heal cuts and new wounds without pain.

CAROB-TREE

It is called in shops, *xylocaracta*, carob, and carobs.

DESCRIPTION This fruit grows upon a great tree, whose branches are small and covered with a red bark; the leaves are long, and spread abroad after the manner of ashen leaves, consisting of six or seven small leaves growing by a rib, one against another, of a sad dark green colour above, and of a light green underneath; the fruit is in certain crooked cods or husks, sometimes of a foot and a half long, and as broad as one's thumb; sweet in taste; in the husk is contained seed, which is large, plain, and of a chestnut colour.

PLACE This plant grows in Spain, Italy, and other hot countries.

GOVERNMENT AND VIRTUES The fruit of the carob-tree is hot and dry, and astringent, especially when it is fresh and green; somewhat subject to the influence of Saturn: the fresh and green carobs do gently loose the belly, but are hard of digestion, and if eaten in great quantity, hurtful to the stomach; but being dried they stop fluxes of the belly.

CARRAWAY

DESCRIPTION   It bears divers stalks of fine-cut leaves lying upon the ground, somewhat like the leaves of carrots, but not bushing so thick, of a little quick taste, from among which rises up a square stalk not so high as the carrot, at whose joints are set the like leaves, but smaller and finer, and at the top small open tufts or umbels of white flowers which turn into small blackish seed, smaller than anise seed, and of a quicker and hotter taste: the root is whitish, small, and long, somewhat like unto a parsnip, but with more wrinkled bark, and much less, of a little hot and quick taste, and stronger than the parsnip; it abides after seed-time.

PLACE   It is usually sown with us in gardens.

TIME   They flower in June and July, and seed quickly after.

GOVERNMENT AND VIRTUES   This is a mercurial plant. Carraway-seed has a moderate sharp quality: the root is better food than the parsnip, and is pleasant and comfortable to the stomach, helping digestion. The seed, bruised and fried, laid hot in a bag or double cloth to the lower parts of the belly, eases the pains of the wind cholic: the roots of carraways, eaten as men eat parsnips, strengthen the stomach of aged people exceedingly; it is fit to be planted in every man's garden. Carraway-comfits, once only dipped in sugar, and half a spoonful of them eaten in a morning fasting, and as many after each meal, is a most admirable remedy for such as are troubled with wind.

CARROT

DESCRIPTION   The wild carrot grows in a manner altogether like the tame, but the leaves and stalks are somewhat whiter and rougher; the stalks bear large tufts of white flowers, with a deep purple spot in the middle, which are contracted together when the seed begins to ripen; so that the middle part being hollow and low, and the outward stalks rising high, makes the whole number to shew like a bird's nest: the root is very small, long, and hard, and quite unfit for meat, being somewhat sharp and strong.

Red carrot

Yellow carrot

PLACE   The wild kind grows in divers parts of this land, plentifully by the field-sides, and in untilled places.

TIME They flower and seed in the end of summer.

GOVERNMENT AND VIRTUES Wild carrots belong to Mercury, and therefore expel wind, and remove stitches in the sides, provoke women's menses, and help to expel and break the stone; the seed also of the same works the like effect, and is good for the dropsy; it helps the cholic, the stone in the kidneys, and the rising of the womb.

CASSIA-FISTULA

It is called cassia in the cane, but is usually known by the general name of cassia-fistula in most countries.

DESCRIPTION The tree which bears the canes, has leaves not much unlike those of the ash-tree; they are great, long, and spread abroad; made of many leaves growing one against another, along by one stem; the fruit is round, long, black, and with woodish husks or cods, most commonly two feet long, and as thick as one's thumb; severed or parted in the inside into divers small cells or chambers, wherein lies flat and brownish seed, laid together with the pulp, which is black, soft, and sweet, and is called the flour, marrow, or cream, of cassia, and is very useful and profitable in medicine.

PLACE It grows in Syria, Arabia, and the East-Indies; and in the West, as Jamaica.

GOVERNMENT AND VIRTUES Cassia is excellent good for those who are troubled with hot agues, the pleurisy, jaundice, or any inflammation of the liver; especially being mixed with waters, drinks, or herbs, that are of a cooling nature. It is good to cleanse the kidneys, it drives forth gravel and the stone, and is a preservative against the stone if drunk in the decoction of liquorice, and parsley roots, or ciches. It is good to gargle with cassia, to assuage and mitigate swellings of the throat, and to dissolve, ripen, and break, imposthumes and tumours.

Avicen writes that cassia, being applied to the part grieved with the gout, assuages the pain.

CEDAR-TREE

There are two kinds hereof, the great cedar-tree and the small cedar; out of the great tree issues a white rosin, called in Latin *cedria*, and *liquor cedrinus*, or liquor of cedar.

PLATE 4
....

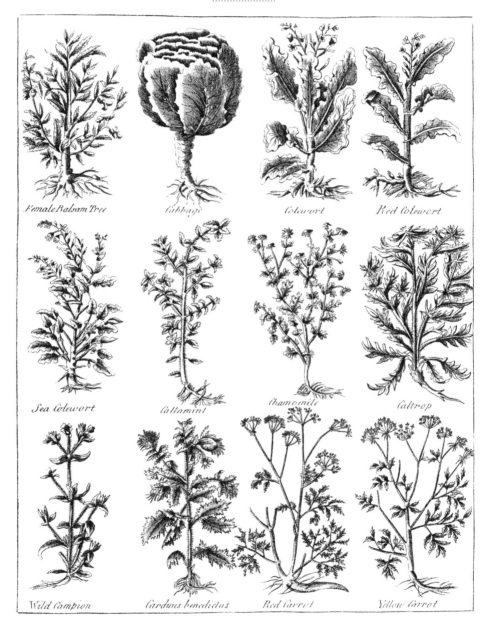

Female Balsam Tree

Cabbage

Colewort

Red Colewort

Sea Colewort

Callamint

Chamomile

Caltrop

Wild Campion

Carduus benedictus

Red Carrot

Yellow Carrot

DESCRIPTION The greater cedar grows very tall, high, great, and thick; the bark from the foot of the stem unto the first branches is rough, and from thence up to the top it is smooth and plain, of a dark blue colour, out of which there drops white rosin of its own kind, which is most odoriferous, or of a sweet smell, and by the heat of the Sun it becomes dry and hard; the limbs and branches of this tree are long, and parted into many other small branches, standing directly one against another, like those of the fir-tree; the said branches are garnished with many small leaves, thick and short, having a sweet savour; the fruit is like that of the fir-tree, but larger, thicker, and harder; the whole tree grows straight up like the fir-tree. Of the smaller cedar there are two kinds; the first kind of small cedar is much like the juniper, but somewhat smaller, the stem is crooked or writhed, and covered with a rough bark; the fruit is round berries, like juniper berries, but somewhat greater; of colour at the first green, then yellow, and at last reddish; and of an indifferent good taste.

The second kind of small cedar grows not high; but remains small and low, like the other; the leaves of this are not prickly, but somewhat round and mossy at the ends, almost like the leaves of tamarisk and savin; the fruit of this kind bears also round berries, which at first are green, afterwards yellow, and, when they are ripe, they become reddish, and are bitter in taste.

PLACE The great cedar grows in Africa and Syria, and upon the mountains of Libanus, Amanus, and Taurus. The second kind grows in Phœnicia, and in certain places of Italy, in Calabria, and also in Languedoc. The third kind grows in Lycia; and is found in certain parts of France, as in Provence and Languedoc.

TIME The great cedar perfects its fruit in two years; and it is never without fruit, which is ripe at the beginning of winter. The small cedar-trees are always green, and loaded with fruit, having at all times upon them fruit both ripe and unripe, as has juniper.

GOVERNMENT AND VIRTUES The great cedar is under the dominion of the Sun, the smaller of Mars; the cedar is hot and dry in the third degree; the rosin or *liquor cedria*, which runs forth of the great cedar-tree, is hot and dry almost in the fourth degree. The fruit of the small cedar is also hot and dry, but more moderately; *cedria*, that is, the liquor or gum of cedar, assuages the toothache, being put into the hollowness of the same. The Ancient Egyptians did use, in times past, to preserve their dead bodies with this *cedria*, for it keeps the same whole, and preserves them from corruption, but it consumes and corrupts living flesh; it kills lice, moths, worms, and all such vermin, so that they will not come near it.

The fruit of the cedar is good to be eaten against the difficulty in passing urine; it provokes urine, and brings down women's menses.

CELANDINE

DESCRIPTION This has divers tender, round, whitish-green, stalks, with greater joints than ordinary in other herbs, as it were knees, very brittle and easy to break, from whence grow branches, with large, tender, long, leaves, divided into many parts, each of them cut in on the edges, set at the joints on both sides of the branches, of a dark bluish-green colour on the upper side, like columbines, and of a more pale bluish-green underneath, full of a yellow sap, when any part is broken, of a bitter taste, and strong scent; at the tops of the branches, which are much divided, grow gold-yellow flowers of four leaves each, after which come small long pods, with blackish seed therein. Its root is somewhat great at the head, shooting forth divers long roots, and small strings, reddish on the outside, and yellow within, and is full of a yellow sap.

PLACE It grows in many places, by old walls, by the hedges and ways sides in untilled places; and being once planted in a garden, especially in a shady place, it will remain there.

TIME They flower all the summer long, and the seed ripens in the mean time.

GOVERNMENT AND VIRTUES This is an herb of the Sun, and under the celestial Lion. The herb with the roots bruised, and bathed with oil of camomile, and applied to the navel, takes away the griping pains in the belly and bowels, and all the pains of the womb, and applied to women's breasts, stays the over-much flowing of their menses; the juice or decoction of the herb, gargled between the teeth that ache, eases the pain. The juice mixed with some powder of brimstone, is not only good against the itch, but takes away all discolouring of the skin whatsoever, and, if it chance that in a tender body it causes any itching or inflammation, it is helped.

SMALLER CELANDINE

It is usually known by the name of pilewort, and fogwort.

DESCRIPTION This celandine, or pilewort, spreads many round pale green leaves, set on weak and trailing branches, which lie upon the ground, and are flat, smooth, and somewhat shining, and in some places, though seldom, marked with black spots, each standing on a long footstalk, among which rise small yellow flowers, consisting of nine or ten small narrow leaves, upon slender footstalks very like a crowfoot, whereunto the seed is not unlike, being many small ones set together upon a head: the root is composed of many small kernels like grains of corn, some twice as long others, of a whitish colour, with some fibres at the end of them.

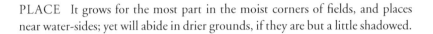

PLACE It grows for the most part in the moist corners of fields, and places near water-sides; yet will abide in drier grounds, if they are but a little shadowed.

TIME It flowers about March or April, and is quite gone in May, so that it cannot be found until it springs again.

GOVERNMENT AND VIRTUES It is under the dominion of Mars; and behold here another verification of that learning of the ancients, *viz.* that the virtue of an herb may be known by its signature; for, if you dig up the root of it, you shall see the perfect image of that disease which is commonly called the piles. The decoction of the leaves and roots does wonderfully help the piles, as also kernels by the ears and throat, called the king's evil, or any other hard wens or tumours. Pilewort made into an oil ointment, or plaster, readily cures both the piles and the king's-evil.

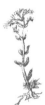

ORDINARY SMALLER CENTAURY

DESCRIPTION This grows up most usually with but one round and somewhat crested stalk, about a foot high, or better, branching forth at the top into many sprigs, and some also from the joints of the stalks below; the flowers, that stand at the tops as it were in an umbel or tuft, are of a pale red, tending to a carnation colour, consisting of five, sometimes six, small leaves, very like those of St John's wort, opening themselves in the day-time, and closing at night; after which comes the seed in little short husks, in form like wheat-corns: the leaves are small and somewhat round: the root is small and hard, perishing every year. The whole plant is of an exceeding bitter taste.

There is another sort of centaury in all things like the former, save only that it bears white flowers.

PLACE They grow generally in fields, pastures, and woods; but that with the white flowers not so frequently as the other.

TIME They flower in July, or thereabouts, and seed within a month after.

GOVERNMENT AND VIRTUES They are under the dominion of the Sun, as appears in that their flowers open and shut as the Sun either shews or hides his face. The decoction is very effectual in all pains of the joints, as the gout, cramps, or convulsions. It is good both for green and fresh wounds, as also for ulcers and sores, to close up the one and cleanse the other; especially if the green herb be bruised, and laid thereon. There is besides these another small centaury, which bears a yellow flower; in all other respects it is like the former, save that the leaves are bigger, and of a darker green, and the stalk passes through the midst of them, as it does in the herb thoroughwax.

CHERRY-TREE

PLACE For the place of its growth, it is afforded room in every orchard.

GOVERNMENT AND VIRTUES It is a tree of Venus. Cherries, as they are of different tastes, so they are of divers qualities; the sweet pass through the stomach and belly more speedily, but are of little nourishment: the tart or sour are more pleasing to a hot stomach, procuring appetite to meat, and help to cut tough phlegm and gross humours; but, when these are dried, they are more binding than when they are fresh, being cooling in hot diseases, and welcome to the stomach. The gum of the cherry-tree, dissolved in wine, is good for a cough, and hoarseness of the throat; it provokes the appetite, and helps to break and expel the stone. Black cherries bruised with the stones, and distilled, the water thereof is much used to break the stone, expel gravel, and break wind.

WINTER CHERRIES

DESCRIPTION The winter cherry has a running or creeping root in the ground, generally of the size of one's little finger, shooting forth at several joints, in several places, whereby it quickly spreads over a great compass of ground; the stalk rises not above a yard high, whereon are set many broad and long green leaves, somewhat like nightshade, but larger; at the joints whereof come forth whitish flowers made of five leaves each, which after turns into green berries, enclosed with a thin skin, which change to reddish when they grow ripe, the berry likewise being reddish and as large as a cherry, wherein are contained many flat yellowish seeds, lying within the pulp, which, being gathered and strung up, are kept all the year, to be used upon occasion.

PLACE They do not grow naturally in this land, but are cherished in gardens for their virtues.

TIME They flower not until the middle or latter end of July, and the fruit is ripe about the end of August, or beginning of September.

GOVERNMENT AND VIRTUES This is also a plant of Venus. The leaves, being cooling, may be used in inflammations; but are not opening as the berries and fruit are, which, by drawing down the urine, provoke it to be voided plentifully when it is stopped, or grown hot, sharp, or painful, in the passage; it is good also to expel the stone and gravel out of the kidneys, and bladder: the distilled water of the fruit, or the leaves together with them, or the berries green or dry, distilled with a little milk, and drunk morning and evening with a little sugar, is effectual against the heat and sharpness of the urine. The decoction of the berries in wine and water is the most usual way.

PLATE 5

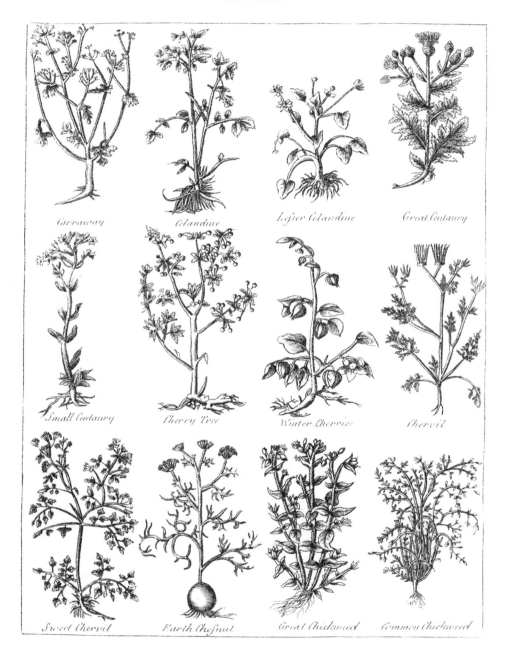

Carraway

Celandine

Lesser Celandine

Great Centaury

Small Centaury

Cherry Tree

Winter Cherries

Chervil

Sweet Chervil

Earth Chesnut

Great Chickweed

Common Chickweed

CHERVIL

It is called cerefolium, mirrhis, and mirtha, chervil, sweet chervil, and sweet cicely.

DESCRIPTION The garden chervil at first resembles parsley, but, after it is more grown, the leaves are much cut and jagged, resembling hemlock, being a little hairy, and of a whitish-green colour, sometimes turning reddish in the summer, as do the stalks also; it rises a little more than half a foot high, bearing white flowers in spiked tusts, which turn into long and round seeds, pointed at the ends, and blackish when they are ripe, of a sweet taste, but no smell, though the herb itself smells reasonably well: the root is small and long, and perishes every year, and must be sown in the spring for seed, and after July for autumn salad.

The wild chervil grows two or three feet high, with yellow stalks and joints set with broader and more hairy leaves, divided into sundry parts, nicked about the edges, and of a dark green colour, which likewise grows reddish with the stalks; at the tops whereof stand small white tusts of flowers, and afterwards smaller and longer seed: the root is white, hard, and endures long. This has little or no scent.

PLACE The first is sown in gardens for a salad-herb; the second grows wild in the meadows of this land; and by hedge-sides, and on heaths.

TIME They flower and seed early, and thereupon are sown again at the end of the summer.

GOVERNMENT AND VIRTUES The garden chervil, being eaten, does moderately warm the stomach, and is a certain remedy to dissolve congealed or clotted blood in the body. The juice or distilled water thereof being drunk, and the bruised leaves laid to the place; being taken either in meat or drink, it is held good to provoke urine, and expel the stone in the kidneys, to bring down women's menses, and to help the pleurisy. The wild chervil, bruised and applied, dissolves swellings in any part of the body.

SWEET CHERVIL

Called by some sweet cicely.

DESCRIPTION It grows very much like the greater hemlock, having large spread leaves, cut into divers parts, but of a fresher green colour than the hemlock, tasting as sweet as the aniseed; the stalk rises up a yard high, or more, being crested or hollow, having the leaves at the joints, but less, and at the tops

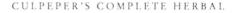

of the branched stalks umbels or tufts of white flowers; after which come large and long crested, black, shining, seed, pointed at both ends, tasting quick, yet sweet and pleasant: the root is great and white, growing deep in the ground, and spreading sundry long branches therein, in taste and smell stronger than the leaves or seed, and continuing many years.

PLACE It grows in gardens.

GOVERNMENT AND VIRTUES These are all three of them of that nature of Jupiter, and under his dominion. This whole plant, besides its pleasantness in salads, has also its physical virtues; the root boiled and eaten with oil and vinegar, or without oil, does much please and warm a cold stomach, oppressed with wind or phlegm, or those that have the phthysic or consumption of the lungs. The same, drunk with wine, provokes women's menses, and expels the after-birth, procures an appetite to meat, and expels wind; the juice is good to heal ulcers; the candied roots hereof are held as effectual as angelica to preserve from infection in the time of plague, and to warm and comfort a cold weak stomach. It is so harmless, that you cannot make use of it amiss.

CHESTNUT-TREE

GOVERNMENT AND VIRTUES The tree is under the dominion of Jupiter, and therefore the fruit must needs breed good blood, and yield commendable nourishment to the body; yet, if eaten overmuch, they make the blood thick, procure the headache, and bind the body; the inner skin that covers the nut, is of so binding a quality, that a scruple of it being taken by a man, or ten grains by a child, soon stops any flux whatsoever: the whole nut being dried and beaten into powder, and a drachm taken at a time, is a good remedy to stop the terms in women. If you dry chestnuts, and beat the kernels into powder, both the barks being taken away, and make it up into an electuary with honey, so have you an admirable remedy for the cough.

EARTH CHESTNUTS

They are called also earth-nuts, ground-nuts, cipper-nuts, and in Sussex they are called pig-nuts.

GOVERNMENT AND VIRTUES They are something hot and dry in quality; under the dominion of Venus; they provoke lust exceedingly; the seed is excellent good to provoke urine, and so also is the root, but does not perform it so forcibly as the seed. The root being dried and beaten into powder, and the powder made into an electuary, is a remedy for spitting and pissing blood.

CHICH PEASE

It is also called by some cicers.

DESCRIPTION The garden sorts, whether red, black, or white, bring forth stalks a yard long, whereon grow many small and almost round leaves, dented about the edges, set on both sides of a middle rib; at the joints come forth one or two flowers upon sharp footstalks, pease-fashion, either whitish or purplish red, lighter or deeper, according as the pease that follow will be, that are contained in small, thick, and short, pods, wherein lie one or two pease, though usually more, a little pointed at the lower end, and almost round at the head, yet a little cornered or sharp. The root is small, and perishes yearly.

PLACE AND TIME They are sown in gardens, or in fields, as pease, being sown later than pease, and gathered at the same time with them, or presently after.

GOVERNMENT AND VIRTUES They are both under the dominion of Venus. They are no less windy than beans, but nourish more; they are thought to increase sperm; they have a cleansing faculty, whereby they break the stone in the kidneys. The white cicers are used more for meat than medicine, yet have they the same effect, and are thought more powerful to increase milk and seed.

The wild cicers are so much more powerful than the garden kinds, by how much they exceed them in heat and dryness, whereby they are more effectual in opening obstructions, and breaking the stone.

CHICKWEED

PLACE These are usually found in moist and watery places, by wood-sides, and elsewhere.

Great chickweed

TIME They flower about June, and their seed is ripe in July.

Common chickweed

GOVERNMENT AND VIRTUES It is a fine, soft, pleasing, herb, under the dominion of the Moon. It is found to be as effectual as purslain to all the purposes whereunto it serves, except for meat only. The herb bruised, or the juice applied, with cloths or sponges dipped therein, to the region of the liver, does wonderfully temper the heat of the liver, and is effectual for all imposthumes and swellings whatsoever; the same helps cramps, convulsions, and palsies: the juice or distilled water is of good use for all heat and redness in the eyes, to drop some of it into them; as also into the ears to ease the pains in them, and is of good effect to ease the pains and heat and sharpness of blood in the piles, and all pains of the body in general that proceed from heat; it is used also in ulcers

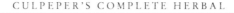

and sores. The leaves boiled with marshmallows, and made into a poultice with fenugreek and linseed, applied to swellings or imposthumes, ripens and breaks them, or assuages the swellings and eases the pains; it helps the sinews when they are shrunk by cramps or otherwise.

CINQUEFOIL

It is called in some countries, five-fingered grass, or five-leaved grass.

White cinquefoil

Red cinquefoil

DESCRIPTION   This spreads and creeps far upon the ground, with long slender strings like strawberries, which take root again and shoot forth many leaves made of five parts, and sometimes of seven, dented about the edges and somewhat hard. The stalks are slender, leaning downwards, and bear many small yellow flowers thereon, with some yellow threads in the middle, standing about a smooth green head; which when it is ripe is a little rough, and contains small brownish seed. The root is of a blackish-brown colour, seldom so big as one's little finger, but growing long with some threads thereat: and by the small strings it quickly spreads over the ground.

PLACE   It grows by wood-sides, hedge-sides, the pathways in fields, and in the borders and corners of them, almost in every part of this kingdom.

TIME   It flowers in summer, some sooner, some later.

GOVERNMENT AND VIRTUES   This is an herb of Jupiter, and therefore strengthens the parts of the body that he rules. It is an especial herb used in all inflammations and fevers: as also for all lotions, gargles, and the like, for sore mouths. The juice hereof drunk about four ounces at a time, for certain days together, cures the quinsey and the yellow jaundice. The roots boiled in milk, and drunk, is a most effectual remedy for all fluxes in man or woman, whether the whites or reds, also the bloody flux. The roots boiled in vinegar, and the decoction thereof held in the mouth, eases the pains of the toothache. The juice or decoction taken with a little honey, helps the hoarseness of the throat, and is very good for the cough of the lungs. The root boiled in vinegar, helps all knots, kernels, hard swellings, and lumps, growing in any part of the flesh, being thereto applied; as also all inflammations. The same also boiled in wine, and applied to any painful or aching joints, or the gout in the hands or feet, or the hip-gout, called the sciatica, and the decoction thereof drunk at the same time, does cure them, and eases violent pains in the bowels. The roots are likewise effectual to help ruptures or burstings, being used with other things available to that purpose, taken either inwardly or outwardly, or both.

CISTUS

Common male cistus

Common female cistus

Of this there are two sorts, the first called *cistus non ladanisera*, because it bears no *ladanum*; the other is a plant of a woody substance, upon which is found that fat liquor or gum, called *ladanum*. The first kind, which yields no *ladanum*, it also of two sorts, *viz.* male and female. The male bears red flowers, the female white; in all things else the one is like the other; out of the root of the female cistus is drawn forth a sap or liquor called *hippocristis*. The second kind of cistus is called also *ledum* and *ladum*; the fat liquor which is gathered from it is called *ladanum*, and in shops *lapdanum*.

DESCRIPTION The first kind of cistus, which bears no *ladanum*, has round hairy stalks, and stems with knotted joints, and full of branches; the leaves are roundish, and covered with a cotton of soft hair, not much unlike the leaves of sage, but shorter and rounder; the flowers grow at the tops of the stalks, of the fashion of a single rose, whereof the male kind is of colour red, and the female white; at the last they change into knops or husks wherein the seed is contained.

There is found a certain excrescence or out-growing, about the root of this plant, which is of colour sometimes yellow, sometimes white, and sometimes green; out of which is artificially drawn a certain juice, which in shops is called *hypocistis*, and is used in medicine.

The second kind of cistus, which is also called *ledum*, is a plant of a woody substance, growing like a little tree or shrub, with soft leaves, in figure not much unlike the others, but longer and browner; upon the leaves of this plant is found that fat substance called *ladanum*, which is generally about midsummer and the hottest days.

PLACE The first kind of cistus grows in Italy, Sicily, Candia, Cyprus, Languedoc, and other hot countries, in rough and untilled places. The second kind grows also in Crete, Cyprus, and Languedoc.

TIME The first kind of cistus flowers in June, and sometimes sooner. The second kind of cistus flowers and brings forth seed in the spring time, and immediately after the leaves fall off, and about midsummer there come new leaves again: upon which leaves in the hottest days, is found a certain fatness, which is diligently gathered and dried, and makes that gum which is called *lapdanum*.

GOVERNMENT AND VIRTUES These plants are governed by Jupiter; the flowers and leaves of cistus are dry in the second degree, and somewhat astringent; that which grows about the roots, is of like temperature but more astringent; *lapdanum* is hot in the second degree almost, and is somewhat dry and astringent. The flowers of cistus boiled in wine and drunk, stop the lask, and all issues of blood. *Hypocistus* stops all fluxes of the belly, and is of a stronger operation than the flowers and leaves of cistus; wherefore it cures the bloody flux, and the immoderate overflowing of women's menses. *Ladanum* is very good against the hardness of the matrix or womb; laid to in manner of a pessary; it draws down the secundine or after-birth, when it is laid upon quick coals, and the fumigation or smoke thereof be received up into the matrix; the same applied to the head with myrrh, or oil of myrrh, cures the scurf thereof.

CIVES

They are also called rush-leeks, chives, civet, and sweth.

TEMPERATURE AND VIRTUES They are indeed a kind of leeks, hot and dry in the fourth degree as they are, and also under the dominion of Mars; if they are eaten raw they send up very hurtful vapours to the brain, causing troublesome sleep, and spoiling the eye-sight; yet of them prepared by the art of the alchemist may be made an excellent remedy for stoppage of urine.

CLARY

Or, more properly, clear-eye.

DESCRIPTION Our ordinary garden clary has four-square stalks, with broad, rough, wrinkled, whitish, or hairy green, leaves, somewhat evenly cut on the edges, and of a strong sweet scent, growing some near the ground, and some by couples upon stalks: the flowers grow at certain distances with two small leaves at the joints under them, somewhat like the flowers of sage, but smaller, and of a whitish-blue colour: the seed is brownish and somewhat flat, or not so round as the wild: the roots are blackish, and do not spread far; it perishes after the seeding time. It is usually sown, for it seldom rises of its own sowing.

PLACE This grows in gardens.

TIME It grows in June and July, some a little later than others, and their seed is ripe in August, or thereabout.

GOVERNMENT AND VIRTUES It is under the dominion of the Moon. The mucilage of the seed made with water, and applied to tumours or swellings, disperses and takes them away; it also draws forth splinters, thorns, or other things, gotten into the flesh. The powder of the dried root put into the nose provokes sneezing, and thereby purges the head and brain of much rheum. The juice of the herb put into ale or beer, and drunk, brings down women's menses, and expels the after-birth.

WILD CLARY

Wild clary is often, though I think imprudently, called *Christ's eye*, because it cures the diseases of the eyes.

DESCRIPTION It is like the other clary, but less, with many stalks about a foot and a half high; the stalks are square and somewhat hairy; the flowers of a bluish colour.

PLACE It grows commonly in this kingdom, in barren places; you may find it plentifully if you look in the fields near Gray's Inn, and the fields near Chelsea.

TIME They flower from the beginning of June to the latter end of August.

GOVERNMENT AND VIRTUES It is something hotter and drier than the garden clary, yet nevertheless under the dominion of the Moon, as well as that the seeds of it being beaten to powder and drunk in wine is an admirable help to provoke lust; a decoction of the leaves being drunk warms the stomach, and it is a wonder if it should not, the stomach being under Cancer the house of the Moon. It helps digestion, scatters congealed blood in any part of the body, and helps dimness of sight; the distilled water thereof cleanses the eyes of redness, waterishness, and heat.

CLEAVERS

It is also called aparine, goose-share, and goose-grass.

DESCRIPTION The common cleavers has divers very rough square stalks, not so big as the tag of a point, but rising up to be two or three yards high sometimes, if it meets with any tall bushes or trees whereon it may climb, yet without any claspers; or else much lower, and lying upon the ground full of joints, and at every one of them shoots forth a branch, besides the leaves thereat, which are usually fix, set in a round compass like a star, or the rowel of a spur: from between the leaves of the joints towards the tops of the branches, come forth very small white flowers at every end upon small thready footstalks, which after they are fallen, there do shew two small, round, rough, seeds; and these, when they are ripe, grow hard and whitish, having a little hole on the side somewhat like unto a navel. Both stalks, leaves, and seeds, are so rough, that they will cleave unto any thing that shall touch them. Its root is small and thready, spreading much in the ground, but dies every year.

PLACE It grows by the hedge and ditch sides, in many places of this land.

TIME It flowers in June and July, and the seed is ripe, and falls again, about the end of July or August, from whence it springs up again, and not from the old roots.

GOVERNMENT AND VIRTUES It is under the dominion of the Moon. It is familiarly taken in broth to keep those lean and lank that are apt to grow fat. The juice of the leaves, or the leaves a little bruised, and applied to any bleeding wound, stays the bleeding; the juice is also very good to close up the lips of green wounds.

CLOWN'S WOUNDWORT

DESCRIPTION It grows up sometimes to three or four feet high, but usually about two feet, with square, green, rough, stalks, but slender, jointed somewhat far asunder, and two very long, and somewhat narrow, dark green leaves, bluntly dented about the edges, and ending in a long point. The flowers stand toward the tops, compassing the stalks at the joints with the leaves, and end likewise in a spiked top, having long and much open gaping hoods, of a purplish-red colour with whitish spots in them, standing in somewhat rough husks, wherein afterwards stand blackish round seeds. The root is composed of many long strings, with some tuberous long knobs growing among them, of a pale yellowish or whitish colour, yet at some times of the year these knobby roots in many places are not seen in the plant: the whole plant smells somewhat strongly.

PLACE It grows in sundry counties of this land, both north and west, and frequently by path-sides in the fields near about London, and within three or four miles distance about it, yet usually grows in or near ditches.

TIME It flowers in June and July, and the seed is ripe soon after.

GOVERNMENT AND VIRTUES It is under the dominion of the planet Saturn. It is singularly effectual in all fresh and green wounds, and therefore bears not this name for nought. And is very available in staunching of blood. A syrup made of the juice is inferior to none for inward wounds, and ruptures of veins: ruptures are excellently and speedily cured by taking now and then a little of the syrup, and applying an ointment or plaster of the herb to the place.

COCKLE

It is called also nigel-weed, and field-nigella.

DESCRIPTION   It has straight, slender, hairy stems, the leaves are also long, narrow, hairy, and greyish; the flowers are of a brown-purple colour, changing towards red, divided into five small leaves, not much differing from the proportion of wild campions; after which there grows round cups, wherein is contained plenty of seed, of a black-brown colour.

PLACE   It is frequent amongst corn, wheat, rye, and barley.

TIME   It flowers in May, June, and July.

GOVERNMENT AND VIRTUES   This is of a Saturnine quality, causes giddiness of the head, and stupifies if it gets amongst the corn to be made with it into bread, and howsoever taken, it is dangerous and hurtful.

COCK'S HEAD

Otherwise called red sitchling, or medick fetch.

DESCRIPTION   This has divers weak but rough stalks, half a yard long, leaning downwards, beset with winged leaves, longer and more pointed than those of lentils, and whitish underneath; from the tops of those stalks arise up other slender stalks, naked without leaves unto the tops, where there grow many small flowers in manner of a spike, of a pale-reddish colour, with some blueness among them; after which rise up in their places, round, rough, and somewhat flat, heads. The root is tough and somewhat woody, yet lives and shoots afresh every year.

PLACE   It grows under hedges, and sometimes in the open fields, in divers places of this land.

TIME   They flower all the months of July and August, and the seed ripens in the mean while.

GOVERNMENT AND VIRTUES   It is under the dominion of Venus. The green leaves bruised and laid as a plaster, disperse knots, nodes, or kernels, in the flesh: and, if when it is dry it be taken in wine, it helps the difficulty in passing urine; and, being anointed with oil, it provokes sweat.

COCOA-NUT TREE

DESCRIPTION AND NAMES   This grows to be a large timber-tree, the body covered with a smooth bark; bare or naked, without any branch, to a great

PLATE 6

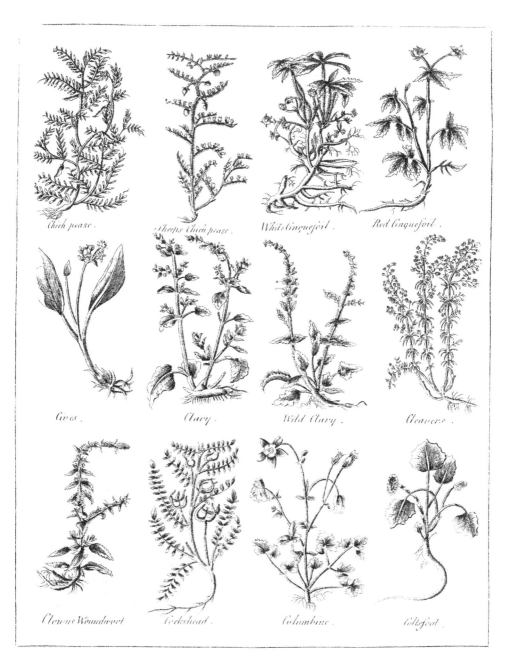

Chich pease.   Sheeps Chich pease.   White Cinquefoil.   Red Cinquefoil.

Cives.   Clary.   Wild Clary.   Cleavers.

Clowns Woundwort.   Cockshead.   Columbine.   Coltsfoot.

height and towards the top it spreads out into sundry great arms, which bow themselves almost round; with large leaves on them like the date-tree leaf, but larger, whose middle rib is very great, and abiding always green, and with fruit also, continually one succeeding another: from between the lower boughs come forth smaller stalks, hanging down, and bearing sundry flowers on them, like those of the chestnut tree; after which come large three-square fruit or nuts, ten or twelve and sometimes twenty thereon together, as big as one's head, or as a small pompion, almost round, but a little smaller at the end, covered with a hard, tough, ash-coloured, thick bark, an inch thick in some places, and within it a hard, woody, brownish, shell, but which becomes black when polished; having at the head or top thereof three holes, somewhat resembling the nose and eyes of a monkey; between which outer bark and this shell grow many gross threads or hairs; within the wooden shell there is a white kernel cleaving close to the side thereof, as sweet as an almond, with a fine sweet water in the middle as pleasant as milk, which will grow less pleasant, or consume, either by over ripeness or long keeping. This tree is called by the Indians *maro*, in Malacca *trican*, and in other places by several other appellations. The timber of this tree is solid and firm, black and shining, like the walnut-tree, and fit for any building; and Garcias saith, it is of two sorts, the one to bear fruit, the other to attract the liquor which issues therefrom, when the branches are cut, or when it is bored, and received into something tied thereunto for that purpose, which liquor they call in their language *sura*; and it shews like unto troubled wine, but in taste like new sweet wine, which being boiled they call *orraque*; and being distilled it yields a spirit like unto our *aqua vitæ*, and it is used for the same purpose as we do ours, and will burn like it: they call it *fula*, and being set in the Sun it will become good vinegar, and that which runs last, being set in the Sun to grow hard, or boiled to hardness, will become sugar, which they call *jagra*. Of the inner kernel, while it is fresh, they make bread; the fresher the nuts are, the sweeter is the meat thereof.

GOVERNMENT AND VIRTUES This is a solar plant; the fruit or kernel of the cocoa-nut does nourish very much, and is good for lean bodies; they increase the natural seed, and are good to mollify the hoarseness of the throat.

COFFEE

This is reported to be the berries of certain shrubs or bushes growing in Arabia, and from thence into Turkey, and other parts. It is said of itself to be insipid, having neither scent nor taste; but being pounded and baked, as they do prepare it to make the coffee-liquor with, it then stinks most loathsomely, which is an argument of some Saturnine quality in it: the propugners for this filthy drink affirm that it causes watchfulness; (so does the stinking hemlock and henbane in their first operation if unhappily taken into the body, but their worse effects soon follow;) they also say it makes them sober when they are drunk. If there had been any worth in it, some of the ancient Arabian physicians would have recorded it; but there is no mention made of any medicinal use thereof, by any author, either ancient or modern.

COLOQUINTIDA

It is also called, wild-bitter-gourd, and the fruit coloquint-apple.

DESCRIPTION Coloquintida creeps with its branches along by the ground, with rough hairy leaves, of a greyish colour, much cloven or cut; the flowers are bleak or pale; the fruit round, of a green colour at the beginning, and afterwards yellow; the bark thereof is neither thick nor hard, the inner part of the pulp is open and spongy, full of grey seed, in taste very bitter; the which is dried and kept for medicinal use.

PLACE Coloquintida grows in Italy and Spain, from which places the dried fruit is brought unto us.

TIME Coloquintida brings forth its fruit in September.

NATURE AND VIRTUES It is under the planetary influence of Mars; of temperature hot and dry in the third degree; the white or inward pith or pulp of the apple, taken about the weight of a scruple, opens the belly mightily, and purges gross phlegm and choleric humours; but if taken in two great a quantity, it causes blood to come forth. Coloquintida, if administered by an unskilful hand, is very dangerous and hurtful to the stomach and liver, and troubles the bowels and entrails.

COLTSFOOT

Called also cough-wort, foal's foot, horse hoof, and bull's foot.

DESCRIPTION This shoots up a slender stalk with small yellowish flowers, somewhat early, which fall away quickly; after they are past, come up somewhat round leaves, sometimes dented a little about the edges, much less, thicker, and greener, than those of the butter-bur; with a little down or freeze over the green leaf on the upper side, which may be rubbed away, and whitish or mealy underneath. The root is small and white, spreading much under ground, so that where it takes it will hardly be driven away again, if any little piece be abiding therein; and from thence spring fresh leaves.

PLACE It grows as well in wet grounds as in drier places.

TIME It flowers in the end of February, the leaves beginning to appear in March.

GOVERNMENT AND VIRTUES The plant is under Venus. The fresh leaves, or juice, or a syrup made thereof, is good for a hot dry cough, for wheezings and shortness of breath: the dry leaves are best for those that have thin rheums, and distillations upon their lungs, causing a cough, for which also the dried leaves taken as tobacco, or the root, is very good. The distilled water hereof simply, or with elderflowers and nightshade, is a singular remedy against all hot agues, to drink two ounces at a time, and apply cloths wet therein to the head and stomach; which also does much good being applied to any hot swellings or inflammations; it helps burnings, and is singular good to take away weals and small pushes that arise through heat.

COLUMBINES

TIME They flower in May, and abide not for the most part when June is past, perfecting their seed in the mean time.

GOVERNMENT AND VIRTUES It is also an herb of Venus. The leaves of columbines are commonly used in lotions with good success for sore mouths and throats; Tragus saith, that a drachm of the seed taken in wine, with a little saffron, opens obstructions of the liver, and is good for the yellow jaundice, if the party after the taking thereof be laid to sweat well in his bed: the seed also taken in wine causes a speedy delivery of women in child-birth.

COMFREY

DESCRIPTION The common great comfrey has divers very large and hairy green leaves, lying on the ground, so hairy or prickly, that if they touch any tender part of the hands, face, or body, it will cause it to itch: the stalk that rises up from among them, being two or three feet high, hollowed, and cornered, as also very hairy, having many such-like leaves as grow below, but runs less and less up to the top. At the joints of the stalks it is divided into many branches, with some leaves thereon; and at the ends stand many flowers in order one above another, which are somewhat long and hollow like the finger of a glove, of a pale-whitish colour, after which come small black seed. The roots are great and long, spreading great thick branches under ground, black on the outside and whitish within, short or easy to break, and full of glutinous or clammy juice, of little or no taste.

PLATE 7

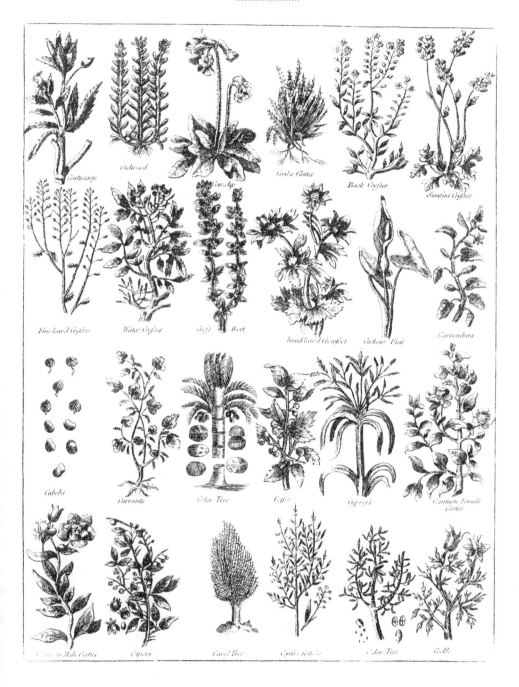

Costmary | Gutweed | Cowslip | Coleseed Garlic Cresses | Bank Cresses | Swatica Cresses

Fine leav'd Cresses | Water Cresses | Flea Wort | broad leav'd Crowfoot | Cuckow Pint | Cucumbers

Cubebs | Currants | Cedar Tree | Coffee | Cypress | Common Female Cistus

Common Male Cistus | Capers | Carol Tree | Cassia fistula | Cedar Tree | Cockle

There is another sort in all things like this, save only it is somewhat less, and bears flowers of a pale purple colour.

PLACE They grow by ditches and water-sides, and in fields that are moist, for therein they chiefly delight to grow: the first generally through all the land, and the other not quite so common.

TIME They flower in June and July, and give their seed in August.

GOVERNMENT AND VIRTUES This is also an herb of Saturn. What was spoken of clown's woundwort may be said of this; the great comfrey helps those that make a bloody urine; the root boiled in water or wine, and the decoction drunk, helps the ulcers of the lungs; it stays the defluxions of rheum from the head upon the lungs, the fluxes of blood or humours by the belly, and women's immoderate menses.

The root being outwardly applied, helps fresh wounds or cuts immediately, being bruised and laid thereunto. It is good to be applied to women's breasts that grow sore by the abundance of milk coming into them. The roots of comfrey taken fresh, beaten small, and spread upon leather, and laid upon any place troubled with the gout, do presently give ease of the pains; and applied in the same manner, give ease to pained joints.

CORAL

There are several kinds of coral, but the red and the white, especially the red, is most in use. There are also several sorts of black coral, called *antipathes*; and there is a kind of coral which is black, rough, and bristly, and is called *sambeggia*.

DESCRIPTION These plants, although their hard substance makes them seem rather to be stones, yet they are vegetables. The great red coral, which is the best, grows upon rocks in the sea, like unto a shrub, with arms and branches, which shoot forth into sprigs, some large and some small, of a pale red colour for the most part, when it is taken out of the water, but when it is polished it is very fair, and of a beautiful red colour; whilst it is in water it is soft and pliable, but, being taken out and kept dry a while, it becomes of a hard stony substance.

PLACE The corals are found in the isles of Sardinia, and divers other places.

CORAL-WORT

It is also called by some, tooth-wort, toothed violet, dog-teeth violet, and *dentaris*.

DESCRIPTION This shoots forth one or two winged leaves upon long brownish footstalks, which are doubled down at their first coming out of the ground: when they are fully opened they consist of seven leaves, most commonly of a sad-green colour, dented about the edges, set on both sides the middle rib one against another, as the leaves of the ash-tree; the stalk bears no leaves on the lower half of it, the upper half bears sometimes three or four, each consisting of five leaves, sometimes but of three; on the top stand four or five flowers upon short foot-stalks, with long husks; the flowers are very like those of the stock gilliflower, of a pale purplish colour, consisting of four leaves apiece, after which come small cods which contain the seed: the root is very smooth, white, and shining; it does not grow downwards, but creeping along under the upper crust of the ground, and consists of divers small round knobs, set together: towards the top of the stalk, there grow small single leaves, by each of which comes a small round cloven bulb, which when it is ripe, if it be set in the ground, it will grow to be a root, and is esteemed a good way of cultivating the herb.

PLACE It grows near Mayfield in Sussex, in a wood called High-reed, and in another wood there also, called Fox-holes.

TIME They flower from the latter end of April to the middle of May, and before the middle of July they are gone and not to be found.

GOVERNMENT AND VIRTUES It is under the dominion of the Moon. It cleanses the bladder, expels gravel and the stone; it eases pains in the sides and bowels; by taking a drachm of the powder of the root every morning in wine it is excellent good for ruptures, as also to stop fluxes: an ointment made of it is exceeding good for wounds and ulcers.

CORIANDER

It is called in shops *coriandrum*, in English coriander, and in some counties colyander.

DESCRIPTION This bears a round stalk, full of branches, each about a foot and a half long; the leaves are jagged and cut, the under leaves that spring up first, are almost like the leaves of chervil or parsley, and the upper leaves are not much unlike the same, or rather like to fumitory leaves, but a great deal tenderer, and more jagged; the flowers are white, and grow in round tuffets, the seed is all round, and hollow within, and of a very pleasant scent when it is dry; the root is hard, and of a woody substance.

PLACE It is sown in gardens, and loves a good soil.

TIME It flowers in July and August, and the seed is ripe shortly after.

GOVERNMENT AND VIRTUES The green plant is cold and dry, of a Saturnine quality; but the sweet savouring seed is of a warm temperature, and useful for many purposes. The seed of coriander being prepared, and taken alone, or covered with sugar, after meals, closes up the mouth of the stomach.

CORNEL-TREE

It is called of some, long cherry, or long cherry-tree.

DESCRIPTION The cornel-tree sometimes grows up to a reasonable bigness, like other trees, and sometimes it is but low, and grows like to a shrub or hedgebush, as divers other small trees do; the wood or timber of this tree is very hard; the flowers are of a faint yellowish colour, the fruit is very red, and somewhat long, almost like an olive, but smaller, with a long little stone or kernel inclosed therein, like the stone of an olive-berry.

PLACE The cornel-tree is in this country to be found no where but in gardens and orchards, where it is planted.

GOVERNMENT AND VIRTUES It cures the falling sickness, and gripings in the belly or bowels; it helps those that have loose or weak sinews, and pains of the sciatica or hip-gout.

COSTMARY

Called also alecost or balsam herb.

TIME It flowers in June and July.

GOVERNMENT AND VIRTUES It is under the dominion of Jupiter. It opens obstructions, and is a wonderful help to all sorts of dry agues. It is astringent to the stomach, and strengthens the liver, and all the other inward parts, and if taken in whey works the more effectually.

COWSLIPS

Known also by the name of peagles.

TIME They flower in April and May.

GOVERNMENT AND VIRTUES Venus lays claim to the herb as her own, and it is under the sign Aries, and our city dames know well enough the ointment or distilled water of it adds beauty. The flowers are held to be more effectual than the leaves, and the roots of little use. An ointment being made with them adds beauty exceedingly; they remedy all infirmities of the head coming of heat and wind; the roots ease pains in the back and bladder. The leaves are good in wounds, and the flowers take away trembling. Because they remedy the palsies, the Greeks gave them the name of *paralysis*.

CRAB'S CLAWS

Called also water fengreen, knight's pond-water, water housleek, pondweed, and fresh-water soldier.

DESCRIPTION It has sundry long narrow leaves, with sharp prickles on the edges of them, also very sharp pointed; the stalks which bear flowers seldom grow so high as the leaves, bearing a forked head like a crab's claw, out of which comes a white flower, consisting of three leaves, with divers yellowish hairy threads in the middle: it takes root in the mud, in the bottom of the water.

PLACE It grows plentifully in the fens of Lincolnshire.

TIME It flowers in June, and usually from thence till August.

GOVERNMENT AND VIRTUES It is a plant under the dominion of Venus, and therefore assuages inflammations and swellings in wounds; an ointment made of it is excellent good to heal them: there is scarce a better remedy growing than this for such as have bruised their kidneys. A drachm of the powder of the herb taken every morning is a good remedy to stop women's menses.

BLACK CRESSES

DESCRIPTION They have long leaves deeply cut and jagged on both sides, not much unlike wild mustard; the stalks are small, very limber though very tough; you may twist them round as you may a willow before they break. The flowers are very small and yellow, after which come small cods which contain the seed.

PLACE It is a common herb, grows usually by the way sides, and sometimes upon mud walls about London.

TIME It flowers in June and July, and the seed is ripe in August and September.

GOVERNMENT AND VIRTUES It is under the dominion of Mars, and is a plant of a hot and biting nature: the truth is, the seed of black cresses strengthen the brain, exceedingly: they are excellent good to stay those rheums which fall down from the head upon the lungs. You may beat the seed into powder if you please, and make it up into an electuary with honey, so have you an excellent remedy by you for the cough, yellow jaundice, and sciatica. The herb boiled into a poultice is an excellent remedy for inflammation.

SCIATICA CRESSES

DESCRIPTION These are of two kinds; the first rises up with a round stalk about two feet high, spread into divers branches, whose lower leaves are somewhat larger than the upper, yet all of them cut or torn on the edges, somewhat like garden cresses, but smaller: the flowers are small and white, growing on the tops of the branches, where afterwards grow husks, with smallish-brown seed therein, very strong and sharp in taste, more than the cresses of the garden. The root is long, white, and woody.

The other sort has the lower leaves whole, somewhat long and broad, not torn at all, but only somewhat deeply dented about the edges toward the ends, but those that grow higher up are less. The flowers and seed are like the former, and so is the root likewise: and both root and seed as sharp as it.

PLACE These grow by the way-sides in untilled places, and by the sides of old walls.

TIME They flower in the end of June, and their seed is ripe in July.

GOVERNMENT AND VIRTUES It is a Saturnine plant: the leaves but especially the roots taken fresh in the summer time, beaten and made into a poultice or salve with hog's grease, and applied to the places pained with the sciatica, the place afterwards bathed and then wrapped with wool or skins after they have sweat a little, will assuredly cure not only the same disease in the hips, huckle-bone, or other of the joints, as gout in the hands or feet, but all other old griefs of the body. Cresses, either boiled or eaten in salads, are very wholesome.

WATER-CRESSES

DESCRIPTION Our ordinary water-cresses spread forth with many weak, hollow, sappy, stalks, shooting out fibres at the joints, and upwards long winged leaves, made of sundry broad, sappy, and almost round, leaves, of a brownish-green colour: the flowers are many and white, standing on long footstalks, after which come small yellow seed, contained in small long pods like horns, the whole plant abides green in the winter, and tastes somewhat hot and sharp.

PLACE They grow for the most part in the small standing waters, yet sometimes in small rivulets of running water.

TIME They flower and seed in the beginning of summer.

GOVERNMENT AND VIRTUES It is an herb under the dominion of the Moon. It is more powerful against the scurvy, and to cleanse the blood and humours, than brooklime, and serves in all the other uses in which brooklime is available; as to break the stone, and provoke women's menses. The leaves bruised, or the juice, mixed with vinegar, and the sore part of the head bathed therewith, is very good for those that have the lethargy.

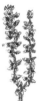

CROSS-WORT

DESCRIPTION Common cross-wort grows with square hairy brown stalks little above a foot high, having four small, broad, and pointed, hairy, yet smooth, green leaves, growing at every joint, each against other crossways, which has caused the name. Toward the tops of the stalks at the joints, with the leaves in three or four rows downward, stand small pale-yellow flowers, after which come small blackish round seeds, four for the most part set in every husk; the root is very small, and full of fibres or threads, taking good hold of the ground, and spreading with the branches a great deal of ground, which perish not in winter, although the leaves die every year, and spring again anew.

PLACE It grows in moist grounds, as well meadows as untilled places about London, in Hampstead church-yard, at Wye in Kent, and sundry other places.

TIME It flowers from May all the summer long, in one place or another, as they are more open to the Sun; the seed ripens soon after.

GOVERNMENT AND VIRTUES It is under the dominion of Saturn. This is a singular good wound-herb, and is used inwardly, not only to stay bleeding of wounds, but to consolidate them, as it does outwardly any green wound, which it quickly dries up and heals. The decoction of the herb in wine, helps to expectorate phlegm out of the chest, and is good for obstructions in the breast, stomach, or bowels, and helps a decayed appetite. It is also good to wash any wound or sore with, to cleanse and heal it.

CROWFOOT

Many are the names this furious biting herb has obtained; it is called frog's foot, from the Greek name *barrakion*, crowfoot, gold-knobs, gold-cups, king's-knob, baffiners, troil-flowers, polts, locket-goulions, and butter-flowers.

DESCRIPTION The most common crowfoot has many dark green leaves, cut into divers parts, in taste biting and sharp, biting and blistering the tongue; it bears many flowers, and those of a bright resplendent yellow colour. I do not remember that I ever saw any thing yellower. Virgins in ancient times used to make powder of them to furrow bride-beds. After the flowers come small heads, somewhat spiked and rugged like a pine-apple.

PLACE They grow very common every where; unless you turn your head into a hedge, you cannot but see them as you walk.

TIME They flower in May and June, even till September.

GOVERNMENT AND VIRTUES This fiery and hot-spirited herb of Mars, is no way fit to be given inwardly, but the herb being bruised and mixed with a little mustard, draws a blister.

CUBEBS

Cubebs are small berries, somewhat sweet, about the bigness of pepper-corns, but not so black nor solid, but more rugged or crested, being either hollow or having a kernel within, of a hot taste, but not so fiery as pepper; and having each a short stalk on them like a tail: these grow on trees less than apple-trees, with leaves narrower than those of pepper; the flower is sweet, and the fruit grows clustering together. The Arabians call them *quabebe*, and *quabebe chini*: they grow plentifully in Java; they are used to warm and strengthen the stomach, when it is overcome with phlegm or wind; they cleanse the breast of thick tough humours, and help the spleen. Being chewed in the mouth with mastic, they draw rheum from the head, and strengthen the brain and memory.

CUCKOW-POINT

It is called alron, janus, and barba-aron, calves-foot, ramp, starch-wort, cuckow-pintle, priest's-pintle, and wake-robin.

DESCRIPTION This shoots forth three, four, or five, leaves at the most, from one root, every one whereof is somewhat large and long, broad at the bottom, next the stalk, and forked, but ending in a point, without a cut on the edges, of a full green colour, each standing upon a thick round stalk, of a handful breadth long, or more, among which, after two or three months that they begin to wither, rises up a bare, round, whitish-green, stalk, spotted and streaked with purple, somewhat higher than the leaves; at the top whereof stands a long hollow house or husk, close at the bottom, but open from the middle upwards ending in a point; in the middle whereof stands the small long pestle or clapper, smaller at the bottom than at the top, of a dark purple colour, as the husk is on the inside, though green without; which after it has so abided for some time, the husk with the clapper decays, and the foot at bottom thereof grows to be a small long bunch of berries, green at the first and of a yellowish-red colour when they are ripe, of the size of a hasel-nut kernel, which abides thereon almost until winter; the root is round, and somewhat long, for the most part lying along, the leaves shooting forth at the bigger end, which, when it bears its berries, are somewhat wrinkled and loose, another growing under it, which is solid and firm, with many small threads hanging thereat. The whole plant is of a very sharp biting taste, pricking the tongue as nettles do the hands, and so abides for a great while without alteration. The root hereof was anciently used instead of starch to starch linen.

PLACE   These grow frequently under almost every hedge-side in many places of this land.

TIME   They shoot forth leaves in the spring, and continue only until the middle of summer, or somewhat later; their husks appearing before they fall away, and their fruit shewing in April.

GOVERNMENT AND VIRTUES   It is under the dominion of Mars. The green leaves bruised, and laid upon any boil, does very wonderfully help to draw forth the poison. A drachm of the powder of the dried root taken with twice as much sugar does wonderfully help those that are pursy or short-winded, as also those that have a cough; it breaks, digests, and rids away, phlegm from the stomach, chest, and lungs. The milk wherein the root has been boiled is effectual also for the same purpose. The said powder taken in wine or other drink, or the juice of the berries, or the powder of them, or the wine wherein they have been boiled, brings down women's menses, and purges them effectually after child-bearing, to bring away the after-birth: taken with sheep's milk, it heals the inward ulcers of the bowels.

CUCUMBERS

According to the pronunciation of the vulgar, cowcumbers.

GOVERNMENT AND VIRTUES They are under the dominion of the Moon. The juice of cucumbers, the face being washed with it, cleanses the skin, and is excellent good for hot rheum in the eyes; the seed is excellent to provoke urine, and cleanse the passages thereof when they are stopped; neither do I think there is a better remedy for ulcers in the bladder, than cucumbers are; the usual course is to use the seeds in emulsions, as they make almond-milk; but a better way by far (in my opinion) is this: when the season of the year is, take the cucumbers and bruise them well, and distil the water from them, and let such as are troubled with ulcers in their bladders drink no other drink.

CUDWEED

Besides cudweed, it is also called cottonweed, chaffweed, dwarf cotton, and petty cotton.

DESCRIPTION The common cudweed rises up with one stalk, though sometimes two or three, thick set on all sides with small, long, and narrow, whitish or woody, leaves, from the middle of the stalk almost up to the top; with every leaf stands a small flower, of a dun or brownish-yellow colour, or not so yellow as others; in which herbs, after the flowers are fallen, come small seed wrapped up with the down therein, and is carried away with the wind. The root is small and thready.

There are other sorts hereof, which are somewhat less than the former, not much different, save only that the stalk and leaves are shorter, and the flowers are paler, and more open.

PLACE They grow in dry, barren, sandy, and gravelly, grounds, in most places of this land.

TIME They flower about July, some earlier and some later, and their seed is ripe in August.

GOVERNMENT AND VIRTUES Venus is lady of it. The plants are all astringent, or binding, and drying, and therefore profitable for defluxions of rheum from the head, and to stay fluxes of blood wheresoever. The green leaves bruised and laid to any green wound, will stay the bleeding.

RED, WHITE, AND BLACK CURRANTS

The Latin names for currants are *ribes*, and *ribes fructu rubro*, the red currant, *albo* white, and *nigro* black.

DESCRIPTION   The red-currant bush has a stalk covered with a thin brownish bark outwards, and greenish underneath; the leaves are of a blackish green, cut on the edges into five parts, much like a vine-leaf, but smaller; the flowers come forth at the joints of the leaves, many together on a long stalk, hanging down about a finger's length; of an herby colour, after which come round berries, green at the first, but red when they are ripe: of a pleasant tart taste, wherein is small seed. The root is woody and spreading. There is another sort hereof, whose berries are twice as large as the former, and of a better relish.

The white-currant tree has a taller and straighter stem than the red, a whiter bark, and smaller leaves, but has such-like berries upon long stalks, of the same bigness as the first, but of a shining transparent whiteness, and of a more pleasant taste than the former.

The black-currant rises higher than the last, and is thicker set with branches round about, and more pliant, the younger covered with a pale, and the elder with a browner, bark; the leaves are smaller than those of the former, and often with fewer cuts therein: the flowers are alike, but of a greenish-purple colour, which produce small black berries; the leaves and fruit have an unpleasant smell, but yet are wholesome, though not palatable.

PLACE   All these sorts of currants grow plentifully in England, in gardens where they are planted; they have been found growing naturally wild in Savoy and Switzerland, as Gesner saith; and some in Austria, saith Clusius: they grow in great abundance in Candia, and other places in the Straights, from whence in great quantities they are brought dried unto us.

TIME   They flower and bear fruit in June, July, and August.

GOVERNMENT AND VIRTUES   Currants are under the influence of the benevolent planet Venus; they are of a most temperate refreshing nature; the red and white currants are good to cool and refresh faintings of the stomach, to quench thirst, and stir up an appetite, and therefore are profitable in hot and sharp agues.

CYPRESS-TREE

It has no other name in English, but this tree is called *cupressus* in Latin; and the nuts or fruit thereof, *nuces cupressi*; in English, cypress-nuts.

DESCRIPTION   The cypress-tree has a thick, strait, long, stem; upon which grow many slender branches; which do not spread abroad, but grow up in length towards the top, so that the cypress-tree is not broad, but narrow, growing to a great height; the bark of the cypress-tree is brown, the timber yellowish, hard, thick, and close, and when it is dry of a pleasant smell, especially if it be set near the fire. Cypress-tree has no particular leaves, but the branches, instead of leaves, bring forth short twigs, cut and snipped in many places, as if they were set about with many small leaves; the fruit is round, almost as big as a prune or plum, which being ripe does open in divers places, and has in it a flat greyish seed.

PLACE The cypress-tree delights in dry, hilly, and mountainous, places, in hot countries.

TIME The cypress-tree is always green; the fruit is ripe in September, at the beginning of winter.

GOVERNMENT AND VIRTUES Saturn rules this plant; the leaves and fruit are dry in the third degree, without any manifest heat, and very astringent; the fruit of cypress, taken into the body, stops looseness and the bloody-flux; the decoction of the same, made with water, has the same virtue. The oil, in which the fruit or leaves of cypress have been boiled, does strengthen the stomach. The leaves of cypress, boiled in sweet wine or mead, help the difficulty in passing urine, and issue of the bladder; the same, beaten very small and applied, close up green wounds, and stop the bleeding thereof; the leaves and fruit of cypress, being infused in vinegar, and the hair washed therewith, make it black.

WHITE DAFFODIL

It is called narcissus, and primrose-pearls.

KINDS There are several kinds hereof, one with a crimson or red-purple circle in the middle of the flower, and another having a yellow circle, resembling a coronet, or cup, in the middle of the flower. There is another kind that is yellow in the middle, and another sort which bears double flowers.

DESCRIPTION The first kind of daffodil, or narcissus, has small narrow leaves like leek blades, with a crested, bare, naked, stalk, without leaves, of a foot or nine inches long, with a flower at the top, growing out of a certain film or skin, generally growing singly, or alone, though sometimes two together, consisting of six little white leaves; in the middle whereof is a small round wrinkled hoop or cup, bordered about the brim with a certain round edge, wherein are contained several small threads or stems, with yellowish tips hanging thereon; after the flowers appear angled husks, wherein grow black seeds; the root is round and bulbous, not much unlike an onion.

The other narcissus, with the yellow cup or circle in the middle, has blades longer and broader, and not so green as those of the first; the stalks are longer and thicker, and upon every one of them stands three or four flowers like unto

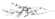
the first, except that they are yellow in the middle. There is another kind that is yellow in the middle, and bears many more flowers, which are smaller than those before described.

PLACE   The two first kinds grow plentifully in many places of France, as Burgundy, Languedoc, &c. in meadows and pastures; but in this country they grow only in gardens where they are planted.

TIME   They flower chiefly in March and April, though some of them bloom not until the beginning of May.

TEMPERATURE AND VIRTUES   Venus challenges the dominion over these plants. The root of it is hot and dry in the third degree; the which root, pounded with a little honey, is good to be applied to burnings or scaldings, and cures sinews that are hurt or sprained, and is good to help dislocations, or members out of joint, being applied thereto. It cleanses ulcers, and ripens and breaks hard imposthumes, if it be mixed with the meal of vetches and honey, and used in the manner of a poultice; and, being mixed with the meal of juray and honey, it draws forth thorns and splinters.

YELLOW DAFFODIL

This kind of daffodil is also called Lide-lily, because it flowers in March, which month in some countries is called Lide, and they are likewise known by the name of daffydown-dillies.

DESCRIPTION   It has long, narrow, green leaves; the stalks are round, upon which grow yellow flowers, of an unpleasant smell; after which come round knobs or husks, like little heads, wherein the seed is contained; it has abundance of roots, which grow thick together, and increase by new sprigs and blades, whereby it spreads and increases itself under ground, so that the increase of this plant is very rapid.

PLACE   It does not grow naturally in this country, but in gardens where it is planted.

TIME   Daffodils flower in March and April, and the seed ripens soon after.

GOVERNMENT AND VIRTUES   Yellow daffodils are under the dominion of Mars, and the roots hereof are hot and dry almost in the third degree. A plaster made of the roots, with parched barley-meal, dissolves hard swellings and imposthumes, being applied thereto.

DAISIES

GOVERNMENT AND VIRTUES The herb is under the sign Cancer, and under the dominion of Venus. The greater wild daisy is a wound-herb of good respect, often used in those drinks or salves that are for wounds, either inward or outward; the juice or distilled water of these, or the small daisies, does much temper the heat of choler, and refreshes the liver and other inward parts. A decoction made of them, and drunk, helps to cure ulcers and pustules in the mouth or tongue. The leaves bruised and applied to the testicles, or to any other parts that are swollen and hot, does dissolve it and temper the heat. A decoction made hereof with walwort and agrimony gives great ease to those who are troubled with the palsy, sciatica, or gout; the same also disperses and dissolves the knots or kernels that grow in the flesh of any part of the body. An ointment made hereof does wonderfully help all wounds that have inflammations about them, or are kept long from healing; and such are those, for the most part, that happen to the joints of the arms and legs.

DANDELION

Vulgarly called piss-a-beds.

DESCRIPTION It is well known to have many long and deeply-gashed leaves lying on the ground, round about the head of the root; the ends of each gash or jag on both sides, looking downwards towards the root, the middle rib being white, which broken, yields abundance of bitter milk, but the root much more. From among the leaves, which always abide green, arise many slender, weak, naked, footstalks, every one of them bearing at the top one large yellow flower, consisting of many rows of yellow leaves, broad at the points, and nicked in, with a deep spot of yellow in the middle; which growing ripe, the green husk wherein the flower stood, turns itself down to the stalk, and the head of down becomes as round as a ball, with long reddish seed underneath, bearing a part of the down on the head of every one, which together is blown away with the wind, or may at once be blown away with one's mouth. The root growing downwards exceeding deep, which being broken off within the ground, will, notwithstanding, shoot forth again; and will hardly be destroyed when it has once taken deep root in the ground.

PLACE It grows frequent in all meadows and pasture grounds.

TIME It flowers in one place or other almost all the year long.

GOVERNMENT AND VIRTUES It is under the dominion of Venus. It is of an opening and cleansing quality, and therefore very effectual for the obstructions of the liver, gall, and spleen, and the diseases that arise from them. It wonderfully opens the passages of urine, both in young and old. It helps also to procure rest and sleep to bodies distempered by the heat of ague fits, or otherwise; the distilled water is effectual to drink in fevers, and to wash the sores. You see here what virtues this common herb has, and that is the reason the French and Dutch so often eat them in the spring.

DARNEL

it is also called juray, and wray; in Sussex they call it crop, it being a pestilent enemy amongst corn.

DESCRIPTION This has all the winter long, sundry long, fat, and rough, leaves, which when the stalk rises, which is slender and jointed, are narrower, but still rough; on the top grows a long spike, composed of many heads, set one above another, containing two or three husks, with sharp but short beards or hawns at the ends; the seed is easily shaken out of the ears, the husk itself being somewhat tough.

PLACE The country husbandmen know this too well to grow among their corn; or in the borders and pathways of other fields that are fallow.

GOVERNMENT AND VIRTUES It is a plant of Saturn. The meal of darnel is very good to cleanse the skin, if it be used with salt and raddish-roots. And, being used with quick brimstone and vinegar, it dissolves knots and kernels; a decoction thereof made with water and honey, and the place bathed therewith, is profitable for the sciatica. Darnel meal applied in a poultice, draws forth splinters from the flesh; the red darnel boiled in red wine, and taken, stays the lask and all other fluxes.

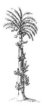

DATE-TREE

This is likewise called palm-tree, and the fruit is called dates, or fruit of the palm-tree.

DESCRIPTION It grows to be a large tree, with a straight thick trunk, covered with a scaly bark; at the top whereof grow many long branches, bearing a vast number of long, straight, narrow, leaves, or twigs like reeds, so that the whole tree appears to be nothing but a bundle of reed-leaves; amongst the branches grows the fruit, clustering together at the first, and wrapped in a certain long and broad covering, like a pillow, which afterwards opens and shows the fruit standing along on certain small sprigs, growing out of a flat yellow branch; the fruit is long and round, containing within it a long and hard stone. Of this tree there are two kinds, the male and female; the male tree brings forth flowers only, which vanish away as soon as the blossom is full; and the female bears the fruit, and brings it to perfection and ripeness.

PLACE The date-tree grows in Africa, Arabia, India, Syria, Judæa, and other eastern countries.

TIME It continues always green, and bears its flowers in the spring. In hot countries the fruit is ripe in autumn.

GOVERNMENT AND VIRTUES The branches and leaves are cold and astringent, the fruit is also somewhat astringent, but hot and dry almost in the second degree; especially before it is thoroughly ripe. Dry dates being administered inwardly or applied outwardly, strengthen the weakness of the liver and spleen. The leaves and branches are good to heal green wounds, and refresh and cool hot inflammations.

DEVIL'S BIT

DESCRIPTION This rises up with a round, green, smooth, stalk, about two feet high, set with divers long and somewhat narrow, smooth, dark green leaves, somewhat snipt about the edges, for the most part; being else all whole, and not divided at all, or but very seldom, even to the tops of the branches, which yet are smaller than those below, with one rib only in the middle; at the end of each branch stands a round head of many flowers set together in the same manner, or more neatly than the scabious, and of a more bluish-purple colour; which being past, there follows seed that falls away. The root is somewhat thick, but short and blackish, with many strings, abiding after seed-time many years. There are two other sorts hereof, in nothing unlike the former, save that one bears white, and the other blush-coloured, flowers.

PLACE The first grows as well in dry meadows and fields, as moist, in many places of this land; but the other two are more rare and hard to meet with; yet are both found growing wild about Appledore, near Rye, in Kent.

TIME They flower usually about August, and the seed is ripe in September.

GOVERNMENT AND VIRTUES The decoction of the herb, with honey of roses put therein, is very effectual to help the inveterate tumours and swellings of the throat, by often gargling the mouth therewith. It helps also to procure women's menses, and eases all pains of the womb and the bowels.

DICTAMNUM OF CANDY

It is observed by Dioscorides, that there are three kinds hereof; the first whereof is the right dictamnum, the second is the bastard dictamnum, and the third is another kind, bearing both flowers and seed; it is called also dittany of Crete, and in the shops *diptanum*.

DESCRIPTION The first kind, which is the right dictamnum, is a hot and sharp plant, much resembling penny-royal, except that this has larger leaves, somewhat hoary or mossy, with a certain fine down, or woolly white cotton; at the top of the stalks or branches grow certain small spiky tufts, hanging by small stems, greater and thicker than the ears or spiky tufts of wild marjoram, and are somewhat of a red colour, in which there grow small flowers. The second kind, called bastard dictamnum, is very much like the first, except in taste; it does not bite or hurt the tongue, neither is it so hot. It has round, soft, woolly, stalks, with knots and joints, at each of which joints there stand two leaves somewhat round, not much unlike the leaves of penny-royal, but that they are larger; the flowers are of a light blue, compassing the stalk, at certain spaces like garlands, and like the flowers of penny-royal and hoarhound; the root is of a woody substance. The third kind is like the second in figure, saving that its leaves are greener and more hoary; covered with a fine, white, soft, hair, almost like the leaves of water-mint; the whole plant has a good and pleasant smell, as it were betwixt the scent of water-mint and sage, as saith Dioscorides.

PLACE The first kind, or the right dictamnum, comes from Crete, now called Candia, an island in the Mediterranean sea, formerly belonging to the Venetians, but now in possession of the Turks. The other two kinds are not confined to Candia only, but grow also in many other hot countries.

GOVERNMENT AND VIRTUES The right dictamnum is hot and dry, and of subtil parts; the other two kinds are also hot and dry, but not quite so hot as the first; they are all under Venus. The juice is of singular efficacy against all kinds of wounds, if dropped or poured therein. The bastard dictamnum has the same virtues as the first, though not quite so powerful in its operations. The third kind is very profitable, compounded with medicines, drinks, and plasters, against stingings.

FALSE DICTAMNUM

This herb is called in Latin *tragium*, and by some fraxinella; some apothecaries do use the root hereof instead of the right dictamnum, from whence it is called bastard or false dictamnum.

DESCRIPTION This plant somewhat resembles *lentisms* or *licoras*, both in leaves and branches; it has round, blackish, rough, stalks, bearing on the tops thereof fair flowers, of a bluish colour, which on the upper part have four or five leaves, and on the lower part it has small long threads, crooking or hanging down almost like a beard. After the flowers are gone, in the place of each come four or five cods, somewhat rough without, slippery or slimy in handling, and of a strong smell, not unlike that of a goat; in which is contained a black, plain, shining, seed. The roots are long and white, sometimes as thick as one's finger, and generally grow one against the other.

PLACE It grows on the isle of Candia, and is sometimes found in the gardens of curious botanists.

TIME It flowers in June and July.

GOVERNMENT AND VIRTUES This plant is also under the dominion of Venus. It is hot almost in the third degree, and of subtil parts; the seed, taken to the quantity of a drachm, is good against the difficulty in passing urine; it is good against the stone in the bladder, breaking and bringing it forth, and brings down the terms of women; the leaves and juice have similar virtues, and, being externally applied, draw out thorns and splinters.

DILL

DESCRIPTION The common dill grows up with seldom more than-one stalk, neither so high, nor so great usually, as fennel; being round, and with fewer joints thereon; whose leaves are sadder, and somewhat long, and so like fennel that it deceives many, but harder in handling, and somewhat thicker, and of a stronger unpleasant smell; the tops of the stalks have four branches, and smaller umbels of yellow flowers, which turn into small seed flatter and thinner than fennel seed. The root is small and woody, perishing every year after it has borne seed; and is unprofitable, being never put to any use.

PLACE It is most usually sown in gardens, and grounds for that purpose, and is also found wild with us in some places.

GOVERNMENT AND VIRTUES Mercury has the dominion of the plant. The dill being boiled, and drunk, is good to ease swellings and pains. The seed is of more use than the leaves, and is used in medicines that serve to expel wind, and the pains proceeding therefrom. The seed being toasted or fried, and used in oils and plasters, dissolves the imposthumes in the fundament, and dries up all moist ulcers. The oil made of dill is effectual to warm, to dissolve humours and imposthumes, to ease pains, and to procure rest. The decoction of dill, be it herb or seed (only if you boil the seed, you must bruise it) in white wine, being drunk, is an excellent remedy to expel wind, and also to provoke the terms.

DOCK

GOVERNMENT AND VIRTUES All docks are under Jupiter; of which the red dock, commonly called bloodwort, cleanses the blood and strengthens the liver; but the yellow dock root is best to be taken when either the blood or liver is afflicted by choler. All of them have a kind of cooling drying quality, the sorrels being most cold, and the bloodworts most drying; of the burdock I have spoken already by itself. The seed of most of the kinds, whether of the garden or field, do stay lasks or fluxes of all sort. The distilled water of the herb and roots cleanses the skin. All docks being boiled with meat, make it boil the sooner; besides bloodwort is exceeding strengthening to the liver, and procures good blood, being as wholesome a pot-herb as any that grows in a garden.

DODDER OF THYME

Called also epithimum, also other dodders.

DESCRIPTION This first from seed gives roots in the ground, which shoot forth threads or strings, grosser or finer, according to the property of the plant whereto it belongs, as also the climate; creeping and spreading on whatever it happens to fasten. These strings have no leaves at all upon them, but wind and entwine themselves so thick, that it not only takes away all comfort of the Sun, but is ready to choke or strangle whatever plant it chances to cleave to. After these strings are risen to that height that they may draw nourishment from the plant, they seem to be broken off from the ground, either by the strength of their rising, or withered by the heat of the Sun; upon these strings are found clusters of small heads or husks, out of which comes whitish flowers, which afterwards give small pale-coloured seed, somewhat flat, and twice as big as poppy-seed. It generally participates of the nature of the plant which it climbs upon; but the dodder of thyme is accounted the best, and is the only true epithimum.

GOVERNMENT AND VIRTUES All dodders are under Saturn. The dodder which grows upon thyme is generally much hotter than that which grows upon colder herbs. This is accounted the most effectual for melancholic diseases, and to purge black or burnt choler, which is the cause of many diseases of the head and brain, as also for the trembling of the heart, faintings, and swoonings, and is helpful in all diseases and griefs of the spleen.

DOG'S GRASS

Known also by the name of quich-grass or couch-grass.

DESCRIPTION   It is well known that this grass creeps far about under ground, with long, white, jointed roots, having small fibres at each joint, very sweet in taste, as the rest of the herb is, and interlacing one another; from whence shoot forth many fair, long, grassy leaves, small at the ends, and cutting or sharp on the edges. The stalks are joined like corn, with the like leaves on them, and a long spiked head with a long husk containing hard rough seed.

PLACE   It grows commonly in this kingdom, particularly in ploughed ground, being very troublesome both to husbandmen and gardeners to weed out of their grounds.

GOVERNMENT AND VIRTUES   It is a gentle remedy under the dominion of Jupiter. This is the most medicinal of all the quich grasses: being boiled and drunk, it opens obstructions of the liver and gall, and the stopping of the urine, and eases the griping pains of the belly, and inflammations, wastes the matter of the stone in the bladder, and also the ulcers thereof. The roots bruised and applied, do consolidate wounds. The seed does most powerfully expel urine, and stays the lask and vomiting.

DOUBLE-TONGUE

There are found two kinds hereof; it is called double-tongue, horse-tongue, and laurel of Alexandria.

DESCRIPTION   Double-tongue has round stalks, like those of Solomon's seal, about a foot and a half high, upon each side whereof grow thick brownish leaves, not much unlike bay-leaves, upon which there grows, in the middle of every leaf, another small leaf, fashioned like a tongue; and betwixt the small and large leaves there grow round red berries, as big as a pea; the root is tender, white, long, and of a pleasant smell.
    There is also another kind of double-tongue, which also brings forth its fruit upon the leaves, and is like the first in stalks, leaves, fruit, and roots, except that the great leaves and berries grow alone, without the addition of the small leaf.

PLACE   It grows in Hungary and Austria, and in the woods and forests in Italy; but is scarcely ever seen in England, unless planted for curiosity.

TIME   The seed of this herb is generally ripe in September.

GOVERNMENT AND VIRTUES Double-tongue is an herb of Venus. The leaves and roots thereof are much esteemed for assuaging swellings of the throat, uvula, and kernels under the tongue; as also against the ulcers and sores of the same, being taken as a gargle. This herb is good for the diseases of the womb. The root of laurel of Alexandria, boiled in wine and drunk, helps the difficulty in passing urine, procures easy delivery, and expels the secundine.

DOVE'S FOOT

Called also crane's bill.

DESCRIPTION This bath divers small, round, pale green leaves, cut in about the edges, much like mallows, standing upon long, reddish, hairy stalks, lying in a round compass upon the ground; among which rise up two or three, or more, reddish, jointed, slender, weak, and hairy stalks, with some such-like leaves thereon, but smaller, and deeper cut toward the tops, where grow many very small bright red flowers of five leaves each; after which comes small heads, with small short beaks pointing forth, as all other sorts of these herbs do.

PLACE It grows in pasture-grounds, and by the path-sides in many places, and is sometimes found growing in gardens.

TIME It flowers in June, July, and August, sometimes earlier and sometimes later, and the seed is ripe quickly after.

GOVERNMENT AND VIRTUES It is a gentle, though martial, plant. It has been found by experience to be singularly good for the wind cholic, and pains thereof; as also to expel the stone and gravel in the kidneys. Green wounds are quickly healed by bruising the herb, and applying it to the part affected.

DOWN, OR COTTON-THISTLE

DESCRIPTION This has many large leaves lying on the ground, somewhat cut in, and as it were crumpled on the edges, of a green colour on the upper side, but covered with long hairy wool, or cottony down, set with very sharp and piercing prickles; from the middle of its heads of flowers come forth many purplish or crimson threads, and sometimes (though but very seldom) white ones. The seed that followeth in the heads, lying in a great deal of fine white down, is somewhat large, long, and round, like the seed of lady's thistle, but somewhat paler. The root is large and thick, spreading much, and usually dies after seed-time.

PLACE It grows on divers ditches, banks, and in corn-fields, and highways, in almost every part of this kingdom.

TIME It flowers and bears seed about the end of summer, at the time of the flowering and seeding of other thistles.

GOVERNMENT AND VIRTUES Mars owns this plant. Galen saith, that the root and leaves of this plant are of an heating quality, and good for such persons as have their bodies drawn together by spasms or convulsions, as also for children that have the rickets.

DRAGONS

GOVERNMENT AND VIRTUES The plant is under the dominion of Mars, and is not without its noxious qualities. To use herbs of this description, the safest way is to press out the juice and distil it in a glass-still in sand; it scours and cleanses the internal as well as external parts of the body exceedingly; an ointment of it is very good to heal wounds and ulcers.

DUCK'S MEAT

This is so well known to swim on the top of standing-waters, as ponds, pools, ditches, &c. that it is needless further to describe it.

GOVERNMENT AND VIRTUES Cancer claims the herb, and the Moon is the lady of it. It is effectual to help inflammations, as also the gout, either applied by itself, or in a poultice with barley-meal. The distilled water hereof is held in high estimation for its virtues against all inward inflammations.

DUNCH-DOWN

It is called dunch-down, because, if the down thereof happens to get into the ears, it causes deafness. It is called in Latin *typha palustris*, and in English reed-mace and water-torch; the leaves of it are called mat-weed, because mats are made therewith.

DESCRIPTION This herb has long, rough, thick, and almost three-square, leaves, filled within with a soft pith or marrow; among the leaves sometimes grows up a long, smooth, naked, stalk, without knots or joints, not hollow within, having at the top a grey or russet long knap or ear, which is round, soft, thick, and smooth, and seems to be nothing else but a thrum of russet wool or flocks, set thick and thronged together; which, as it ripens, is turned into down, and carried away with the wind. This down or cotton is so fine, that in some countries they fill cushions and beds with it.

DWARF PLANE-TREE

In Latin this tree is called *platanus orientalis vera*.

GOVERNMENT AND VIRTUES The leaves boiled in wine, and used in the manner of an ointment, stop fluxions of the eyes; the bark boiled in vinegar, is used for pains of the teeth; but its use in physic is now become obsolete.

EGLANTINE

This is the better known by its common name, sweet brier, and is called in some counties wild brier, and pimpernel-rose. The Latins call it *cynorrhodon*, and the Greek *rodon agrion*. Another species of eglantine is the dog-rose, and all other wild roses.

TIME AND PLACE The sweet brier from its fragrant and pleasant smell, is cultivated in most gardens and pleasure grounds. It grows likewise wild in the borders of fields, and in woods, in almost every part of this kingdom; but not by far so plentifully as the dog-rose. It begins to shoot forth its buds early in the spring, and flourishes and flowers during the time of all the other rose-trees.

GOVERNMENT AND VIRTUES Sweet-briar is under the dominion of Jupiter, and the dog-rose is under the Moon. The leaves of the flowers are not so efficacious in medicine as rose-leaves, which, being also more abundant, are always used in preference. The spongy apples or balls which are found upon the eglantine, if pounded to a paste, and mixed with honey and wood ashes, are an excellent remedy for the alopecia, or falling off of the hair.

The red berries which succeed the flowers, called hips, if made into a conserve, and eaten occasionally, gently bind the belly, and sharpen the appetite. The powder of the dried pulp is an excellent remedy for the whites; and, if mixed with the powder of the balls, and given in small quantities, is an excellent remedy for the cholic.

ELDER-TREE

I consider it needless to trouble my readers with a description of this tree, since there is scarce a school-boy but can point it out; shall therefore proceed to the:

PLATE 8

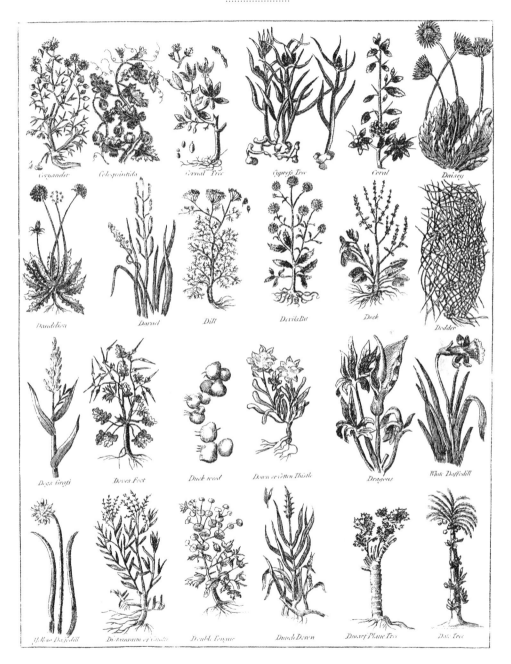

Coriander   Coloquintida   Cornal Tree   Cypress Tree   Coral   Daisey

Dandelion   Darnel   Dill   DevilsBit   Dock   Dodder

Dogs Grass   Doves Foot   Duck weed   Down or cotton Thistle   Dragons   White Daffodill

Y. Rose Daffodill   Dictamnum et Cinara   Double Tongue   Dutch Down   Dwarf Plane Tree   Date Tree

DWARF-ELDER

Called also dead-wort and wall-wort.

DESCRIPTION This herb springs fresh from the ground every spring; its leaves and stalks perishing at the approach of winter. It is like the common-elder both in form and quality, rising up with a square, rough, hairy, stalk, about four feet high, though sometimes higher: the winged leaves are somewhat narrower than of that aforementioned; but in other respects not unlike them; the flowers are white dashed with purple, standing in umbels, resembling those of the former except in smell, these being the most pleasant; after the flowers come small blackish berries, full of juice whilst they are fresh, containing small hard kernels, or seed. The root does creep under the upper crust of the ground, springing in divers places, and being in general about the size of a person's finger.

PLACE It grows wild in many parts of the kingdom, and is with difficulty erazed from the place where it once takes root.

TIME Most of the elder-trees flower in June, and their fruit is ripe in August, but the dwarf kind or wall-wort flowers somewhat later, and its fruit is not ripe till September.

GOVERNMENT AND VIRTUES Both the common and dwarf-elders are under the dominion of Venus. The first shoots of the common-elder boiled like asparagus, or the young leaves and stalks boiled in fat broth, expel phlegm and choler; the middle or inward bark boiled in water, and drunk, purges exceedingly; and the berries, either green or dry, are often given with good success for the dropsy. The decoction of the root mollifies the hardness of the womb, and brings down the menses; the berries boiled in wine perform the same effect, and the hair of the head washed therewith is made black.

ELECAMPANE

DESCRIPTION This shoots forth many large leaves, long and broad, lying near the ground, small at both ends, somewhat soft in handling, of a whitish green on the upper side and grey underneath, each set upon a short footstalk; from among these rise up divers great and strong hairy stalks, three or four feet high, with some leaves thereon, compassing them about at the lower ends, and are branched toward the tops, bearing several large flowers, like those of the corn marygold, both the border of the leaves and the middle thrum being yellow; this is followed by a down, with long, small, brownish, seed among it, which is carried away with the wind. The root is large and thick, branching forth many ways, blackish on the outside, and white within, of a very bitter taste, and strong but pleasant smell, especially when they are dried; it is the only part of the plant which has any smell.

PLACE It grows in moist grounds and shadowy places oftener than in the dry and open borders of fields and lanes, and other waste places, almost in every county of this kingdom.

TIME It flowers in June and July, and the seed is ripe in August. The roots are gathered for medicinal purposes, as well in the spring, before the leaves come forth, as in autumn or winter.

GOVERNMENT AND VIRTUES It is a plant under the dominion of Mercury. The fresh root of elecampane preserved with sugar, or made into a syrup, or conserve, is very good to warm a cold and windy stomach; also to help a cough, shortness of breath, and wheezing in the lungs. The dry root made into powder, mixed with sugar and taken, answers the same purposes, and is also profitable to those who have their urine stopped; likewise to prevent the stoppages of the menstrua, the pains of the womb, and of the stone in the kidneys, or bladder.

ELM-TREE

This tree is so well known, growing generally in most counties of this kingdom, that it would be needless to describe it.

GOVERNMENT AND VIRTUES It is a cold and Saturnine plant. The leaves hereof, bruised and applied, heal green wounds, being bound thereon with its own bark; the decoction of the leaves, bark, or root, heals broken bones by bathing the part affected therewith; the water that is found in the bladders on the leaves, while it is fresh, is a good wash for cleansing the skin, and making it fair. The bark ground with brine or pickle, until it comes to the thickness of a poultice, and laid on the place painted with the gout, gives great ease; and the decoction of the bark in water is exceeding good to bathe such places as have been burned with fire.

ENDIVE

DESCRIPTION Common garden endive bears a longer and larger leaf than succory, and abides but one year, quickly running up to stalk and seed, and then perishing; it has blue flowers, and the seed is so much like that of succory, it is hard to distinguish them.

PLATE 9

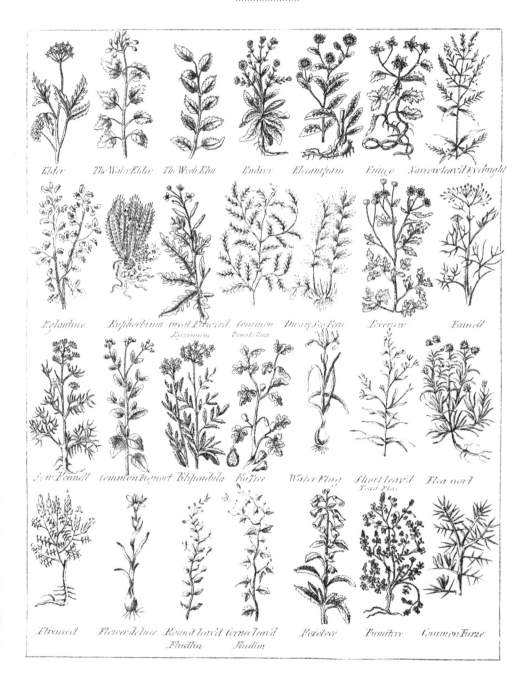

Elder   The Water Elder   The Wych Elm   Endive   Elecampane   Eringo   Narrow leav'd Everlasting

Eglantine   Euphorbium   Great Flixweed   Common   Dwarf Sea Fern   Evergreen   Fennel
       Everyman   Female Fern

Sow Fennel   Common Figwort   Filipendula   Fox Tree   Water Flag   Short leav'd   Flea wort
       Toad Flax

Flaxweed   Flower de luce   Round leav'd   Corner leav'd   Foxglove   Fumitory   Common Furze
       Fluellin   Fluellin

GOVERNMENT AND VIRTUES It is a fine, cooling, cleansing, plant; the decoction of the leaves, or the juice, or the distilled water, of endive, serves well to cool the excessive heat of the liver and stomach, as also the hot fits of agues, and other inflammations; it cools the heat and sharpness of the urine, and the excoriations in the urinary parts: the seed has the same properties, though rather more powerful. The syrup of it is a fine cooling medicine for fevers.

ERINGO

Known also by the name of sea-holly.

DESCRIPTION The leaves of this plant are nearly round, deeply dented about the edges, hard, and sharp pointed, a little crumpled, and of a bluish-green colour each having a long footstalk; the leaves, when young, are neither so hard nor prickly as when come to its maturity. The stalk is round and strong, somewhat crested with joints, bearing leaves thereat, which are more divided, sharp, and prickly, than those before mentioned; from these joints it also branches forth many ways, each bearing on the top several bluish, round, prickley, heads, with many small jagged, prickly, leaves under them, standing like a star, which are sometimes of a greenish or white colour. The root grows very long, sometimes to the length of eight or ten feet, set with rings or circles toward the upper part, but smooth and without joints downwards, brownish on the outside, but very white within, with a pith in the middle, of a pleasant taste, but much more so when carefully preserved and candied with sugar.

PLACE It is found on the sea-coasts, and in almost every part of this kingdom bordering on the sea.

TIME It flowers at the latter end of the summer, and gives its seed about a month after.

GOVERNMENT AND VIRTUES The plant is hot and moist, and under the sign Libra. It helps the yellow jaundice, the dropsy, the pains in the loins, expels the stone, and procures women's menses. The decoction taken for fifteen days, on going to bed and in the morning fasting, helps the difficulty in passing urine, and all defects of the kidneys.

ERYSIMUM

DESCRIPTION this plant has long leaves deeply cut or jagged on the edges, not much unlike the leaves of wild mustard; the stalks are small, slender, and pliant, and will twist and wind like the withy. Upon each of these stalks grow many yellow flowers; which are followed by long slender husks, containing seed of a sharp biting taste; the root is very long and thick, with many small strings or threads hanging thereto.

PLACE It delights in stony untilled places, and is to be found in most of the bye-paths and bank-sides in this kingdom.

TIME It generally flowers in the months of June and July, though their blossoms are sometimes seen later in the year.

GOVERNMENT AND VIRTUES The seed of this plant taken with honey ripens and causes the evacuation of phlegm; it is also good against shortness of breath, and is effectual in removing an old cough. If the seed be steeped in fair water and then dried by the fire, it is good for the gripings of the belly. An ointment made of the seed consumes and wastes hard swellings and impostumes.

EUPHORBIUM, OR GUM-THISTLE

This plant is so well known, and so common in every part of this kingdom, that any description of it would be altogether superfluous.

PLACE They grow in most fields and meadows throughout this kingdom, and particularly in grounds sewed with corn.

TIME They flower from the beginning of June until the end of September; and the seed progressively ripens from the end of June to the beginning of November.

GOVERNMENT AND VIRTUES This plant is under the dominion of the planet Mars, and partakes more of his fiery nature than any of the other thistles. It is hot and dry in the fourth degree. A plaster made of it, with twelve times as much oil, and a little wax, heals all aches of the joints, lameness, palsies, cramps, and shrinkings of the sinews. The pills of euphorbium greatly help dropsies, pains in the loins, and gouts. The simple oil of this plant has the same virtues as that of castor, but is much stronger.

EYE-BRIGHT

DESCRIPTION Common eye-bright is a small low herb, rising up usually with but one blackish-green stalk, about a span high, spread from the bottom into sundry branches, whereon are set small, and almost round, yet pointed, dark green leaves; they are finely snipped about the edges, two always set together, and very thick; at the joints with the leaves, from the middle upwards, come forth small white flowers, striped with purple and yellow, after which follow small round heads containing very small seed; the root is long, small, and thready at the end.

PLACE It grows in meadows and grassy places.

GOVERNMENT AND VIRTUES It is under the sign Virgo, and Sol claims the dominion over it. The juice of this herb, taken in white wine or broth, or dropped into the eyes for several days together, helps all the infirmities of them. Some make a conserve of the flowers for the aforesaid purpose.

FEATHERFEW

DESCRIPTION Common featherfew has many large, fresh, green, leaves, very much torn or cut on the edges; the stalks are hard and round, set with many such-like leaves, but somewhat smaller; at the tops stand many single flowers, each upon a small footstalk; they consist of many small white leaves, standing round a yellow thrum. The root is somewhat hard and short, with many strong fibres.

PLACE There are some places in this kingdom where it grows wild; but it is generally a garden plant.

TIME It flowers in the months of June and July.

GOVERNMENT AND VIRTUES This herb is governed by Venus. A decoction of the flowers in wine, with a little nutmeg or mace therein, drunk several times a day, is an approved provocative of women's menses, as also a great help to expel the after-birth. The decoction, mixed with sugar or honey, is good to help a cough, to cleanse the chest or stomach of phlegm, and to expel the stone. The powder of the herb taken in wine, with some oxymel, purges both choler and phlegm, and is good for those who are short-winded, or are troubled with melancholy or lowness of spirits; it is effectual in removing all pains of the head arising from a cold, the herb being bruised, and applied to the crown thereof. The decoction thereof drunk warm, and the herb bruised with a few grains of bay-salt, and applied to the wrists, will prevent the return of ague-fits.

FENNEL

Every garden affords this so plentifully, that it needs no description.

GOVERNMENT AND VIRTUES It is governed by Mercury, under Virgo, and bears antipathy to Pisces. It is exceeding good to be boiled with fish, as it consumes the phlegmatic humour arising therefrom. The leaves and seed boiled in barley-water, and drunk, are good to increase milk and make it more wholesome. The seed is of great use in medicines given to help bring down the menses, and cleanse the parts after delivery. The roots are good to be put into broths that are taken to cleanse the blood, to open obstructions of the liver.

SOW-FENNEL

Besides the common English names of sow-fennel, hogs' fennel, hoar-strong, hoar-strang, sulphur-wort, and brimstone-wort, it is called in Latin *peucidanum*.

DESCRIPTION The common sow-fennel has many branched stalks of thick and somewhat long leaves, three of which generally grow together; the stalk is straight and crested, with joints thereon, somewhat less than the common fennel, and branching forth at the top several small sprays with tufts of yellow flowers, after which comes flat, thin, and yellowish, seed, rather larger than that of the former. The root grows great and deep, with many fibres hanging thereto, of a strong smell, and yields a yellowish clammy juice, almost like a gum.

PLACE It grows plentifully in the low salt marshes near Feversham in Kent.

TIME It flowers and seeds in July and August.

GOVERNMENT AND VIRTUES This also is an herb of Mercury. The juice dissolved in wine, or put into an egg, is good for a cough, or shortness of breath, and to expel wind; it purges the belly gently, helps the hardness of the spleen, gives ease to pregnant women, and also to the pains of the bladder, and womb. A little of the juice dissolved in wine, and dropped into the ears, eases the pains thereof, or, put into an hollow tooth, eases the tooth-ache.

FENUGREEK

It is called in Latin *foenum græcum*, or otherwise greek-hay.

DESCRIPTION It grows up with tender stalks, round, blackish, hollow, and full of branches; the leaves are divided into three parts, like those of trefoil; the flowers are pale or whitish, not much unlike the blossoms of lupines, but smaller. After these are fallen away, there follow long cods or husks, crooked and sharp-pointed, wherein is contained the seed, which is of a yellowish colour. The root is full of small hanging hairs.

PLACE It very seldom grows in this kingdom, unless planted in the gardens of botanists.

TIME It blossoms in July, and the seed is ripe in August.

GOVERNMENT AND VIRTUES Fenugreek-seed is hot in the second degree, and dry in the first, and under the influence of the planet Mercury. The seed is only used in medicine. The decoction or broth of the seed, drunk with a little vinegar, expels and purges all superfluous humours which cleave to the bowels; the same decoction first made with dates is of a softening and dissolving nature, therefore the meal thereof being boiled in mead or honey-water, does consume, soften, and dissolve, hard swellings and imposthumes; also a paste made thereof with saltpetre and vinegar, does soften and waste the hardness and swelling of the spleen. The decoction of fenugreek is an excellent wash for the head.

FERN

DESCRIPTION Of this there are two kinds principally to be treated of; *viz.* the male and female. The female grows higher than the male, but the leaves thereof are less, and more divided or dented, but of the same smell as that of the male. The virtues of each are the same.

PLACE They grow on heaths and in shady places near the hedge-sides in most parts of this kingdom.

TIME They flower and seed at midsummer.

GOVERNMENT AND VIRTUES It is under the dominion of Mercury, both the male and female. The roots of both these sorts of ferns, being bruised and boiled in mead, or honey-water, and drunk, abate the swelling and hardness of the spleen. The green leaves, eaten, cause abortion, consequently are unfit for the use of pregnant women. The roots bruised, and boiled in oil, make a very profitable ointment to heal wounds, or draw forth thorns from the flesh.

WATER-FERN

It is called osmond-royal.

DESCRIPTION This shoots forth in the spring-time; it has several rough hard stalks, half-round, or flattish on one side, and hollow; they are about two feet high, having many branches of winged yellowish-green leaves on all sides,

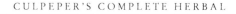

set one against another, longer, narrower, and not nicked on the edges; from the top of some of these stalks grows forth a long bush of small and more yellowish-green scaly aglets, set in the same manner on the stalks as the leaves are; these are supposed to be the flowers and seed. The root is rough, thick, and scaly, having a white pith in the middle which is called the heart thereof.

PLACE   It grows in moors, bogs, and watery places, in many parts of this kingdom.

TIME   It is green all the summer, but the root lives during the winter.

GOVERNMENT AND VIRTUES   Saturn owns this plant. It has all the virtues of the former ferns, though much more effectual in its operations than either, and is a singular remedy for wounds, bruises, &c. The decoction drunk, or boiled down to an oil or ointment, and applied, is also good for bruises, and gives much ease to the cholic and in splenetic diseases. Of the ashes of these ferns, with water, are made balls (particularly in Warwickshire and Staffordshire) with which, being dried in the sun, they wash their clothes instead of soap; but before they use them they put them into a fire till they are red-hot, and then they will easily powder. This fern also is used in Sussex to burn lime, the flame being very fit for that purpose. The juice of the root is good for burns. The ashes cast upon stones, instead of nitre, make glass of a green colour.

FIG-TREE

To give a description of a tree so well known to almost every body who lives in this kingdom were needless; I shall therefore only observe, that it is much fitter for medicinal purposes than any other.

GOVERNMENT AND VIRTUES   The tree is under the dominion of Jupiter. The milk that issues from the leaves or branches when they are broken, being dropped upon warts, takes them away; the decoction of the leaves is exceeding good to wash sore heads with. A decoction of the leaves taken inwardly, or rather the syrup of them, dissolves congealed blood caused by falls or bruises, and is good for the bloody flux. A syrup of the green fruit, is very good for coughs, hoarseness, shortness of breath, and all diseases of the breast and lungs; it is equally efficacious for the dropsy and falling sickness.

FIG-WORT

Called also throat-wort.

DESCRIPTION Common great fig-wort shoots forth several great, strong, hard, square, brown, stalks, three or four feet high, whereon grow large, hard, and dark green, leaves, two on a joint, being larger and harder than nettle leaves, but do not sting; at the tops of the stalks stand many purple flowers, set in husks, not unlike those of water-betony, which are followed by round heads with a small point in the middle, containing small brownish seed. The root is large, white, and thick, shooting forth many branches under the upper crust of the earth, which abides many years, but the leaves perish annually.

PLACE It grows frequently in moist and shady places, and in the bottoms of fields and meadows.

TIME It flowers about July, and the seed ripens about a month after the flowers are fallen.

GOVERNMENT AND VIRTUES Venus claims dominion over this herb. The decoction of the herb taken inwardly, and the bruised herb applied outwardly, dissolves clotted and congealed blood coming from any wound and is no less effectual in removing knots, kernels, bunches, and wens, growing in the flesh; it is good also for the hæmorrhoids. An ointment made hereof may be used for the above purposes when the fresh herb is not to be had.

FILAPENDULA

It is by some called dropwort.

DESCRIPTION It shoots forth many leaves of various sizes, growing on each side of a rib, and much dented on the edges, somewhat resembling wild tansy or agrimony, but feeling much harder; among these rise up one or more stalks, two or three feet high, spreading into many other branches, each bearing several white sweet-smelling flowers, consisting of five leaves apiece, with small threads in the middle; they stand together in a tuft or umbel, each upon a small footstalk, and are succeeded by round chaffy heads, like buttons, which contain the seed. The root consists of many tuberous pieces, fastened together by many small, long, blackish, strings, which run from one to another.

PLACE It grows in many places of this kingdom, in the corners of dry fields and meadows, and also by hedge-sides.

TIME They flower in June and July, and their seed is ripe in August.

GOVERNMENT AND VIRTUES It is under the dominion of Venus. It is very effectual to open the urinary passages, and to help the difficulty in passing urine, and all other pains of the bladder. The roots made into powder, and mixed with honey after the manner of an electuary, are good to be taken by those whose stomachs are swollen, and expelling the wind. It is called drop-wort, because it gives ease to those who evacuate their water by drops.

FIR-TREE

This tree is called in Latin *abies*, by the Dutch, *mastboom*, because of its utility in making masts for ships, and the liquid or clear rosin that issues from the bark of the young trees, is generally known to us by the name of Venice turpentine.

DESCRIPTION   The fir-tree is large, high, and long, and continues always green; it grows much higher than the pine or pitch-tree; the stalk is very even and straight, plain beneath and without joints, but upwards it grows with joints and knobs; upon these joints grow the branches, bearing leaves almost like a yew, but smaller, longer, and sharper at the ends, of a bluish-green colour, the fruit is like the pineapple, but smaller, and narrower, not hanging down, but growing straight upward. From out of the bark of the young trees, is gathered a fair liquid rosin, clear and shining, in taste bitter, almost like to citron-peel or lemon-peel condited. There is also found upon this tree, a white rosin or gum, somewhat like that which the pine and pitch-trees produce.

PLACE   It grows upon the high mountains in Greece, Italy, Spain, and France, and in many places of Germany and Norway; from whence the timber thereof is imported into this kingdom, for the purposes of building, &c.

GOVERNMENT AND VIRTUES   It is under the dominion of Mars. The liquid or clear rosin is hot and dry in the second degree, of a sharp quality, and of a digestive or cleansing nature; this liquid taken, to the quantity of half an ounce, looses the belly and cleanses the kidneys and bladder, provokes urine, expels the stone and gravel, and is good to be taken often by those who are troubled with the gout; the same taken with nutmeg and sugar, about the quantity of a nut, helps the difficulty in passing urine. It is also an excellent remedy for green wounds, for it cleanses and heals speedily.

FISTIC-NUTS

These nuts are also called in shops *pistacia*, pistacies, and fistici.

DESCRIPTION   The tree bearing these nuts, has long great leaves, spread abroad, consisting of five, seven, or more, leaves, growing one against another, upon a reddish rib or sinew, whereof the last, which is alone at the top of the

PLATE 10

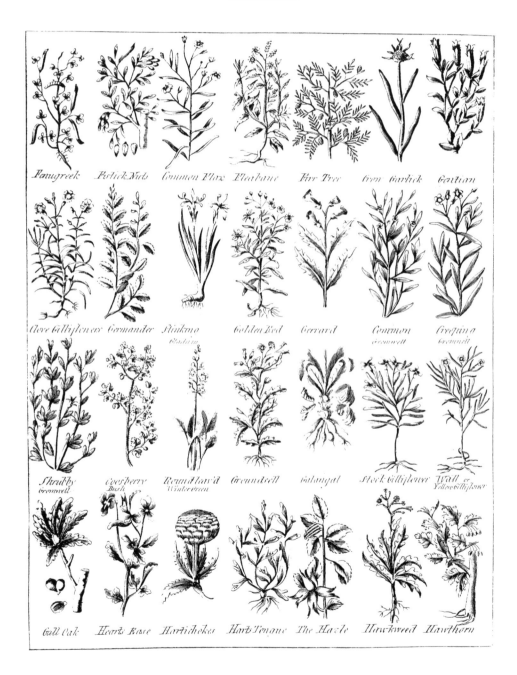

Faugreek   Fistick Nuts   Common Flax   Fleabane   Firr Tree   From Garlick   Gentian

Clove Gilliflowers   Germander   Plantino Gladwin   Golden Rod   Gerrard   Common Gromwell   Creeping Gromwell

Shrubby Gromwell   Goosberry Bush   Round leav'd Winter Green   Groundsell   Galangal   Stock Gilliflower   Wall or Yellow Gilliflower

Gall Oak   Hearts Ease   Hartichokes   Harts Tongue   The Hazle   Hawkweed   Hawthorn leaf, is much the largest; the fruit is much like the hasel-nuts, or kernels of the pine-apple.

PLACE This tree is a stranger in this country, but is a native of Syria and other eastern countries.

GOVERNMENT AND VIRTUES Fistic-nuts are under the influence of Jupiter. They are of a mean or temperate heat, and somewhat astringent; they are good to open stoppages and obstructions of the liver, and for strengthening the same; they are also good for the stomach, they open the pipes of the breast and lungs, and being eaten either alone or with sugar, are exceeding good for the phthysic and shortness of breath.

FLAX

It is called in Latin *linum*, by which name it is well known in shops; also lin, whence the cloth that is made thereof is called linen-cloth; its seed is called linseed, and the oil produced therefrom linseed-oil.

DESCRIPTION Flax has a tender stalk, covered with sharp narrow leaves, parted at the top into small short branches, which bring forth fair blue flowers; these are succeeded by round knobs or buttons, containing a blackish, large, fat, and shining, seed.

PLACE It is cultivated in this country, and sown in fine moist fertile grounds, especially such as lie low.

TIME It flowers in May and June, and ripens soon after.

GOVERNMENT AND VIRTUES It is under the dominion of Venus; the seed of this plant, being only used in medicine, is hot in the first degree, and temperately moist and dry. The seed, or linseed, being boiled in water and applied as a poultice or plaster, softens cold tumours or swellings. Linseed pounded with figs is good to ripen and bring to a head boils and other swellings; also to draw forth thorns and splinters, being mixed with the root of wild cucumber. The seed mixed with honey, and taken as an electuary, cleanses the breast, and helps the cough; compounded with raisins, it is good for such as are consumptive, or troubled with hectic fevers.

FLAX-WEED

Called likewise toad-flax.

DESCRIPTION Our common flax-weed has many stalks, thick set with long and narrow blue or ash-coloured leaves, and bearing from the middle upward a vast number of pale yellow flowers, of a strong unpleasant smell, with deeper yellow mouths, and blackish flat seed in round heads. The root is somewhat woody and white, especially the chief branch of it, which spreads itself many ways, having several fibres hanging thereto.

PLACE This grows in every part of this kingdom, and is to be found by the way-sides in meadows, banks, and borders.

TIME It blossoms in summer, and the seed is ripe usually about the middle or latter end of August.

GOVERNMENT AND VIRTUES Mars owns this herb. It is frequently used to expel the abundunce of those watery humours by urine which cause the dropsy. The decoction of the herb, with the leaves and flowers in wine, does somewhat move the belly downwards, opens obstructions of the liver, helps the yellow jaundice, provokes women's menses, and drives forth the after-birth.

FLEABANE

It is called also in English mullet, and in Latin *conyza*.

GOVERNMENT AND VIRTUES It is hot and dry in the third degree. The herb being spread under foot, or burnt and smoked in any place, will destroy fleas and gnats. An ointment of the root and leaves is used with success for the itch.

FLEAWORT

DESCRIPTION The ordinary fleawort rises up with a stalk about two feet high, though sometimes higher; full of joints and branches on every side, quite up to the top; at each of the joints grow two small, long, and narrow, whitish-green leaves, which are somewhat hairy. At the tops of the branches stand several small, short, scaly or chaffy heads, out of which come forth small whitish-yellow threads, somewhat like those of the plantane herbs, which are the blossoms of flowers. The seed contained in those heads, is small and shining, and very much resembles fleas, both in size and colour, whilst it is fresh, but turns black as its age advances. The root is short, white, hard, and woody, perishing every year, and rising from its own seed, which it promiscuously sheds.

There is another sort hereof, differing not from the former in the manner of its growth, but the stalks and branches are somewhat greater, bending down towards the ground; the leaves are rather larger, the heads a little less, and the seed very much alike. The root and leaves abide all the year, and do not perish in the winter season like the former.

PLACE The first grows only in gardens, but the second plentifully in fields and pastures near the sea.

TIME They flower in July, or thereabouts.

GOVERNMENT AND VIRTUES The herb is cold and dry, and of a Saturnine quality. The mucilage of the seed made with rose-water, and a little sugar-candy added thereto, is very good in all hot agues and burning fevers and inflammations; also to allay the thirst, and lenify the dryness and roughness of the tongue and throat. It helps hoarseness of the voice, diseases of the breast and lungs, caused by heat or sharp salt humours, and also the pleurisy. The mucilage of the seed made with plantane-water, with the yolk of an egg and a little populeon added thereto, is a safe and sure remedy for the sharpness, prickings, and pains, of the hæmorrhoids, or piles, if it be laid on a cloth and bound thereto. It heals inflammations in all parts of the body, and the pains arising therefrom, as the head-ache, &c. It eases the pains of imposthumes, swellings, and breakings out of the skin; as also the pains of the joints, gout, sciatica, and dislocated members. It is a good remedy for sore breasts and nipples of women.

FLIXWEED

DESCRIPTION It rises up with a round, upright, hard, stalk, four or five feet high, spreading into several branches, whereon grow many greyish-green leaves very finely cut, and severed into a number of short and almost round parts. The flowers are very small and yellow, growing spike-fashion, after which come very long small pods, containing yellowish seed. The root is long and woody, perishing every year.

There is another sort of this plant, differing from the former only in the leaves, these being somewhat broader; both kinds are of a very disagreeable smell, and of a biting taste.

PLACE They grow wild in fields and by hedge-sides and highways; also among rubbish, and other places.

TIME They flower and seed in June and July.

GOVERNMENT AND VIRTUES This herb is also Saturnine. The herb and seed is of excellent use to stay the flux and lask of the belly, being taken in water wherein gads of heated steel have been often quenched; and is no less effectual for these purposes than plantane or comfrey, and to restrain any other flux of blood, either in man or woman. Syrups, ointments, and plasters, of it, are truly valuable household medicines.

FLOWER-DE-LUCE

It also bears the name of yellow water-flag.

DESCRIPTION There are other flower-de-luces, from which this herb differs chiefly in the leaves; those of this plant are much longer and narrower, and of a sad green colour; in other respects there is little or no difference. The leaves all grow together, from the middle of which rises the stalk, bearing on the top small yellow flowers, with three falling leaves, and other three arched that cover their bottoms; but, instead of the three upright leaves which are in the other kinds, in this there are substituted three very short leaves, which are followed by long triangular heads, each containing large and flattish seed. The root is long and slender, of a pale-brownish colour on the outside, and of a hoary lightish colour within, having many hard fibres thereat, and of a harsh taste.

PLACE It usually grows in watery ditches, ponds, lakes, and moor-sides, which are filled with standing or running waters.

TIME It flowers in July, and the seed is ripe in August.

GOVERNMENT AND VIRTUES It is under the dominion of the Moon. The root is of a very astringent, cooling, and drying, nature, and thereby helps all lasks and fluxes, whether of blood or humours, as bleeding at the mouth, nose, or other parts, and the immoderate flooding of women's menses. The distilled water of the whole herb, flowers, and roots, is a sovereign remedy for weak eyes, being either dropped therein or cloths or sponges wet therewith and applied to the forehead; being also fomented on swellings and inflammations and cankers incident to women's breasts, also ulcers in the privy parts of either sex, it is very profitable. An ointment made of the flowers is better for these external applications.

FLUELLIN

DESCRIPTION It shoots forth many long branches, partly lying upon the ground, and partly standing upright, set with almost round leaves, yet a little pointed, and sometimes bordering upon an oval shape, placed without order, somewhat hoary, and of a greenish-white colour; from the joints to the tops of the stalks, grow with the leaves, upon small short footstalks, small flowers, one

Round-leaved fluellin

Corner-leaved fluellin

at each place, opening like snap-dragons, or rather like toad-flax, with the upper part of a yellow colour, and the under of a purplish, with a small heel or spur behind; after these come small round heads, containing small black seed. The root is small and thready, perishing annually, and rising again of its own sowing.

There is another sort which has longer branches, wholly trailing upon the ground, two or three feet long, and sometimes not quite so thick set with leaves, which also grow upon small footstalks; they are rather larger than the former, and sometimes jagged on the edges, but the lower part being the broadest, and terminating in a small point, its shape does not bear the most distant resemblance to that of the ear of most animals; it is somewhat hairy, but not hoary, and of a better green than the first. The flowers come forth like those aforementioned, but the colour of the upper part is rather white than yellow, and the purple not so fair; the flower is every way larger, as are the seeds and seed-vessels. The root is like the other, and perishes yearly.

PLACE They grow in the borders and other parts of corn-fields and fertile grounds, especially near South-fleet in Kent; and at Buckworth, Hamerton, and Rickmansworth, in Huntingdonshire; and in many other places.

TIME They are in bloom about June or July, and the whole plant is dry and perished before September.

GOVERNMENT AND VIRTUES It is a lunar herb. The leaves bruised and applied with barley meal to watering eyes that are hot and inflamed by defluxions from the head, helps them exceedingly; as also the flooding of blood and humours.

FOXGLOVE

DESCRIPTION It has many long and broad leaves lying upon the ground, dented about the edges, a little soft or woolly, and of a hoary green colour; among these grow up several stalks, but generally one which bears the aforesaid leaves from the bottom to the middle upwards, from whence to the top it is set with large and long, hollow, reddish-purple, flowers, being a little longer at the lower edge, and spotted with white on the inside; there are threads also in the middle, from whence rise round heads, pointed sharp at the ends, and containing small brown seed therein; they grow one above another, with small green leaves thereat, hanging their heads downward, and each turning the same way. The roots consist of small fibres, among which are some of a tolerable size. The blossoms are without smell, and the leaves are of a bitter hot taste.

PLACE It grows in dry sandy places, and as well on high as low grounds; also under the hedge-sides, in almost every part of this kingdom.

TIME It seldom flowers before July, and the seed is ripe in August.

GOVERNMENT AND VIRTUES This herb is under the dominion of Venus. It is of a gentle cleansing nature, and is frequently used to heal fresh or green wounds, by bruising the leaves and binding them thereon, and the juice thereof is also used for sores, to cleanse, dry, and heal, them. The decoction made with sugar or honey, is effectual in cleansing and purging the body, both upwards and downwards, of tough phlegm and clammy humours, and to open obstructions of the liver and spleen.

FUMITORY

DESCRIPTION Our common fumitory is a tender sappy herb, sending forth from one square, slender, weak, stalk, and leaning downwards on all sides, many branches two or three feet long, with leaves thereon of whitish or rather bluish, sea-green leaves, finely cut and jagged; at the tops of the branches stand many small flowers, one above another, forming a kind of spike, of a reddish-purple colour, with whitish berries; these are succeeded by small round husks, which contain the seed. Its root is yellow, small, and not very long, full of juice while it is green, but perishes as the seed ripens. In some parts of Cornwall there is a species of this plant which bears white blossoms.

PLACE It grows generally in corn-fields and cultivated grounds, and is also a garden plant.

TIME It flowers in May, and the seed ripens soon after.

GOVERNMENT AND VIRTUES Saturn claims dominion over this herb. The syrup or juice made hereof, or the decoction made in whey, with some other purging or opening herbs and roots added thereto, is very effectual for the liver and spleen, opening the obstructions thereof, and clarifying the blood. It cures the yellow jaundice, and expels it by urine, which it procures in abundance. The powder of the dried herb given for some time together, cures melancholy, but the seed is most effectual.

The distilled water of the herb is also of good effect in the former diseases, being taken with good treacle; or gargled with a little water and honey of roses, it helps the sores of the mouth and throat.

FURZE-BUSH

It is so well known by this name, as also of goss, or whins, that a minute description would be totally useless.

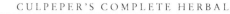

PLACE It is known to grow on dry barren heaths, and other waste, gravelly, and sandy, ground.

TIME They flower in the summer months.

GOVERNMENT AND VIRTUES Mars owns this herb. It is hot and dry, and good to open obstructions of the liver and spleen. A decoction made with the flowers, is effectual against the jaundice, as also to provoke urine, and cleanse the kidneys from the gravel and stone.

GALINGAL

DESCRIPTION It has long, hard, and narrow leaves; the stalk is triangular, about a foot and a half high, bearing on the upper part several small leaves, from among which grow spiky tops and white seed; the root is long, consists of many threads, which are much tangled one within the other.

PLACE It grows in low and moist grounds; it is seldom seen in this kingdom, unless such as is planted in gardens.

TIME This herb brings forth its spiky tops and seed, together with its leaves, in June and July.

GOVERNMENT AND VIRTUES It is a plant of Mars, and the root is hot and dry in the third degree. The roots boiled, and the decoction drunk, provoke urine, bring down the menses, expel the stone, and are good for those who are troubled with the dropsy; the same is also good for the cough. The powder of the root dries up and heals sores of the mouth and is an excellent ingredient for hot ointments.

GALL-OAK

DESCRIPTION The strong gall-oak, so named from the fruit it bears, does not grow so large nor high as other oaks, but shorter and very crooked, with fair spreading branches; on these grow long leaves, very much cut in on the edges, and hoary underneath; this tree flowers and bears acorns, as also a round woody substance, which is called a gall, and the timber is of a very hard substance. There are several kinds of gall-oaks, some of them are much shorter than others, bearing leaves more or less cut or jagged on the edges, and producing a greater quantity of galls, and no acorns at all; some bear large galls, others small, some knobbed or bunched, and others smooth; each are of different colours, some white, others red, yellow, and green.

PLACE These oaks grow frequently in Italy, Spain, and other hot countries.

TIME They shoot forth their long catkins or blossoms early in the spring, which fall away for the most part before the leaves appear. The acorns are very seldom ripe before October.

GOVERNMENT AND VIRTUES I shall here explain the use, virtues, and temperament, of the galls of these foreign trees only, as their acorns differ but little from those produced by our English oaks.

The small gall, called *omphacitis*, is dry in the third degree, and cold in the second; Saturnine, and of a sour harsh nature. It is effectual in drawing together and fastening loose and faint parts, as the overgrowing of the flesh; it expels and dries up rheums and other fluxes, especially those that fall upon the gums, almonds of the throat, and other places of the mouth.

The other whiter gall does also bind and dry, but not so much as the former; it is good against the dysentery or bloody flux. The decoction of them in water remedies the falling of the womb, or the galls being boiled and bruised, and applied to the fundament when fallen, or to any swelling or inflammation, will prove a certain cure. The coals of burned galls, when quenched in wine or vinegar, are good to staunch bleeding in any place. They will dye the hair black, and are one of the chief ingredients for making ink; they are likewise used by dyers for making black dye.

The oak apple is much of the nature of galls, though inferior in quality, but may be substituted for them with success to help rheums, fluxes, and other such-like painful distempers.

GARLIC

GOVERNMENT AND VIRTUES Mars owns this herb. It provokes urine and women's menses; it kills worms in children, cuts and brings forth tough phlegm, purges the head, helps the lethargy, and is a good preservative against, and a remedy for, any plague-sore, or ulcer; it takes away spots and blemishes of the skin, eases pains of the ears, and ripens and breaks imposthumes and other swellings. It has been noticed that onions are equally effectual for the said purposes, but garlic has many peculiar virtues which the onion cannot boast of; for instance, it has a special quality to remove all inconveniences proceeding from corrupt agues or mineral vapours, or from drinking stagnated or unclean water; as also by taking of wolf-bane, henbane, hemlock, or other poisonous herbs. It is also exceeding good in hydropic diseases, the jaundice, falling sickness, cramps, convulsions, the piles or hæmorrhoids, and other cold diseases. However, having shewed its many virtues, it is also necessary that its vices should not be concealed; its heat is very vehement, and every thing of that description naturally conveys ill vapours to the brain; in choleric cases it adds fuel to the fire; in men oppressed with melancholy, it extenuates the humour, and confounds the idea with strange visions and fancies, and therefore ought to be taken with the strictest care by those whose ill-disposition of body will not admit of a liberal application. A few cummin seeds, or a green bean or two being chewed after eating garlic, will entirely remove the disagreeable smell of the breath proceeding therefrom.

GENTIAN

Called also felwort and baldmony. It is acknowledged that the gentian used by us some years ago, was imported from beyond the sea, but we have since happily found that our own country is by no means deficient of those blessings which can contribute to the health of man. There are two sorts of gentian in the growth of this kingdom, which have been proved by the experience of the most able physicians, to be rather of superior excellence to that of the foreign herb.

DESCRIPTION The greater of the two has many long and small roots, which grow deep in the ground, and abide all the winter. The stalks grow several together, of a brownish-green colour, which are sometimes two feet high, especially if the soil is good, having many long, narrow, dark green, leaves, set by couples up to the top; the flowers are long and hollow, of a brightish-purple colour, and ending in five corners.

The smaller kind grows up with several stalks, not quite a foot high, parted into many branches, whereon grow two or three small leaves together, not unlike those of the lesser centaury, of a whitish-green colour; on the top of the stalks grow divers perfect blue flowers, standing in long husks, but not so big as the other. The root is very small and thready.

PLACE The former grows in many places in the east and west countries, as at Longfield near Gravesend, also at Cobham, Lellingstone, and in the chalk pits adjacent to Dartford in Kent. The second kind grows also in many places in Kent, as about Southfleet and Longfield, and upon the barren hills in Bedfordshire. It is likewise found not far from St Alban's, upon a piece of waste ground on the road from Dunstable towards Gorhambury.

TIME They bloom in August, and shed their seed soon after.

GOVERNMENT AND VIRTUES They are under the dominion of Mars. They resist putrefaction, poison, and pestilence; nor is there a more excellent herb for strengthening the stomach, and helping digestion; it preserves the heart, and prevents fainting and swooning. The powder of the dried roots opens the obstructions of the liver, and restores lost appetite. Steeped in wine and drunk, it refreshes such as are weary with travelling; it helps stitches and griping pains in the sides, and is an excellent remedy for such as are bruised by falls; it provokes urine and the terms exceedingly, consequently should be avoided by pregnant women. The decoction is very profitable for those who are troubled with cramps and convulsions; also it breaks the stone, and is a great help for ruptures. It is good for cold diseases, and to expel tough phlegm, and cure all scabs, itch, and fretting sores and ulcers. It is an admirable remedy to destroy the worms in the body, by taking half a drachm of the powder in the morning in any convenient liquor, and is equally good for the king's evil. To help agues of all sorts, the yellow jaundice, and the bots in cattle, there is no herb superior to this. When kine are bitten on the udder by any venomous beast, if the affected parts are washed with a decoction hereof, it will prove a certain cure.

GERMANDER

DESCRIPTION Common germander shoots forth many stalks, with small and somewhat round leaves, dented on the edges; the flowers stand at the tops, of a deep-purple colour. The root is composed of many springs, which shoot forth a great way round about, soon overspreading the adjacent ground.

PLACE It grows usually in gardens.

TIME It flowers in June and July, and the seed is ripe in August.

GOVERNMENT AND VIRTUES It is an herb under the dominion of Mercury. It strengthens the brain and apprehension exceedingly, and relieves them when drooping; taken with honey, it is a remedy for coughs, hardness of the spleen, and difficulty of urine; or made into a decoction and drunk, it helps those who are troubled with the dropsy, especially if taken at the beginning of the disorder. It also brings down women's menses; used with honey, it cleanses ulcers, and made into an oil, and the eyes anointed therewith, takes away the moisture and dimness of them, and is good for the pains of the sides and cramps. The decoction thereof taken for some days together, drives away and cures both the tertian and quartan agues; it is also good against all diseases of the brain, as continual head-ache, falling sickness, melancholy, drowsiness and dullness of the spirits, convulsions and palsy.

CLOVE GILLIFLOWERS

GOVERNMENT AND VIRTUES They are temperate flowers, of the nature and under the dominion of Jupiter; no excess, neither in heat, cold, dryness, nor moisture, can be perceived in them. They are great strengtheners of the brain and heart, and will therefore make an excellent cordial for family purposes. Either the conserve or syrup of these flowers taken at intervals, is good to help such whose constitution is inclinable to be consumptive.

STOCK GILLIFLOWERS

There are found two kinds of these flowers the one is called the castle or stock gilliflower, which may be kept both winter and summer; the other is not so large, and is called the small stock gilliflower, which must be annually sown; they are called *leucoion*, and *vioæ albæ*, or white violets, because the leaves are white; the leaves of the flowers are of various colours, and called by some writers *violæ matroniales*, or dames violets.

DESCRIPTION These two plants are not much unlike wall-flowers, but that their leaves are whiter and softer; however, I shall treat of them respectively. The great castle or stock gilliflower bears hard and straight leaves, about two feet long, by far longer and larger than the leaves of wall-flowers. The blossoms are of a fragrant or pleasant smell, somewhat like those of heart's ease, though much larger; sometimes of a white, sometimes of an ash colour, some of a carnation, and others of a scarlet and purple colour. These are followed by long husks, containing flat and large seeds. The small stock gilliflower has stalks somewhat like the former, with whitish, woolly, soft, leaves; the flowers are of a fine fragrant smell, and of various colours, followed by seeded cods, and in every respect like the first, except being smaller. It is about a foot high, and perishes yearly.

PLACE They are sown and planted in most of our English flower-gardens, but are seldom found growing wild.

TIME The great castle gilliflower blossoms in March and April, the second year after it is sown; but the smaller kind flowers in July and August, the same year in which it is first sown.

GOVERNMENT AND VIRTUES They are of temperature hot and dry, of a similar nature with the yellow or wall gilliflowers, and are plants of Mercury. The flowers of the stock gilliflower, boiled in water and drunk, are good to remove all difficulty of breathing, and help the cough; they also provoke the menses and urine.

WALL, OR YELLOW GILLIFLOWERS

This flower is supposed to be of the violet species. It is a small bush or shrub, called in Latin *leucocia lutea*, and by the apothecaries *keyri*, in English yellow and wall gilliflowers.

DESCRIPTION   The yellow wall gilliflower is green both winter and summer; the stalks thereof are hard, and of a woody substance, and full of branches; the leaves are thick set thereon, long, narrow, and green; on the tops of the stalks grow the flowers, which are of a very fair yellow colour, of a strong but pleasant smell, and every flower is divided into four small leaves; after these are past, there come cods or husks, which contain large, flat, and yellow, seed.

PLACE   It grows in great quantities on the ruined walls of stone buildings, and is very often planted in gardens, though the garden kinds are generally double flowered, which gives them a peculiar beauty the other cannot boast of.

TIME   It generally flowers in March, April, and May.

GOVERNMENT AND VIRTUES   They are hot and dry plants of the Sun, whose influence they are under, being of subtile parts. Being dried, and boiled in water, it provokes urine, and brings down the terms; a plaster, made of the blossoms with oil and wax, is good to heal chaps of the fundament, and the falling down of the same; or, mingled with honey, cures ulcers and sores of the mouth. Two drachms of the seed taken in wine is a sure specific for bringing down the menstrua; or a pessary made of the same, and conveyed into the matrix, answers the same purpose.

STINKING GLADWIN

DESCRIPTION   This is a species of the flower-de-luce, having several leaves growing from the root, very much resembling those of the flower-de-luce, but that they are sharper edged and thicker in the middle, of a deeper green colour, narrower and sharper pointed, and of a strong disagreeable smell if they are pressed between the fingers: in the middle rises up a reasonable-sized stalk, about a yard high, bearing three or four flowers at the top, made somewhat like those of the flower-de-luce, with three upright leaves, of a dead purplish ash-colour, with veins in them of a different colour, the other three leaves do not fall down, neither are the three small ones so finely arched, nor do they cover those at the lower part; in these particulars it differs somewhat from that aforesaid. These are succeeded by three-square hard husks, opening wide into three parts when they are ripe, wherein lie reddish seed, which in time turns black. The root is like that of the flower-de-luce, but reddish on the outside and whitish within, of a very sharp and hot taste, and of an exceeding disagreeable smell.

PLACE   This plant grows as well on the upland grounds as in woods and moist shadowy places, as also by the sea-side, in many parts of this kingdom, and is often cultivated in gardens.

TIME It blossoms in July, and the seed is ripe in August and September; yet the husks when they are ripe, will open themselves, and contain their seed two or three months before they shed it.

GOVERNMENT AND VIRTUES It is supposed to be under the dominion of Saturn. A decoction of the roots, purges corrupt phlegm and choler, but when wanted to operate more gently, a few slices of the roots infused in ale, will answer the purpose, though those whose stomachs will not admit of this, make use of the leaves only. The juice hereof snuffed up the nostrils, causes sneezing, and thereby draws from the head much corruption; or the powder thereof used the same way, produces the like effect.

The powder drunk in wine, helps those who are troubled with cramps and convulsions, or with the gout or sciatica, and eases the gripings of the belly; it helps the difficulty in passing urine, and cleanses, purges, and stays, the sharp and evil humours which cause long fluxes. The root boiled in wine and drunk, does effectually procure women's menses, and, used as a pessary, works the same effect; but causes abortion in women with child. Half a drachm of the seed beaten to powder and taken in wine, does speedily cause an evacuation of urine; or taken with vinegar, dissolves the hardness and swellings of the spleen. The root is very effectual in all wounds, and particularly those of the head; as also to draw forth splinters, thorns, broken bones, or any other thing sticking in the flesh, by being used with a little verdigrease and honey, together with the great centaury root.

GOLDEN ROD

DESCRIPTION It grows up with brownish, small, round stalks, two feet high and sometimes more; having thereon many narrow and long dark green leaves, generally plain on the edges, and are sometimes, though very rarely found with white strakes or spots thereon; the stalks are divided towards the top into many small branches, bearing thereon small yellow flowers, all which are turned one way; these, being ripe, are succeeded by a kind of down, which is carried away by the wind. The root consists of many small fibres, which grow but a little beneath the surface of the ground; it lives for some years, shooting forth new branches each year, which perish at the approach of winter.

PLACE It grows in the open places of woods and coppices, both in moist and dry grounds, in many parts of this kingdom.

TIME It flowers about the month of July.

GOVERNMENT AND VIRTUES Venus claims dominion over this herb. It is spoken of by Arnoldus de Villa Nova as a most excellent remedy for the stone in the kidneys, as also to expel the gravel by urine. The decoction of the herb, either green or dry, or the distilled water thereof, is very effectual for inward bruises, likewise for staying the floodings of the body, as fluxes of humours, bloody fluxes, and the immoderate menses of women. It is a sovereign wound herb, whereby green wounds and old ulcers are speedily cured; it is of particular efficacy in all lotions for sores or ulcers in the mouth, throat, or privities, of either sex. A decoction is serviceable to fasten the teeth when loose.

GOOSEBERRY-BUSH

Called also feap-berry, and, in Sussex, dewberry-bush, and likewise in many places wine berry.

GOVERNMENT AND VIRTUES They are under the dominion of Venus. The berries, whilst they are unripe, being scalded or baked, are good to procure the return of a lost appetite, especially if the cause proceeds from a stomach afflicted with choleric humours. They are exceeding good to stay the longing of pregnant women. The decoction of the leaves of the tree cools hot swellings and inflammations, as also the St Anthony's fire. The ripe gooseberries, being eaten, are an excellent remedy to allay the violent heat of the stomach and liver; and the young and tender leaves break the stone and expel the gravel both from the bladder and kidneys.

GOUT-HERB

This herb is also frequently called herb gerrard.

DESCRIPTION It is very low, seldom rising more than half a yard high; it consists of several leaves which stand on brownish-green stalks, generally three together, snipped on the edges, and of a strong unpleasant smell. The umbels of flowers are white, and the seed blackish; the root runs deep into the earth, and soon spreads itself over a great deal of ground.

PLACE It grows by hedge and wall sides, and often in the borders and corners of fields, and sometimes in gardens.

TIME It flowers in July, seeding about the latter end of the same month.

GOVERNMENT AND VIRTUES Saturn is the ruler of this plant. It is probable it took the name of gout-herb from its peculiar virtues in healing the cold gout and sciatica, as it has been found by experience to be a most admirable remedy for these disorders; as also joint aches, and other cold disorders. It is even affirmed, that the very carrying of it about in the pocket will defend the bearer from any attack of the aforesaid complaint.

WINTER-GREEN

DESCRIPTION It shoots forth seven, eight, or nine, leaves, from a small, brownish, creeping root, each standing upon a long footstalk; they are nearly as broad as they are long, round pointed, of a sad-green colour, hard in handling, and somewhat like the leaf of a pear-tree. From among these rises up a slender weak stalk, standing upright, bearing at the top many small, white, and sweet-smelling, flowers, laid open like a star, consisting of five round pointed leaves, with many yellow threads standing in the middle, surrounding a green head, having a longish tube with them, which in time proves to be the seed vessel; when ripe it is of a five square shape, with a small point, containing seed as small as dust.

PLACE It grows but seldom in fields, but frequently in woods in the northern counties in this kingdom, as Yorkshire, Lancashire, &c.

TIME It flowers in June and July, shedding its seed soon after.

GOVERNMENT AND VIRTUES Winter-green is under the dominion of Saturn, and is an excellent remedy for the speedy healing of green wounds, the leaves being bruised and applied, or the juice of them is equally effectual. The herb boiled in wine and water, and drunk by those who are troubled with ulcers, wonderfully helps them. It stays all fluxes, whether of blood or humours, as the lask, bloody flux, immoderate menstrua, and bleeding of wounds, and takes away such inflammations as rise from the pains of the heart.

GROMEL

Of this I shall briefly describe three kinds, which are chiefly used medicinally; the virtues of each are the same, but different in the manner of their growth.

Common gromel

DESCRIPTION The greater gromel rises up with slender, hard, and hairy stalks, trailing and taking root as it lies on the ground; it spreads itself by several small branches, whereon grow hairy dark-green leaves. At the joints, with the leaves, grow many small blue flowers, which are succeeded by hard stony, roundish, seed. The root is round and woody, and lives during the winter, shooting forth fresh herbage every spring.

Shrubby gromel

The small wild gromel grows up with several straight, hard, branched, stalks, two or three feet high, full of joints, bearing at each, small, long, hard,

Creeping gromel

and rough, leaves, very much like the former, but less. Among these leaves grow small white blossoms, which are followed by greyish round seed like the first. The root is not very large, but exceedingly thready.

The garden gromel has many upright, slender, woody, hairy, stalks, brown, and crested, with but few branches, bearing leaves like the former; the flowers are white, after which come rough brown husks, containing white, hard, round, seed, shining like pearls, and greater than either of the former. The root is like that of the first, with many branches and strings thereat, and of long duration.

PLACE The two first grow wild in barren and untilled places. The last is a nursling in the gardens of the curious.

TIME They all flower from midsummer till September, and the seed ripens quickly after.

GOVERNMENT AND VIRTUES The dominion over these herbs is wholly claimed by Venus. They are of singular force in breaking the stone and expelling gravel, either in the reins or bladder; as also to provoke urine, and help the difficulty in passing urine. The seed is most effectual for the above purposes, being bruised and boiled in white wine, or other convenient liquor; the powder of the seed is equally efficacious. Two drachms of the seed in powder taken with breast-milk, will procure a speedy delivery to women afflicted with hard travail, and that cannot be delivered. The herb itself (when the seed is not to be had) either boiled, or the juice thereof drunk, will answer all the aforesaid purposes, though not so powerful in its operation.

GROUNDSEL

DESCRIPTION Our common groundsel has a round, green, and somewhat brownish, stalk, spreading towards the top several branches, set with long and somewhat narrow green leaves, cut in on the edges, not much unlike the oak leaves, but less, and round at the ends; at the tops of the branches stand many small green heads, out of which grow yellow threads or thrums, which are the flowers: these continue many days thus blown before they are turned into down, which with the seed is carried away by the wind. Its root is small and thready, soon perishing, and as soon rising again from its own sowing.

PLACE It grows almost every where, as well on the tops of walls as among all kinds of rubbish and rude grounds, but especially in gardens.

TIME It may be seen in bloom at almost any time of the year, and, if permitted to occupy good ground, each plant will spring and seed at least twice in a year.

GOVERNMENT AND VIRTUES The herb is influenced by Venus. It is a universal medicine for all diseases proceeding from heat, in whatever part of the body they may chance to happen; it is a safe and gentle purge for a foul stomach, operating each way. It is of a moist and cold nature, consequently causes expulsion, and represses the heat caused by the motion of the internal parts, through the effects of an emetic or other medicine. This herb preserved either as a syrup, an ointment, or distilled water, is a medicine unrivalled in its efficacy for the cure of all hot diseases, both for its safety and speed. A drachm given in oxymel, after using a little exercise, provokes urine, and expels the gravel from the reins and kidneys; also it helps the sciatica, cholic, and pains of the belly. The people in Lincolnshire use this externally against pains and swellings; and, as they affirm, with great success.

HART'S TONGUE

DESCRIPTION It consists of several leaves rising from the root, every one separately, folding themselves in their first springing and spreading; when at their full growth, they are about a foot long, smooth and green, but hard and sappy in the middle, streaked on the back athwart on both sides of the middle rib, with small and somewhat long brownish marks; the bottoms of the leaves are a little bowed on each side of the middle rib, and somewhat small at the end. The root is composed of many black threads, which are much entangled together.

TIME It is green all the winter, having new leaves every year.

GOVERNMENT AND VIRTUES Jupiter claims dominion over this herb. It is a singular remedy to strengthen the liver when weak, and ease it when afflicted; it is esteemed for its efficacy in removing the hardness and stoppings of the spleen and liver; also against the heat of the liver and stomach, as well as the lask and bloody flux. The distilled water is good for the passions of the heart, and gargled in the mouth will stay the hiccough, help the falling of the palate, and stop the bleeding of the gums.

HAWK-WEED

DESCRIPTION It has many large leaves lying on the ground, having many deep gashes on the edges, somewhat like those of the sow-thistle; from among these rises up a hollow rough stalk, two or three feet high, branched from the middle upwards. On these are set, at every joint, several leaves cut but very little on the edges, bearing at the top many pale yellow flowers, consisting of small narrow leaves, broad pointed, and nicked in on the edges, set in a double

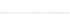

row, and sometimes more, the outside leaves being the largest. These flowers are turned into down, bearing small brownish seed, which is blown away with the wind. The root is long and rather large, with many small fibres thereat. The whole plant is full of bitter milk.

PLACE It grows in many places, especially in fields and borders of pathways, in dry grounds.

TIME It blossoms and disperses its down in the summer months.

GOVERNMENT AND VIRTUES Saturn claims dominion over this herb. Dioscorides says, it is cooling, somewhat dry and binding, and therefore good for the heat and gnawings of the stomach, for inflammation and hot ague-fits. The juice thereof, taken in wine, helps digestion, expels wind, prevents clogging the stomach, and causes an easy evacuation of urine. A scruple of the dried juice, taken in wine and vinegar, is profitable for the dropsy; the decoction of the herb, taken with honey, digests thin phlegm in the chest and lungs, and, mixed with hyssop, it helps the cough. The decoction hereof, mixed with that of wild succory made with wine, and taken, helps the wind cholic, and hardness of the spleen, procures rest and sleep, prevents venery, cools heats, purges the stomach, increases blood, and helps all diseases of the reins and bladder. The green herb bruised, and mixed with a little salt, is effectual in helping burns, if it be used before the blisters rise; also inflammations, St Anthony's fire, and all pushes and eruptions, heat and salt phlegm. The same applied with meal and fair water, in the manner of a poultice, to any place affected with convulsions and the cramp, or dislocated members, gives great help and ease. The distilled water cleanses the skin from all blemishes.

HAWTHORN

It is generally a hedge-bush, but, by being carefully pruned and dressed, it will grow to a reasonable height. As for the hawthorn-tree of Glastonbury, which is said to flower yearly on Christmas-day, it rather shews the superstition of those who entertain this opinion than excites wonder on any other account, since the same may be found in many other places of this kingdom; as at a place called Whitegreen, near Namptwich in Cheshire; and also in Romney-marsh. These, if the winter happens to be mild, will be in full bloom about Christmas.

GOVERNMENT AND VIRTUES It is a tree of Mars. The berries, or the seed in the berries, beaten to powder and drunk in wine, are a singular remedy for the stone, and no less effectual for the dropsy. The distilled water of the flowers stays the lask; and the seeds, cleeted from the down, then bruised and boiled in wine, will give instant relief to the tormenting pains of the body.

If cloths and sponges are wet in the distilled water, and applied to any place wherein thorns, splinters, &c, are lodged, it will certainly draw them forth.

HASEL-NUT

GOVERNMENT AND VIRTUES   They are under the dominion of Mercury. The parched kernels made into an electuary, or the milk drawn from the kernels with mead or honeyed water, are very good to help an old cough; and, being parched, and a little pepper added thereto, and taken in drink, digest the distillations of rheum from the head. The dried husks and shells, to the quantity of about two drachms, taken in red wine, stay the lasks, and women's menses; but the red skin which covers the kernel is much more effectual for the latter purpose.

HEART'S EASE

It is called in Sussex pansies, and is so well known by almost every person, that I shall decline troubling my readers with a description of it.

PLACE   Besides those which are cultivated in gardens, they grow wild in barren and unfertile grounds.

TIME   They flower and seed all the time of spring and summer.

GOVERNMENT AND VIRTUES   This is a Saturnine plant. A strong decoction of the herb and flowers is an excellent cure for the veneral disorder; it is also good for convulsions in children, inflammations of the lungs and breast, pleurisy, &c. It will make an excellent syrup for the aforesaid purposes.

HEDGE-HYSSOP

DESCRIPTION   There are several sorts of this plant, the first of which is a native of Italy, and only reared here by the curious. Two or three kinds however grow wild in England, two of which I shall here mention; *viz.* the first is a low smooth plant, not quite a foot high, of a very bitter taste, composed of many square stalks, diversly branched from the bottom to the top; it has many joints, shooting forth at each two small leaves; these are rather broader at the bottom than at the top, a little dented on the edges, of a sad-green colour, and full of veins. The flowers stand also at the joints, being of a fair purple colour with white spots, and made very much like those of dead-nettle; the seed is small and yellow, and the roots spread much under ground. The second seldom grows more than half a foot high, shooting forth several small branches, whereon grow many small leaves set one against the other, somewhat broad, but very short; the flowers are not much unlike the former in shape, but of a pale-reddish colour; the seed is small and yellowish, and the root spreads like that of the first.

PLACE They grow in wet low grounds, and by water-sides, and the latter sort may be found amongst the bogs on Hampstead Heath.

TIME They generally flower in June, July, and August, and the seed ripens presently after.

GOVERNMENT AND VIRTUES They are under the dominion of Mars. They are very unsafe to take inwardly, unless well rectified by an alchemist, and only the purity of them given, as they are violent purgers, especially of choler and phlegm. Being prepared, they are very good for the dropsy, gout, and sciatica.

BLACK HELLEBORE

It is called also fetter-wort, fetter-grass, bear's foot, Christmas-herb, and Christmas-flower.

DESCRIPTION It has many fair green leaves rising from the root, each of them standing about a span high from the ground; the leaves are all divided into seven, eight, or nine, parts, dented from the middle to the point on both sides, and remain green all the winter. About Christmas time, if the weather be somewhat temperate, the flowers appear upon footstalks, each composed of five large round, white leaves, which are sometimes purple toward the edges, with many pale yellow thrums in the middle. The seed is divided into several cells, somewhat like those of columbines, but rather larger; the seed is long and round, and of a black colour. The root consists of numberless blackish strings, all united into one head. There is likewise another species of black hellebore, which frequently grows in woods and forests, very much like this, except that the leaves are smaller and narrower. It perishes in the winter.

PLACE The first is cultivated in gardens; the second is commonly found in the woods in Northamptonshire.

TIME The former blossoms in December and January, and the latter in February and March.

GOVERNMENT AND VIRTUES It is an herb of Saturn, consequently would be taken with greater safety after being purified than when raw. The roots are very effectual against all melancholic diseases, especially such as are of long standing, as quartan agues and madness; it helps the falling sickness, the leprosy, the yellow and black jaundice, the gout, sciatica, and convulsions; or, used as a pessary, provokes the terms exceedingly. The same being beaten to a powder, and strewed upon ulcers, consumes the dead flesh and instantly heals them; it will also help gangrenes by taking inwardly twenty grains thereof corrected with half as much cinnamon. Country people use it for the cure of such beasts as are troubled with the cough, or have taken any poison, by boring a hole through the ear and putting a piece of the root therein.

HEMLOCK

DESCRIPTION The common great hemlock grows up with a green stalk, four or five feet high, and sometimes higher, full of red spots; at the joints are set very large winged leaves, which are divided into many other winged leaves, set one against another, dented on the edges, and of a sad-green colour. The stalks are branched towards the top, each bearing umbels of white flowers, which are followed by whitish flat seed. The root is long, white, hollow, and sometimes crooked, of a very strong, heady, and disagreeable, smell.

PLACE Its growth is not confined to any particular spot in this kingdom, but it may be found by most old walls, hedge-sides, and uncultivated grounds.

TIME It generally flowers and seeds in July.

GOVERNMENT AND VIRTUES Saturn governs this plant. It is exceeding cold, and of a very dangerous quality, consequently must not be applied internally. It is of good effect for inflammations, tumours, and swellings of any part of the body, the privities excepted; also St Anthony's fire, weals, pushes, and ulcers, proceeding from hot sharp humours, by cooling and repelling the heat. The leaves bruised, and laid to the brow or forehead, are good for those whose eyes are red and swelled, and for cleansing them of web or film growing thereon. If the root is roasted in embers, afterwards wrapped in double wet papers, and then applied to any part afflicted with the gout, it will speedily remove the pain thereof. Should any person, unfortunately, through mistake, eat the herbage of this plant instead of parsley, or the root instead of a parsnip (both bearing a great resemblance to each other) it will certainly cause a phrenzy or stupefaction of the senses; I will recommend to the patient the strongest and best wine they can procure, and to drink it immediately, before the ill effects of the herb strike to the heart. If wine cannot be instantly had, Pliny advises to take a good draught of strong vinegar, which he affirms to be a sovereign remedy.

HEMP

It is so common a plant, and so well known by almost every resident of this kingdom, that a description of it would be altogether superfluous.

TIME It is sown about the latter end of March or beginning of April, and is ripe in August and September.

GOVERNMENT AND VIRTUES It is under the dominion of Saturn. The seed consumes wind, but if used too liberally it dries up the natural seed for procreation, though, being boiled in milk, and taken a little at a time, it is a good remedy for a dry cough. An emulsion made of the seed is given with good success for the jaundice, especially in the beginning of the disease, if there be no ague accompanying it, for it opens obstructions of the gall, and causes digestion of choler; it stays lasks and continual fluxes, eases the cholic, allays the troublesome humours of the bowels, and stays bleeding at the mouth, nose, or any other place. The decoction of the root allays inflammations, eases the pains of the gout, the hard tumours or knots in the joints, the pains and shrinkings of the sinews, and the pains of the hips. The fresh juice, mixed with a little oil and butter, is an exceeding good cure for burns.

HEN-BANE

DESCRIPTION The common hen-bane has very large, thick, soft, woolly, leaves, lying upon the ground, much cut or torn on the edges, of a dark, ill, greyish-green, colour; from among these rise up several thick and short stalks, two or three feet high, spread into many smaller branches with less leaves thereon, bearing small yellow flowers, which scarcely appear above the husks; they are usually torn on the one side, ending in five round points growing one above another, of a dead yellowish colour, somewhat paler toward the edges, with many purplish veins, and of a dark yellowish-purple colour at the bottom of the flower, with a small pointel of the same colour in the middle; each of them stands in a hard close husk, somewhat like those of asarabacca, and rather sharp at the top points, containing much small seed, very like poppy seed, but of a dusky greyish colour. The root is large, white, and thick, branching forth many ways under ground, not much unlike a parsnip, except in colour, and is, together with the plant, of a very strong, disagreeable, and offensive, smell.

PLACE It generally grows near pathways, and under the sides of hedges and old walls.

TIME It blossoms in July, and springs annually from its own sowing; though many believe it to flower much earlier.

GOVERNMENT AND VIRTUES It is a Saturnine plant. The leaves are good for cooling hot inflammations in the eyes, or other parts of the body; and, being boiled in wine, and used as a foment, it will assuage all manner of swellings, either in the scrotum, women's breasts, or other parts of the body; also the gout, sciatica, and pains of the joints, if proceeding from a hot cause. Being applied with vinegar to the forehead and temples, it helps the head-ache, and causes those to sleep who are prevented by hot violent fevers.

HERB ROBERT

DESCRIPTION It grows up with a reddish stalk about two feet high, bearing on long and reddish footstalks many leaves, these are divided at the ends into three or five divisions, some cut deeper than others, and also dented on the edges, which oftentimes turn of a reddish colour. At the top of the stalk grow several flowers, each consisting of five leaves, much larger than those of dove's foot, and of a deeper red colour, after which come beak-heads as in others. The root is small and thready, and of an unpleasant smell.

PLACE It may be found almost any where near the waysides, ditch-banks, &c.

TIME It flowers in June and July, and the seed is ripe soon after.

GOVERNMENT AND VIRTUES This herb is under the dominion of Venus. It is esteemed an excellent remedy for the stone, and will stay blood, from whatever cause it might happen to flow; it speedily heals all green wounds, and is effectual in curing ulcers in the privities and other parts.

HERB TRUELOVE

DESCRIPTION Ordinary herb truelove has a small creeping root running under the upper crust of the ground, somewhat like a couch-grass root, but not so white, shooting forth stalks with leaves, some of which carry small berries, and others not; every stalk smooth, without joints, and of a blackish-green colour, rising about half a foot high if it bears berries, but not so high if otherwise; on the top are four leaves set directly one against the other, resembling a cross, or rather a ribbon tied in a truelove's knot, from whence it took its name; these leaves are somewhat like the leaves of nightshade, but a little broader, having sometimes three leaves, sometimes five, and frequently six, some of which are larger than others. From the middle of the four leaves rises up one small slender stalk, about an inch high, bearing on the top a flowerspread open like a star, consisting of four small and long narrow pointed leaves, of a yellowish-green colour, with four smaller ones lying between, and in the middle stands a round, dark, purplish, button or head, compassed about with eight small yellow mealy threads of three colours, which form a beautiful flower; when the other leaves are withered, the button or head in the middle becomes a blackish-purple berry about the size of a grape, full of juice, and contains many white seeds.

PLACE   It grows in woods and coppices, especially about Chislehurst and Maidstone in Kent; and is likewise frequently found in the borders of fields, and other waste grounds.

TIME   They spring up about April or May, and flower soon after; the berries are ripe in the end of May and June.

GOVERNMENT AND VIRTUES   This plant is claimed by Venus. The leaves or berries hereof are effectual to expel poison of all sorts, especially that of the aconites; also the plague, and other pestilential diseases. The roots beaten to powder and taken in wine, give ease to those who are troubled with the cholic; the leaves are exceeding good for green wounds, as also to cleanse and heal up sores and ulcers and speedily allays all inflammations. The leaves or juice applied to nails of the hands or feet that have imposthumes or sores gathered together at the roots or under them, will prove a certain cure in a short time.

HOARHOUND

DESCRIPTION   Common hoarhound grows up with square hoary stalks, about half a yard or two feet high, set at the joints with two round crumpled rough leaves, of a dull hoary-green colour, of a tolerably pleasant smell, but very bitter taste. The flowers are small, white, and gaping, set in rough, hard, prickly husks; these, together with the leaves, surround the joints from the middle of the stalk upwards, and are succeeded by small, round, blackish seed. The root is blackish, hard, and woody, with many strings, and very durable.

PLACE   It is found in most parts of this kingdom, especially in dry grounds, and waste green places.

TIME   It generally blossoms in and about July, and the seed is ripe in August.

GOVERNMENT AND VIRTUES   It is an herb of Mercury. A decoction of the dried herb with the seed, or the juice of the green herb taken with honey, is a certain remedy for those who are short-winded, or have a cough, or are fallen into a consumption, either through long sickness, or thin distillations or rheum upon the lungs. It helps to expectorate tough phlegm from the chest, being taken with the roots of iris, or oris. It brings down the menstrua, expels the after-birth, and gives ease to those who are afflicted with long and painful travail. The leaves used with honey, purge ulcers, and ease the pains of the sides. The juice thereof, used with wine and honey, helps to clear the eyesight, and, snuffed up the nostrils, purges away the yellow jaundice; the same used with a little oil of roses and dropped into the ears, eases the pains thereof. Galen says, it opens obstructions both of the liver and spleen, and purges the breast and lungs of phlegm: or outwardly applied, it both cleanses and digests. There is a syrup made of this plant sold by most apothecaries, which I would recommend as an excellent help to evacuate tough phlegm and cold rheum from the lungs of aged persons, especially those who are asthmatic or short-winded.

HOLLY

Called also holm or hulver-bush.

GOVERNMENT AND VIRTUES This tree is of a Saturnine quality; the berries expel wind, and are therefore esteemed good for removing the pains of the cholic; they are of a strong nature; for, by eating a dozen of them in the morning fasting, when they are ripe, and not dried, they purge the body of gross and clammy phlegm; but, if you dry the berries and beat them into powder, they are binding; they stop fluxes of every kind, as also the terms of women. Both the bark and leaves are exceeding good to be used in fomentations for broken bones and dislocated members.

HONEY-WORT

There are divers species of the honey-wort, namely, the great, small, and rough; as, the greater yellow and red; the greater yellow or purple; and the smaller yellow and white; the flowers of all or either of which the bees are remarkably fond of, and much delighted with.

DESCRIPTION The greater honey-wort grows up upon a thick green stalk, to a moderate height, having many great, deep-pointed, green leaves, placed one above another; towards the top of each stalk come umbels of flowers, thick set, and rising up spiral or crested; mostly of a bright yellow colour; though some are red, others purple, and some perfectly white.

PLACE The honey-worts grow not wild in England, but are cherished up in gardens, and planted in the pleasure-grounds and nurseries of the curious.

TIME They spring up in April, and flower from the latter end of May to August, but perish in the winter.

GOVERNMENT AND VIRTUES Honey-worts are under Mercury. They are of a temperate quality, between cold and hot; but rather inclining to cold, and are somewhat astringent. They stop immoderate fluxes of the belly, and women's menses. The juice of the herb, with a little saffron dissolved in it, is an excellent remedy for weak, watery, or bleary, eyes; and is used to heal ulcers. Some people use it instead of bugloss and borage, in all cases where those herbs are recommended. The flowers are very sweet.

HOPS

The manured hops are so well known, that I shall decline writing its description; shall therefore proceed to that of the wild hops.

DESCRIPTION The wild hop grows up like the tame, twining upon trees and hedges that stand near them; it has rough branches and leaves like the former, but much smaller heads; these heads are so scarce, that one stalk seldom produces more than one or two; – in this the chiefest difference consists.

PLACE They grow on low moist grounds, and are found in most parts of this kingdom.

TIME They spring up in April, and flower about the latter end of June, but the heads are not gathered till the latter end of September.

GOVERNMENT AND VIRTUES It is under the dominion of Mars. This operates in opening obstructions of the liver and spleen, cleansing the blood, loosening the belly, expelling the gravel, and provoking urine; the decoction of the tops of hops, whether tame or wild, works these effects. Half a drachm of the seed in powder, taken in drink, brings down women's menses, and expels urine. A syrup made of the juice and sugar, cures the yellow jaundice, eases the head-ache proceeding from heat, and tempers the heat of the liver and stomach; it is likewise given with good effect to those who are afflicted with long and hot agues. Both the wild and the manured are of one property, and alike effectual in all the aforesaid disorders.

HORSE-TAIL

Of this there are many kinds, but I shall decline troubling my readers with the description of any other than the most eminent.

DESCRIPTION The great horse-tail, at the first springing, has heads somewhat like asparagus, which afterwards grow to be hard, rough, hollow, stalks, jointed in several places, and about a foot high; the lower part appearing to be put into the upper. On each side grows a bush of small, long, rush-like, hard leaves, each part resembling a horse's tail (from whence it took its name). At the tops of the stalks come forth small catkins, somewhat like those of trees. The root creeps under the ground, having many joints.

PLACE This horse-tail (as do most of the other kinds hereof) generally grows in moist and wet grounds.

TIME They spring up in April, and their catkins bloom in July; in August they shed their feed, and then perish, rising afresh every spring.

GOVERNMENT AND VIRTUES Of this herb, the smooth rather than the rough, and the leased rather than the bare, are most physical. Saturn claims dominion over it, yet its qualities are harmless. It is very good to staunch bleedings, either inwardly or outwardly, the juice or decoction thereof being drunk, or externally applied. It stays lasks and fluxes of every kind, either in men or women; suppresses the evacuation of blood through the urinary passages, and quickly heals green wounds. It is an excellent cure for ruptures in children. The decoction, taken in wine, provokes urine, and helps the stone and difficulty in passing urine; and a small quantity of the distilled water thereof, drunk two or three times in a day, eases the disagreeable sensations of the bowels, and is effectual against a cough. By bathing the parts affected with the warm juice or distilled water of this plant, it cures hot inflammations.

HOUND'S TONGUE

DESCRIPTION The great ordinary hound's tongue has many long and somewhat narrow, soft, hairy, darkish-green leaves, lying on the ground, and not much unlike those of bugloss; from among these rises up a rough hairy stalk, about two feet high, with smaller leaves thereon, and branches at the top into many parts, bearing at the foot of each a small leaf; on this branch are many small flowers, which consist of small purplish-red leaves, of a dead colour, scarcely rising out of the husk wherein they stand, with a few threads in the middle. It has sometimes a white flower. After the flowers are fallen, there follow rough flat seeds, with a small pointel in the middle, easily cleaving to any thing it happens to touch. The branch whereon these flowers grow is crooked, or turned inwards, before they are in blossom, but straightens itself as the flowers come to perfection. The root is black, thick, and long, hard to break, and full of clammy juice, smelling somewhat strong and disagreeable, as do also the leaves.

PLACE It grows in most parts of this kingdom, in waste grounds, untilled places, highway-sides, and under hedges.

TIME It generally flowers in the months of May and June, and the seed is ripe shortly after.

GOVERNMENT AND VIRTUES It is a plant under the dominion of Mercury. The root is very effectually used in pills and decoctions, or otherwise, to stay all sharp and thin defluxions of rheums from the head into the eyes or nose, or upon the stomach or lungs, as also for coughs and shortness of breath. The leaves boiled in wine (though many approve of water) with oil and salt added thereto, mollify and open the belly downwards, and help to cure the biting of a mad dog, by applying the leaves to the wound. Bruising the leaves, or the juice of them boiled in hog's lard, and applied, helps to preserve the hair from falling, and eases the pain of a scald or burn; or the bruised leaves, laid to any green wound, speedily heal the same. The root baked in embers, wrapped in paste, or wet papers, or in a wet double cloth, and a suppository made thereof and applied to the fundament, does very effectually help the piles or hæmorrhoids; also the distilled water of the herb and root is used with good effect for all the aforesaid purposes, either taken inwardly or applied outwardly, especially as a wash for wounds and punctures, and particularly ulcers occasioned by the venereal disease.

HOUSELEEK

It is too well known, as well by the name of sengreen as houseleek, to require any description.

PLACE AND TIME It grows commonly on the tops of houses and walls, and flowers in July.

GOVERNMENT AND VIRTUES Jupiter claims dominion over this herb, from which it is fabulously reported, that it preserves whatever it grows upon from fire and lightning. The ordinary houseleek is good for all inward and outward heats, either in the eyes or other parts of the body. A posset made with the juice of houseleek is singularly good in all hot agues, for it cools and tempers the blood and spirits, and quenches thirst; by dropping the juice thereof into the eyes, it cures them of all hot defluxions of sharp and salt rheums, and is equally effectual for all disorders of the ears, being used in the same manner. It stops the immoderate floodings of the menstrua, and helps the humours of the bowels; it cools and abates all hot inflammations; and is a certain ease to those who are afflicted with the gout, when proceeding from a hot cause. By bathing the hands and feet with the juice, and laying the skin of the leaves on them afterwards, it cleanses them of warts and corns; it also eases the head-ache and distempered heat of the brain, occasioned by phrensies or want of sleep, being applied to the temples and forehead. The leaves, bruised and laid upon the crown of the head, stay the bleeding of the nose very quickly. The distilled water of the herb is likewise profitable for all the aforesaid purposes. The leaves, being gently rubbed on any place stung with nettles or bees, do quickly take away the pain, and discharge the blisters proceeding therefrom.

HYSSOP

TEMPERATURE AND VIRTUES The herb is Jupiter's, under the sign Cancer, consequently strengthens such parts of the body as these govern. Dioscorides says, that hyssop boiled with rue and honey, and drunk, helps those who are troubled with coughs, shortness of breath, wheezing, and rheumatic distillation of the lungs; taken with oxymel, it expels gross humours by stool; also with fresh or new figs bruised, it helps to loosen the belly, but more effectually if the root of flower-de-luce be added thereto. It restores the natural colour of the skin when discoloured by the yellow jaundice, and being taken with figs and nitre it helps the dropsy and spleen.

Being boiled in wine, it is good to wash inflammations, and takes away black and blue spots and marks proceeding from blows, bruises, or falls, if applied with warm water. Being boiled with figs, it makes an excellent gargle for the quinsey or swelling in the throat; or boiled in vinegar and gargled in the mouth it cures the tooth-ache.

Bruised and mixed with salt, honey, and cummin-seed, it helps the falling-sickness, and expels tough phlegm, and is effectual in all cold griefs or diseases of the chest and lungs, being taken either as a medicine or syrup. The green herb bruised and a little sugar mixed therewith, will speedily heal up any cut or green wound, being thereto applied.

INDIAN LEAF

It is called by the indians *cadegi indi*, that is, *folium Indum*. It is also called *malabathrum*, and by the East Indians *tamala patra*.

DESCRIPTION They are broad leaves, composed of three ribs, and a little pointed at the ends; amongst these are other leaves which sometimes grow on their branches, two usually at a joint, tasting somewhat hot, like the bay-leaf, as does likewise the bark; among these leaves is sometimes found a small fruit, very much resembling an acorn in the cup; this is probably the fruit of the tree, and gathered with the leaves.

GOVERNMENT AND VIRTUES It is a solar plant; the virtues of it are these: it provokes urine, it warms and strengthens the stomach exceedingly. It is good to put into cordial and stomachic compositions.

IVY

PLACE It may be found upon most old stone walls of churches, houses, and ruinous buildings, and frequently in woods and upon trees.

TIME It flowers in July, but the berries do not ripen till they have felt the winter frosts.

GOVERNMENT AND VIRTUES It is under the dominion of Saturn. It is very pernicious to the nerves and sinews, being taken too liberally, but particularly helpful when externally applied. The fresh leaves of ivy, boiled in vinegar, and applied warm to the sides of those that are troubled with the spleen, ache, or stitch in the sides, give immediate ease; or, used with rose-water and oil of roses to bathe the temples and forehead, ease the head-ache, though of long continuance. It is likewise an excellent cure for green wounds, burnings, scaldings. The juice of the berries or leaves, snuffed up the nose, purges the head and brain of thin rheum which causes defluxions into the eyes and nose. By the continual drinking out of a cup made of ivy, all symptoms of the spleen are entirely erased. The speediest cure for a surfeit by wine, is to drink a draught of the same liquor wherein a handful of bruised ivy-leaves have been boiled.

ST JOHN'S WORT

DESCRIPTION The common St John's wort shoots forth brownish, upright, hard, round, stalks, two feet high, spreading many branches from the sides up to the top, with two small dark-green leaves set one against another, somewhat like those of the smaller centaury, but narrower and full of small holes, which can scarcely be discerned unless held up towards the light. At the tops of the stalks and branches stand yellow flowers, each composed of five leaves, with many yellow threads in the middle, which being bruised, yield a reddish juice like blood; these are succeeded by small round heads containing small blackish seed, smelling like rosin. The root is hard and woody, with many strings and fibres, and of a brownish colour; they live many years, shooting afresh yearly.

PLACE It grows in woods and coppices, as well those that are shady as those that are open and exposed to the sun.

TIME They flower about midsummer, and their seed is ripe in the latter end of July and August.

GOVERNMENT AND VIRTUES It is under the celestial sign Leo, and governed by the Sun. It is by no means the least valuable for its efficacy in the cure of wounds, hurts, or bruises, by being boiled in wine and drunk, if the complaint is inwardly; or, if outwardly, by converting it into an oil, ointment, bath, or lotion. It opens obstructions, dissolves swellings, closes up the lips of wounds. Two drachms of the seed of this herb, beaten to powder, and drunk in a little broth, gently expel choler or congealed blood from the stomach. The decoction of the leaves and seeds, being drunk rather warm before the ague-fits come on, in the course of a little time will entirely remove them. Drinking the decoction of the seed for forty days together helps the sciatica, the falling sickness, and the palsy.

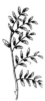

JUJUBE-TREE

Dodoneus says there are two sorts of jujubes, red and white; and of the red three different kinds, *viz.* the greater jujube-tree, called in Latin *ziziphus five jujuba major*; the smaller jujube, called *ziziphus sive jujuba minor*; and the wild jujube-tree.

DESCRIPTION   The greater jujube-tree grows sometimes very high, but oftener spreads itself in breadth, having a crooked body; the wood is hard and whitish, the bark rugged, and the branches great and spreading; the smaller twigs about a foot long, and full of leaves on both sides, one a little above another, and an odd one at the end; these leaves are small, broad, and pointed at the end; finely dented about the edges, with long veins in them, each standing on a long footstalk, smooth, and feel hard. At the foot of every leaf, towards the tops of the twigs, come forth small yellowish flowers, each consisting of five leaves; these are succeeded by the fruit, which is somewhat like a small plum, or olive, but rather long, green, and harsh at the first; afterwards they become yellowish, and when ripe they are of a fine red colour, of a sharp sweetness, and somewhat clammy; flattish next the stalk, containing a stone not unlike that of the olive or Cornelian cherry; and its skin is thicker and harder than that of the plum. The branches are thorny, standing two always at a joint, one whereof is crooked, the other straight: the roots are long and fast in the earth.

The smaller jujube-tree is, in branches, leaves, flowers, and fruit, very much like the former, except that it is every way somewhat smaller; it is also thick set with thorns like the other, but these are rather shorter.

The wild jujube-tree is lower, and more like a shrub, than either of the former, but thicker set with small sharp thorns; the leaves are not unlike, but grow not so thick on a twig, and are smaller; the fruit of this is also red, somewhat less, drier of substance, and of a sharper taste, than the others.

PLACE   The first growth naturally in Africa, Egypt, and most eastern countries; and was, as Pliny observes, conveyed from thence into Italy, where it now grows in great plenty. The other kinds are likewise found in Italy, and in some parts of France; the wild kind growing in the fields and hedges.

PLATE 11

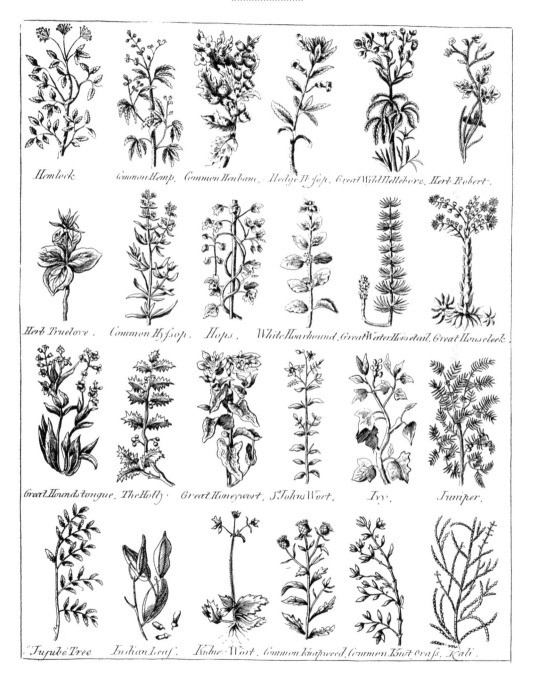

Hemlock.   Common Hemp.   Common Henbane.   Hedge Hyssop.   Great Wild Hellebore.   Herb Robert.

Herb Truelove.   Common Hyssop.   Hops.   White Hoarhound.   Great Water Horsetail.   Great Houseleek.

Great Houndstongue.   The Holly.   Great Honeywort.   St Johns Wort.   Ivy.   Juniper.

Jujube Tree.   Indian Leaf.   Kidney Wort.   Common Knapweed.   Common Knot Grass.   Kali.

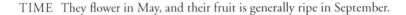

TIME They flower in May, and their fruit is generally ripe in September.

GOVERNMENT AND VIRTUES Venus claims dominion over these. Jujube-berries, when fresh, open the body, purge choler, and cleanse the blood. They are of a temperate quality in heat and moisture; they cool the heat and sharpness of the blood, and therefore are good in hot agues, also to expectorate tough phlegm and other diseases of the chest and lungs, as coughs, shortness of breath, hot distillations, &c. and, being taken in syrups or electuaries, expel the roughness of the throat and breast. They are good to cleanse the reins and bladder, their viscous qualities making the passages slippery, and expelling the gravel and stone with infinitely less pain; and they stay vomiting when caused by sharp humours. They are hard of digestion, being either fresh or dry, and therefore are used in decoctions, syrups, or electuaries. I shall here present my readers with a most valuable receipt for the cure of all sharp humours, ulcers, or inflammations in the kidneys and bladder; and for the stone, jaundice, falling-sickness, and dropsy. – It is thus prepared: Take jujubes, the seed of parsley, fennel, anise, and carraways, of each one ounce; of the roots of parsley, burnet, saxifrage, and carraway, one ounce and a half; let the seed be bruised, and the roots washed and cut small, then infuse them all night in a bottle of white wine, and in the morning boil it in a close earthen vessel until a third part be consumed; strain it, and drink four ounces at a time, the first and last thing morning and evening; abstaining from all other drink for at least three hours. This you will find effectual for the aforesaid disorders.

JUNIPER-BUSH

PLACE They are very plentiful in most woods and commons, particularly upon Warley-common, near Brentwood in Essex; upon Finchley-common, without Highgate; adjacent to the Newfound Wells near Dulwich; upon a common between Mitcham and Croydon; in the highway near Amersham in Buckinghamshire; and in many other places.

TIME The berries are not ripe the first year, but continue green two summers and one winter before they ripen, when they change their colour to black; they are ripe about the fall of the leaf.

GOVERNMENT AND VIRTUES This admirable solar shrub can scarcely be equalled for its virtues. Its berries are hot in the third degree, and dry in the first, being an excellent counter-poison and a great resister of pestilence. It is so powerful a remedy for the dropsy, that, by drinking only the lye made of the ashes of this herb, it cures the disease; it provokes the terms, helps the fits of the womb, strengthens the stomach, and expels wind; indeed there are few better remedies for the wind and cholic, than the chemical oil drawn from the berries; but, as many, in all probability, would be at a loss how to extract this oil, I would advise them to eat ten or a dozen of the ripe berries every morning fasting, as these will occasionally answer the aforesaid purposes; they are also good for a cough, shortness of breath, consumption, pains in the belly, ruptures, cramps, and convulsions; they strengthen the brain, help the memory, fortify the sight by strengthening the optic nerves, and give safe and speedy delivery to women in labour; they are excellent good in all sorts of agues, they help the gout and sciatica, and strengthen all the limbs of the body. The ashes of the wood are a special remedy for the scurvy in the gums, by rubbing them therewith; the berries stay all fluxes, help the hæmorrhoids or piles; they break the stone, procure lost appetite, and are very good for palsies and falling sickness. A lye made of the ashes of the wood, and the body bathed therewith, cures the itch, scabs, and leprosy.

KALI

It is called also glass-wort and salt-wort; there are four kinds of kali described by Parkinson, *viz.* 1. *Kali majus cochleatum*, great glass-wort with snail-like seed. 2. *Kali minus album*, small glass-wort. 3. *Kali Ægyptiacum*, glass-wort of Egypt. And 4. *Kali geniculatum*, *sive salicornia*, jointed glass-wort. I shall only describe the last.

This jointed kali or glass-wort, grows up usually but with one upright, round, thick, and almost transparent, stalk, a foot high or more; thick set, and full of joints or knots, without any leaves at all, but shooting forth joints one out of another, with short cods at the heads of them, and such-like smaller branches on each side, and they are divided into other smaller ones; it is thought to bear neither flower nor seed; the root is small, long, and thready. Some other kinds there are differing somewhat in the form of the joints, and one kind wholly reddish, and differing from the other in nothing else.

The first and third are absolute strangers in our countries, but grow in Syria, Egypt, Italy, and Spain; the second grows, not only in those countries, but in colder climates, upon many places of our own coasts, especially of the West Country. The last generally grows in all countries, in many places of our sea-coast, where the salt-water overflows.

TIME They all flourish in the summer, and those that perish give their seed in August, or later; the last abides all the winter.

GOVERNMENT AND VIRTUES Kali, or glass-wort, all the sorts thereof are under the dominion of Mars; they are all of a cleansing quality, without any great or manifest heat; the powder of any of them, or the juice, which is much better, taken in drink, purges downwards phlegmatic, waterish, and adust, melancholy humours, and therefore is very effectual for the dropsy, to provoke urine, and expel the dead child. It opens stoppings of the liver and spleen, and wastes the hardness thereof; but it must be used with discretion, as a great quantity is dangerous, hurtful, and deadly.

The ashes are very sharp and biting like a caustic, and the lye that is made thereof is so strong, that it will fetch off the skin from the hands or any part of the body, but may be mixed with other more moderate medicines to take away scabs, leprosy, and to cleanse the skin: the powder of stones, and the ashes hereof, being melted, is the matter whereof glass is made, which, when it glows in the furnace, casts up a fat matter on the top, and when it is cold is fat and brittle, and is called sandiver.

KIDNEY-WORT

Called also wall-pennyroyal, and wall-pennywort.

DESCRIPTION It has many thick, flat, and round, leaves, growing from the root, every one having a long footstalk fastened underneath about the middle of it, a little unevenly waved sometimes about the edges, of a pale green colour, and hollow on the upper side, like a saucer. From among these rise one or more tender, hollow, smooth stalks, about half a foot high, bearing thereon two or three small leaves, not round like those below, but somewhat long, and divided on the edges; the tops are sometimes divided into long branches, bearing a number of flowers, set round about a long spike, one above another; they are hollow and shaped like a small bell, and of a whitish-green colour; these are followed by small heads containing very small brownish seed, which, falling on the ground, springs up in great plenty before the winter, if it happens to fall on a moist soil. The root is round and smooth, greyish without and white within, having small fibres at the head of the root and bottom of the stalk.

PLACE It grows in abundance in many parts of this kingdom, particularly the west, upon stone and mud walls, upon rocks and stony ground, at the foot and on trunks of rotten trees.

TIME It usually flowers in the beginning of May, and the seed, ripening quickly after, sheds itself. About the end of the same month the leaves and stalks begin to wither, and remain in that state till September, when the leaves spring up again, and abide green all the winter.

GOVERNMENT AND VIRTUES Venus claims this herb under Libra. The juice or distilled water, being drunk, is very effectual for all inflammations and unnatural heats; also to cool a fainting stomach, a hot liver, or heat in the bowels. The bruised herb or the distilled water thereof, applied to pimples, or other inflammations proceeding from heat, quickly heals the same; it likewise eases the pains of the kidneys occasioned by the fretting of the stone, provokes urine, is available for the dropsy, helps to break the stone, cools inflamed parts, eases the pains of the bowels, and stops the bloody flux. It is a singular remedy for the painful piles, or hæmorrhoidal veins, by bathing the affected parts with the juice thereof, or using it as an ointment; and is effectual in easing pains of the hot gout, the sciatica, and the inflammations and swellings of the scrotum; it cures the kernels or knots in the neck or throat, called the king's evil; it heals kibes and chilblains by washing them with the juice, or anointing them with an ointment made thereof. It is also used in green wounds, to stay the blood and heal them.

KNAP-WEED

DESCRIPTION   The common sort of knap-weed has many long and somewhat broad dark-green leaves, rising from the root, deeply dented about the edges, and sometimes a little rent or torn on both sides in two or three places, and somewhat hairy; from among these grows up a strong round stalk, four or five feet high, which is divided into many branches; at the tops of these stand large green scaly heads, bearing in the middle many dark purplish-red thrums or threads: these are succeeded by black seed, wrapped in down, somewhat like those of the thistle, but smaller. The root is white, hard, and woody, with many fibres annexed thereto; it perishes not, but lives during the winter, shooting forth fresh leaves every spring.

PLACE It grows frequently in fields and meadows, but chiefly in borders and hedges, and may be found on waste grounds.

TIME   It is generally in blossom about June and July, and the seed is ripe shortly after.

GOVERNMENT AND VIRTUES Saturn claims dominion over this herb. It helps to stay fluxes, bleeding at the nose and mouth, or other outward parts, and closes broken blood-vessels; it is good for those who are bruised by a fall, blow, or otherwise; it is very profitable for ruptures, by drinking the decoction of the herbage and root in wine, and applying the same outwardly to the place; it is exceeding good for sores; and is an admirable remedy for a sore throat, swelling of the uvula and jaw, and all green wounds.

KNOT-GRASS

PLACE It grows in almost every part of this kingdom, by the highway-sides, by the footpaths in fields, and by the sides of old walls.

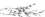

TIME It grows up late in the spring, and remains green till the winter, when all the branches perish.

GOVERNMENT AND VIRTUES Saturn appears to have dominion over this herb, though many are of the opinion it is influenced by the Sun. The juice of the common kind of knot-grass is very effectual to stay bleeding at the mouth and nose, by drinking it in steeled or red wine for the one, or applied to the forehead or squirted up the nostrils for the other. It is no less effectual to stay fluxes of blood and humours, women's menses, and running of the reins. It helps the difficulty in passing urine, and allays the heat proceeding therefrom; and, by taking a drachm of the powder of the herb in wine, for several days together, it powerfully expels the gravel or stone from the kidneys and bladder. Being boiled in wine and drunk, it stays all defluxions of rheumatic humours upon the stomach, and eases the inward pains that proceed from the heat, sharpness, and corruption, of blood, and choler. The distilled water of this herb taken by itself, or with the powder of the plant or seed, will equally answer all the aforesaid purposes, and is held in high estimation for its admirable efficacy in cooling all manner of inflammations, breakings-out, hot swellings and imposthumes, and all kinds of fresh and green wounds, and quickly healing them, being washed therewith. The juice is very good for broken joints and ruptures.

LADIES' MANTLE

DESCRIPTION it has many leaves rising from the root standing upon long hairy footstalks, being almost round, but a little cut in on the edges, into eight or ten parts, more or less, making it seem like a star with so many corners and points, and dented round about, of a light green colour, somewhat hard in handling, as if it were folded or plaited at first, and then crumpled in divers places, and a little hairy, as the stalk is also, which rises up among them to the height of two or three feet, with such-like leaves thereon, but smaller; and, being weak, is not able to stand upright, but bends down to the ground, divided at the top into two or three small branches, with small and yellowish-green heads, and flowers of a whitish colour breaking out of them, which being past, there comes small yellow seed-like poppy-seed; the root is somewhat long and black, with many strings or fibres.

PLACE It grows naturally in many pastures and woodsides, in Hartfordshire, Wiltshire, and Kent, and other places of this land.

TIME It flowers in May and June, and remains green all the winter.

GOVERNMENT AND VIRTUES Venus claims the herb as her own. Ladies mantle is very proper for those wounds that have inflammation, and is very effectual to stay bleedings, vomitings, fluxes of all sorts in men or women, and bruises by falls or otherwise, and helps ruptures; it is also good for some disorders in women's breasts, causing them to grow less and hard, being both inwardly and outwardly applied. The distilled water, taken for twenty days together, helps conception; and a bath, made of the decoction of the herb, will sometimes prevent miscarriages. It is one of the most useful wound-herbs, and therefore highly prized and praised by the Germans, who, in all wounds, inward and outward, drink the decoction thereof, and wash the wounds therewith. It quickly heals green wounds, not suffering any corruption to remain behind.

LADIES' SMOCK, OR CUCKOO-FLOWER

DESCRIPTION The root is composed of many small white threads, from tender dark-green leaves, set one against another, upon a middle rib, the greatest being at the ends, amongst which rise up divers tender, weak, round, green, stalks, somewhat streaked, with longer and smaller leaves upon them; on the tops of which stand flowers, almost like stock gilliflowers, but rounder, and not so long, of a blushing white colour: the seed is reddish, and grows in small pouches, being of a sharp biting taste, and so is the herb.

PLACE They grow in moist places and near to brook sides.

TIME They flower in April or May, and the lower leaves continue green all the year.

GOVERNMENT AND VIRTUES They are under the dominion of the Moon, and very little inferior to water-cresses in all their operations: they are very good for the scurvy: they provoke urine and break the stone, and excellently warm a cold and weak stomach, restoring lost appetite and helping digestion.

LARCH-TREE, AND ITS AGARIC

DESCRIPTION AND NAMES It grows about Italy, and also in Asia. It is called *larix* both in Greek and Latin; and also agaricum, and agaricus; the agaric is an excrescence, or kind of mushroom, that grows on this tree, being within white, soft, and spongy, like a mushroom. The agaric is hot in the first degree, and dry in the second; it has an attenuating cleansing quality, and purges obstructions of the entrails by stool; it purges phlegm, choler, and melancholy, and cleanses the breast, lungs, liver, and reins; provokes urine and the terms; helps pains of the joints, and causes a good colour.

It is not good to be taken alone, without corrigents; therefore the syrup of roses, solutive with agaric, is good to be taken; it cures the yellow jaundice, and is exceeding good for agues coming of thick humours, for which they take pills of hiera with agaric; it may be given with oxymel for agues of all sorts, and gripings of the belly; it is good against shortness of breath, the phthisic, and consumption.

LAVENDER

TIME It flowers about the end of June and the beginning of July.

GOVERNMENT AND VIRTUES Mercury owns the herb, and it carries its effects very potently. Lavender is of special use for pains of the head and brain that proceed of a cold cause, as the apoplexy, falling sickness, the drowsy or sluggish malady, cramps, convulsions, palsies, and often faintings. It strengthens the stomach, and frees the liver and spleen from obstructions, provokes women's menses, and expels the dead child and after-birth. The flowers of lavender steeped in wine are efficacious in obstructions of urine, or for those troubled with the wind or cholic, if the places be bathed therewith. A decoction made with the flowers of lavender, horehound, fennel, and asparagus roots, and a little cinnamon, is used to help the falling-sickness and giddiness of the brain: to gargle the mouth with the decoction thereof is good for the tooth-ache. Two spoonfuls of the distilled water of the flowers taken, help them that have lost their voice; as also the tremblings and passions of the heart, and faintings and swoonings, not only being drunk, but applied to the temples or nostrils; but it is not safe to use it where the body is replete with blood and humours, because of the hot and subtile spirits wherewith it is possessed. The chemical oil drawn from lavender, usually called oil of spike, is of so fierce and piercing a spirit, that it is cautiously to be used, some few drops being sufficient to be given with other things, either inwardly or outwardly.

LAVENDER COTTON

It being a common garden herb, I shall forbear the description; only take notice that it flowers in June and July.

GOVERNMENT AND VIRTUES It is under the dominion of Mercury. It resists poison, putrefaction, and helps the bitings of venomous beasts: a drachm of the powder of the dried leaves, taken every morning fasting, in any convenient vehicle, stops the running of the reins in men, and whites in women: the seed being beaten into powder, and taken as wormseed, kills worms: the like does the herb itself, being boiled in milk, and the milk drunk: scabs and itch are cured by bathing with a decoction of it.

LEMON-TREE, OR LEMONS

There are several sorts of lemons: some great, others small; some having very thick and rugged peels, and some very smooth; some are of a wild juice, others sharp, and some very tart and crabbed; which alterations may be made both by the soil and place where they grow or are planted.

1. The ordinary lemon tree is called *malus limonia acida vulgaris*.

2. *Malus limonia acida*, cortice tenui; the thin-rinded sour lemon.

3. *Malus limonia acida*, fructa rolunda; the sour round lemon.

4. *Malus limonia dulcis major*, the greater sweet lemon.

5. *Malus limonia dulcis minor*, the smaller sweet lemon, or civil lemon.

6. *Malus limonia silvestris minima*; the least wild lemon-tree.

DESCRIPTION

1. The ordinary lemon-tree grows great and high, with great arms and slender branches, long greenish thorns; the leaves are long like unto bay leaves, both dented about the edges, and full of holes; the flowers are white and sweet; the fruit long and round, of a pale yellow colour; and the rind rugged and uneven.

2. All the difference between this and the former is this, that the other is bigger. The rind of this second is of a fine pale yellow colour, smoother than the first-mentioned, and thinner; is full of a pleasant sharp juice, with seeds amongst it, as the other also has.

3. The tree that bears the round lemons is in all things like the last; only in this, that it has few or no thorns upon it; and the fruit is like it, having a thin rind, but is somewhat-rounder, with a small crown at the head.

4. The greater sweet lemon is greater than any of the former described lemons; the rind is more smooth and yellow; and the juice more sweet and pleasant.

5. The civil lemon is of the same size as the thin-rinded sour lemon, and so like, that it is hard, by the outside, to know one from the other; but this has a little deeper-coloured rind, and the juice of a sweet pleasant taste, with a little sharpness.

6. The least wild lemon grows wild in Syria and Egypt, and bears very small fruit, no bigger than a pigeon's egg.

PLACE These lemons are brought from Spain and several of their islands.

TIME They are evergreens, and never without blossoms, green and ripe fruit, throughout the year.

GOVERNMENT AND VIRTUES The lemons are solar, yet of different parts and contrary effects; they are of good use to resist poison, venom, or infection; an ounce and an half of the juice of unripe lemons, drunk in wine, cleanses the kidneys of the stone and gravel.

An antidote against any malignant or contagious disease, is thus prepared: Take four ounces of the pure juice of lemons, steep therein an angle of gold, or the weight thereof in leaf-gold, the space of twenty-four hours; then take out the gold, or draw the juice clear from it, and give some of it in a draught of wine, with a little of the powder of angelica root, unto any infected with the plague, and, if there be any hopes of recovery, it will help them. The juice of sweet lemons is neither so cooling nor operative as the other. The distilled water, drawn from the inner pulp or white substance of the lemons, clears the skin and face from freckles and spots, provokes urine, and expels the stone, by being drunk. The juice of lemons is good for seamen, and others at sea, to put into their beverage, to prevent the scurvy, to which people are much subjected in long voyages; it is likewise very properly used to quench thirst in warm climates.

An excellent remedy for scab and itch: Take a lemon, and cut it through the middle, after putting thereon some powder of brimstone, roast it, either against the fire, or under some embers, as you would do a warden-pear, and therewith rub the parts troubled with itch or scabs.

LENTILES

They are called *lens*, and *lenticula*, in Latin. In some countries of England, where they sow them for meat for their cattle, they call them tills.

There are three sorts. 1. *Lens major*, the greater lentil. 2. *Lens minor*, the smaller lentil. And, 3, *Lens maculata*, the spotted lentil.

DESCRIPTION

1. The greater lentil grows two feet long, with many hard, yet slender and weak, branches, from whence, at several places, shoot forth long stalks of small winged leaves, many on each side of a middle rib, which middle rib ends in a small clasper; between the leaves and the stalks come the flowers, which are small, of a sad reddish colour inclined to purple, almost like the flowers of vetches; standing, for the most part, two at the end of a long foot-stalk; after the flowers are gone, there succeed small, short, flat, pods, wherein is flat, round, smooth, seed, of a pale yellowish ash-colour; the root is fibrous, and dies every winter.
2. The smaller lentil differs from the former only in this, that the stalks, leaves, and seed, are less; the flowers more pale, and the seeds whiter.

The third differs not much from the last; but the seed is spotted with black.

GOVERNMENT AND VIRTUES They are under the dominion of
Saturn; of a mean temperature between heat and cold, and dry in the second

degree. According to Galen, they are somewhat astringent, and bind the body, especially the outward skin. It is of contrary qualities, for the decoction thereof does not bind but loosen the body; therefore, those who would have it bind must throw away the first water and use the second, which stops the lask, and strengthens the stomach and inward parts.

LETTUCE

GOVERNMENT AND VIRTUES The Moon owns it. The juice of lettuce mixed or boiled with oil of roses, and applied to the forehead and temples, procures sleep, and eases the head-ache proceeding from a hot cause; being boiled and eaten, it helps to loosen the belly: it helps digestion, quenches thirst, increases milk in nurses, eases griping pains of the stomach or bowels that come of choler.

It abates bodily lust, being outwardly applied with a little camphire: applied in the same manner to the region of the heart, liver, or reins, or by bathing the said place with the juice or distilled water, wherein some white sanders or red roses are put also, it not only represses the heat and inflammation therein, but comforts and strengthens those parts, and also tempers the heat of urine. Galen advises old men to use it with spices, and, where spices are wanting, to add mint, rocket, and such-like hot herbs, or else citron, lemon, or orange, seeds, to abate the cold of one and heat of the other. The seed and distilled water of the lettuce work the like effects in all things: but the use of lettuce is chiefly forbidden to those that are short-winded, or have any imperfection in their lungs, or spit blood.

LILY OF THE VALLEY

Called also conval-lily, may-lily, and lily constancy.

DESCRIPTION The root is small, and creeps far in the ground, as grass roots do; the leaves are many; amongst which rises up a stalk half a foot high, with many white flowers like little bells, with turned edges, of a strong though pleasing smell; the berries are red, and not much unlike those of asparagus.

PLACE They grow plentifully upon Hampstead Heath, and in various other places in this kingdom.

TIME They flower in May, and the seed is ripe in September.

TEMPERATURE AND VIRTUES It is under the dominion of Mercury, and therefore without doubt, strengthens the brain, renovates a weak memory,

PLATE 12

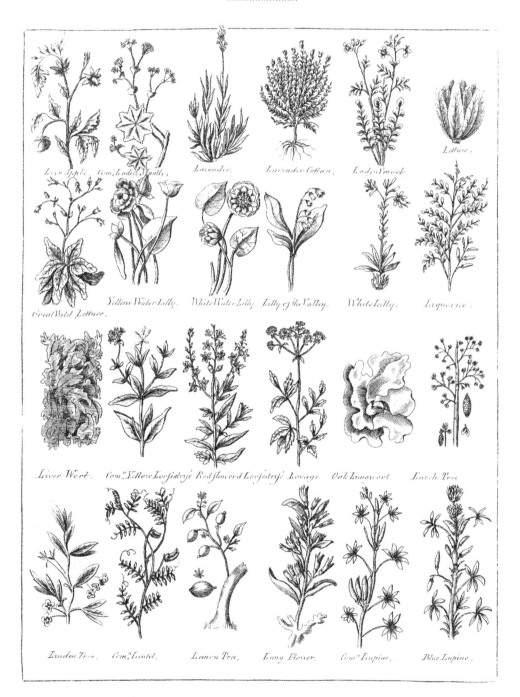

Love Apple. Com: Ladies Mantle. Lavender. Lavender Cotton. Ladys Smock. L. Aloe.

Great Wild Lettuce.

Yellow Water Lilly. White Water Lilly. Lilly of the Valley. White Lilly. Liquorice.

Liver Wort. Com: Yellow Loosestrife Red flower'd Loosestrife Lovage. Oak Lungwort. Larch Tree.

Linden Tree. Com: Lentil. Lemon Tree. Lung Flower. Com: Lupine. Blue Lupine.

and makes it strong again. The distilled water, dropped into the eyes, helps inflammations thereof, as also that infirmity, which they call pin and web: the spirit of the flowers, distilled in wine, helps the palsy.

WATER-LILY

White water-lily

Yellow water-lily

Of this there are two principal noted kinds, *viz.* the white and the yellow.

DESCRIPTION The white lily has very large and thick dark-green leaves lying on the water, sustained by long and thick foot-stalks, that rise from a great, thick, round, and long, tuberous black root, spongy or loose, with many knobs thereon, like eyes, and whitish within, from the midst of which rise other the like thick and great stalks, sustaining one large white flower thereon, green on the outside, but as white as snow within, consisting of divers rows of long and somewhat thick and narrow leaves, smaller and thinner the more inward they be, encompassing a head within, with many yellow threads or thrums in the middle, where, after they are past, stand round poppy-like heads, full of broad, oily, and bitter, seed.

The yellow kind is little different from the former, only it has fewer leaves on the flowers, greater and more shining seed, and a whitish root both within and without: the roots of both being somewhat sweet in taste.

PLACE They are found growing in great pools and standing waters, and sometimes in slow running rivers, and ditches of running water, in sundry places of this land.

TIME They flower most commonly about the end of May, and their seed is ripe in August.

GOVERNMENT AND VIRTUES The herb is under the dominion of the Moon, and therefore cools and moistens like the former. The leaves and flowers of the water-lilies are cold and moist, but the root and seed are cold and dry; the leaves cool all inflammations, and both outward and inward heats of agues, and so do the flowers.

WHITE LILIES

GOVERNMENT AND VIRTUES They are under the dominion of the Moon, and, by antipathy to Mars, expel poison; the juice, being tempered with barley-meal baked, and eaten as ordinary bread, is an excellent cure for the dropsy. An ointment made of the root and hog's-lard is very good for scald heads, and unites the sinews when cut; it has also great virtues in cleansing ulcers; the root, boiled in any convenient decoction, gives speedy delivery to women in travail, and expels the after-birth. The ointment is also extremely good for swellings in the privities and cures burns and scalds.

LINE, OR LINDEN-TREE

Of the line-tree there are accounted two sorts, the male and the female; and of the female also two sorts, the greater and the smaller. It is called in Latin, *tilia*.

DESCRIPTION
1. *Tilia mas*, the male line, grows to be a great tree, with large spreading boughs, but not so much as the female, nor so flexible, but harder and more brittle, and of a thicker bark; the leaves are like unto elder-leaves, but smaller and longer; and on every one, for the most part, grow small bladders full of worms that turn into flies, which, when matured, fly away. This tree seldom bears either flower or fruit; yet, when it does bear, it is round flat husks; many growing close together, each hanging on a long foot-stalk by itself, with a notch or clest at the head or end thereof. The wood hereof is more knotty and yellower than that of the female.

2. *Tilia fœmina major*. The greater female line-tree grows to be a larger tree than the former; is covered with a dark-coloured bark, the next thereunto being very pliable to bend, having some other thin rinds within that; the leaves are fair and broad, with a longer end; dented about the edge; at the end of the branches oftentimes, and at the foot of the leaves, shoot forth long and narrow whitish leaves, along the middle rib whereof springs out a slender long stalk, with divers white flowers thereon; after which follow small berries, where in is contained black round seed; the wood is whitish, smooth, and light.

3. *Tilia fœmina minor*. The smaller linden-tree is like the last in all things, except that it grows smaller in body, leaves, and flowers; the leaves are of a darker green colour, and it bears no fruit after the flowers.

PLACE AND TIME   The greater female kind is planted in many places in this kingdom, and usually flowers in May. The others are seldom to be met with in this island.

GOVERNMENT AND VIRTUES   There is no medicinal use made of the male linden. The female is under the dominion of Venus, of a moderate temperature, and somewhat drying and astringent. The leaves being pounded or bruised, after boiling, and applied to the legs or feet, when swelled with the falling down of humours, does help them; the bark is also effectual.

The flowers of the line-tree and of lily convally distilled together are good against the falling sickness; so likewise is the distilled water of the bark; and is also serviceable against those fretting humours which occasion the bloody flux, and griping in the guts. The water, wherein the inner bark has been steeped till it becomes thick and mucilaginous, and applied with cloths wet therein, helps burnings and scaldings.

LIQUORICE

DESCRIPTION the English liquorice shoots up with several woody stalks, whereon are set, at several distances, many narrow, long, green, leaves, set together on both sides of the stalks, and an odd one at the end, nearly resembling a young ash-tree sprung up from the seed. This by many years continuance in a place without removal, but not else, will bring forth numerous flowers standing together spike-fashion, one above another upon the stalks, in the form of pea-blossoms, but of a very pale blue colour which turn into long, somewhat flat, and smooth, pods, wherein is contained small, round, hard, seed. The root runs down exceeding deep in the ground, with divers other smaller roots and flowers growing with them; they shoot out suckers in every direction, by which means the product is greatly increased. The root is of a brownish colour on the outside, and yellow within.

PLACE It is planted in fields and gardens in divers places of this kingdom, greatly to the profit of the cultivators.

GOVERNMENT AND VIRTUES It is under the dominion of Mercury. Liquorice boiled in clear water, with some maiden-hair and figs, makes a good drink for such as are troubled with a dry cough, hoarseness, wheezing, or shortness of breath, and for all complaints of the breast and lungs, phthisic, or consumptions, caused by the distillation of salt humours on them. It is also good in all pains of the reins, the difficulty in passing urine, and heat of urine. The juice of liquorice is as effectual in all the diseases of the breast and lungs, the reins and bladder, as the decoction.

LIVER-WORT

DESCRIPTION the common liver-wort grows close, and spreads much upon the ground, in moist and shadowy places, with numerous green leaves sticking flat one to another, very unevenly cut in on the edges, and crumpled, from among which arise small slender stalks, an inch or two high at most, bearing small flowers at the tops, somewhat like stars.

GOVERNMENT AND VIRTUES It is under the command of Jupiter, and under the sign Cancer. It is a singular good herb for all diseases of the liver, both to cool and cleanse it, and helps inflammations in any part; it is likewise serviceable in the yellow jaundice; being bruised and boiled in beer, and drunk, it cools the heat of the liver and kidneys, and helps the running of the reins in men and the whites in women; it is a singular remedy to stay the spreading of tetters, ringworms, and other sores and scabs, and is excellent for those whose livers are corrupted by surfeits, which cause their bodies to break out, for it fortifies the liver exceedingly, and makes it impregnable.

LOOSE-STRIFE, OR WILLOW HERB

DESCRIPTION the common yellow loose-strife grows to the height of four or five feet, with great round stalks a little crested, diversely branched, from the middle to the tops, into great and long branches, on all of which, at the joints, there grow long and narrow leaves, but broader below, and usually two at a joint, yet sometimes three or four, somewhat like willow leaves, smooth on the edges; from the upper joints of the branches, and at the tops of them also, stand many yellow flowers of five leaves a piece, with divers yellow threads in the middle, which turn into small round heads, containing small cornered seeds. The root creeps under ground, almost like couch-grass, but greater, and shoots up every spring, with brownish heads, which afterwards grow up into two stalks; it has no scent nor taste, but only astringent.

PLACE It grows in most parts of the kingdom, in moist meadows, and by the sides of water.

TIME It flowers from June to August.

GOVERNMENT AND VIRTUES This herb is good for all manner of bleeding at the mouth or nose, or wounds; all fluxes of the belly, as well as the bloody flux, given either to drink or administered as a clyster; it stays also the abundance of women's menses. It is a singular good herb for green wounds, to stay the bleeding, and quickly closes together the lips of the wound, if the herb be bruised, and the juice only applied. It is often used in gargles for sore mouths, as also for the secret parts. The smoke hereof, on its being burned, drives away flies and gnats, which are used in the night-time to infest the habitations of people dwelling near marshes, and in the fenny countries.

LOOSE-STRIFE, WITH SPIKED HEADS
OF FLOWERS

DESCRIPTION This grows with many woody square stalks, full of joints, about three feet high at least, at every one whereof are two long leaves, shorter, narrower, and of a darker-green colour, than the former, and somewhat brownish. The stalks are branched into many long stems of spiked flowers, half a foot long, growing in bundles one above another, out of small husks very like the spiked heads of lavender, each of which flowers has five round-pointed leaves of a purple-violet colour, or somewhat inclining to redness, in which husks stand small round heads after the flowers are fallen wherein is contained small seed; the root creeps under ground like unto the yellow, but is greater than it; and so are the heads of the leaves when they first appear out of the ground, and more brown than the other.

PLACE It grows usually by rivers, and ditch-sides in wet grounds, as about the ditches at and near Lambeth, and in many other parts of the kingdom.

TIME It flowers in the months of June and July.

GOVERNMENT AND VIRTUES The herb is an herb of the Moon, and under the sign Cancer; it is an excellent preservative of the sight when well; nor is there a better cure for sore eyes than eye-bright taken inwardly, and this used outwardly; it is cold in quality. This herb clears the eyes of dust or any thing which may have got into them, and preserves the sight; it is also a good remedy for wounds and thrusts, being made into an ointment in the following manner: To every ounce of the water add two drachms of May butter without salt, and of sugar and bee's wax the same quantity of each, which must boil gently all together; when thus brought to a proper consistence, let tents be dipped in the ointment after it is cold, and put into the wounds, and the place covered with a linen cloth doubled, on which the ointment may be thinly spread. It likewise cleanses and heals ulcers and sores, by washing them with the water, and laying on them a green leaf or two in the summer, or dry leaves in the winter. This water, when warmed, and used as a gargle, or even drunk sometimes, cures the quinsey, or king's evil in the throat..

LOVAGE

DESCRIPTION it has many long and great stalks, with large winged leaves, divided into many parts like smallage, but much larger and greater, every leaf being cut about the edges, broadest forwards, and smallest at the stalk, of a green colour, smooth and shining: from among which rise up sundry strong hollow green stalks, five or six feet, and sometimes seven or eight feet, high, full of joints, but smaller leaves set on them than grow below; and with them, toward the tops, come forth long branches, bearing at their tops large umbles of yellow flowers, and after them flat brownish seed. The root grows thick, great, and deep, spreading much, and enduring long, of a brownish colour on the outside, and whitish within. The whole plant, and every individual part of it, smells strong and aromatically, and is of an hot, sharp, biting, taste.

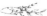

PLACE It is usually planted in gardens, where, if it be suffered, it grows huge and great.

TIME It flowers in the end of July, and seeds in August.

GOVERNMENT AND VIRTUES It is an herb of the Sun, under the sign Taurus. If Saturn offend the throat, this is your cure. It opens, cuts, and digests humours, and mightily provokes women's menses and urine; half a drachm at a time of the dried root in powder, taken in wine, does wonderfully warm a cold stomach, helping digestion, and consuming all raw and superfluous moisture therein; eases all inward gripings and pains, dissolves wind, and resists poison and infection. To drink the decoction of this herb is a well-known remedy for any sort of ague, and greatly helps the pains and torments of the body and bowels occasioned by cold. The seed is effectual to all the purposes aforesaid, except the last, and works more powerfully. The distilled water from the herb helps the quinsey in the throat, if the mouth and throat be gargled and washed therewith; and relieves the pleurisy being drunk three or four times. When dropped into the eyes, it takes away the redness or dimness of them; it also takes away spots or freckles in the face.

LOVE-APPLE

It is also called golden apple, apple of love, and in Latin *poma amoris*.

DESCRIPTION It grows into a tree of a reasonable height, with large dented leaves, cut in upon the edges, and of a pale green colour. The blossoms are large and white, which falling, the fruit follows.

PLACE The tree is a native of Ethiopia; but it is planted in the gardens or nurseries of many of the curious in this kingdom.

TIME They blossom in April and May, and the fruit is ripe in August and September.

GOVERNMENT AND VIRTUES The apples of love are under Venus; yet are they cold and moist in an extreme degree. They are olygotrophic and cacochymic; yet in hot countries, they are eaten as sauce, boiled with pepper, salt, and oil. The juice, boiled in axungia to a salve, heals all inflammations and burnings; and the leaves boiled with oil-olive, till crisped, then strained, and afterwards boiled with wax, rosin, and a little turpentine, to a salve, are an infallible remedy for sores and ulcers of the privities, or for wounds and ulcers in other parts of the body, coming of heat, or viscous humours of the blood.

LUNG-FLOWER

There are several sorts of these plants, generally called autumn gentians.

DESCRIPTION

1. The great autumn gentian rises up, according to the richness of the ground, higher or lower; sometimes two feet high, at others not above one foot; sometimes many, and others fewer, stalks; of a brownish-green colour, with many long and narrow dark-green leaves, set by couples upon them, up to the tops, which seldom branch forth, but bear every one a large hollow flower, in most of them of a deep bluish-purple colour, but in some a little paler, ending in five points. The roots are numerous, small, and long, growing deep into the ground, and abiding all the winter.

2. *Gentianella autumnalis fimbriato flore*; autumn gentian of Naples. This creeps up like couch grass, from a long, yellowish, small, root, shooting forth a few long and narrow leaves, like those of flax, but shorter; but those that grow up to the middle of the stalk are larger, and smaller again from the middle to the top, two set at every joint all along, and striped from every one of the joints, on both sides, to the top of the stalk, which is green, and about a foot high; at the top comes a purplish-green husk, which has four large-pointed leaves that enclose the flower, which is long and writhed before it blows, and of a pale blue colour; but, when it is blown open, it is of a deeper-blue colour, having four leaves somewhat long, and as it were purfled about the edges, with a little hairiness; there is also a small leaf at the bottom of each flower, with a few yellow threads in the middle, standing about a head, which grows to be the seed-vessel, forked into two parts at the head, being greater there than below, and contains in it very small black seed when it is ripe.

3. Autumn gentian, with small centaury leaves, called in Latin *Gentianella autumnalis, centaurea minoris folio*. This rises up with sundry stalks scarce a foot high, parted into many small branches, whereon do stand two leaves together, very like those of the smaller centaury, not so long as either of the former, but a little broader and of a lighter green colour; at the tops of the stalks and branches grow divers blue flowers, set in small long husks half-way rising above the tops of them; the seed is small, and grows in long horned vessels; the root is small and fibrous.

4. There is another sort with small centaury-like flowers, which is more spreading; is small, but has larger leaves and flowers than centaury; of the same colour as the flowers of centaury, yet having more, and lasts longer. The root, however, perishes in winter.

5. Another smaller gentian, with centaury leaves, is very like the last, but smaller, and the stalks much lower, not being above three inches high, having many small branches, whereon are large blue flowers; the seed and vessels, when they are ripe, are like unto the last; the root is also small; but has many more fibres than the others.

PLACE The first is found growing in many parts of Germany, and many other foreign countries; in divers places of this kingdom, *viz.* at Gravesend; near Greenhithe; in a chalk-pit not far from Dartford; and at Cobham; all in Kent: it grows both in wet and dry grounds. The second, upon the hills in Naples, as related by Columna. The third in divers places in Kent, as about Southfleet, and Longfield; also in Bedfordshire; and near Old Verulam in Hartfordshire. The rest are strangers here.

TIME These flower not until August, and thence have the name of autumn gentian.

GOVERNMENT AND VIRTUES These lung-flowers, or autumn gentian, are also under the dominion of Mars, as the gentian or self-wort is; and much of the same temperature in respect to heat and driness; and may be used both inwardly and outwardly as effectually as gentian.

The roots of these gentians, being made into fine powder, and taken in wine, open all obstructions of the liver. It eases pains in the stomach, and helps such as cannot keep or relish their meat, or have lost their appetite. It helps such as are lame in their joints; is effectual for pains, stitches, and prickings, in the sides. The root is likewise held to be good against agues, when taken in any other liquor but wine; the distilled water of the herb is equally useful.

LUNG-WORT

DESCRIPTION This is a kind of moss that grows on sundry sorts of trees, especially oak and beech; with broad, greyish, tough, leaves, diversely folded, crumpled, and gashed in on the edges, and sometimes spotted also with many small spots on the upper side; it was never seen to bear any stalk, or flower at any time.

GOVERNMENT AND VIRTUES Jupiter seems to own this herb, which is greatly used by physicians to help the diseases of the lungs, and for coughs, wheezings, and shortness of breath, which it cures both in man and beast; it is very successfully used in lotions that are taken to stay the moist humours that flow to ulcers, which hinder their healing; as also to wash all other ulcers in the privy parts of man or woman.

LUPINES

There are several kinds of lupines, as, the great white lupine, called *lupinus fativus albus*; the spotted white lupine, called *lupinus alter albus*; and the smallest blue lupine, called *lupinus minimus cœruleus*.

Common lupine

Blue lupine

DESCRIPTION

1. The great white lupine rises up with a strong, upright, round, woolly, stalk, set confusedly with divers soft woolly leaves upon long foot-stalks, each being divided into several parts, narrow, long, and soft, greenish on the upper side, and woolly underneath; the main stalk is divided into two parts, after the flowers are grown from the uppermost joint, and are like unto the great garden bean, but wholly white, without any spot; after the flowers come long, soft, woolly, stalks, containing in them flat white leaves, somewhat yellowish within, of a very bitter taste. The root is long, hard, and fibrous, and perishes every winter.

2. The spotted white lupine differs from the former in the greatness and in the flower, which is spotted with blue on the head of the innermost leaves, and the hollow of the uppermost.

3. The smallest blue lupine is very like the other blue lupine, but smaller, both stalks and leaves; the flowers are blue, and the seed a little spotted.

PLACE They grow naturally wild, but in England only are planted in gardens.

TIME The lupines flower in July and August, and the seed is ripe soon after.

GOVERNMENT AND VIRTUES Lupines are under the dominion of Mars: and have an opening, cleansing, dissolving, and digestive, property; but, if they be steeped in water until they have lost their bitterness, they may be eaten; however, they are very hard to digest, breed gross humours, and pass slowly through the belly, yet do not stop any flux; if they be so steeped, and afterwards dried and taken with vinegar, they provoke appetite. The decoction of lupines, taken with honey, opens obstructions of the liver and spleen, provokes urine and the terms. An ointment of lupines, to beautify and make the face smooth, is made in the following manner: Take the meal of lupines, the gall of a goat or sheep, juice of lemons, and a little alumen saccharinum, and mingle them into the form of a soft ointment.

MADDER

DESCRIPTION Garden-madder shoots forth many very long, weak, four-square, reddish, stalks, trailing on the ground a great way, very rough and hairy, and full of joints, at every one of which come forth divers long and somewhat narrow leaves, standing like a star about the stalks; rough also and hairy, toward the tops whereof come forth many small pale yellow flowers; after which come small round heads, green at first, and reddish afterwards, but black when they are ripe, wherein is contained the seed. The root is not very great, though about a yard long, spreading divers ways, and is of a clear-red colour while it is fresh.

PLACE It is cultivated in gardens or large fields.

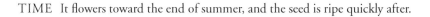

TIME It flowers toward the end of summer, and the seed is ripe quickly after.

GOVERNMENT AND VIRTUES It is an herb of Mars; has an opening quality, but afterwards binds and strengthens; it opens also the obstructions of the spleen, and diminishes the melancholic humour. It is available for the palsy and sciatica; is effectual for inward and outward bruises, and is therefore much used in vulnerary drinks. The root, for all those aforesaid purposes, is to be boiled in wine or water, as the case requires, and some honey or sugar put thereunto afterwards. The seed hereof, taken with vinegar and honey, helps the swelling and hardness of the spleen. The decoction of the leaves and branches is a good fomentation for women to sit over that have not their menses.

MAD-WORT

PLACE It is often sown in gardens. the seed comes from Italy.

TIME It flowers and flourishes in May; the seed is ripe in August.

QUALITIES AND VIRTUES It is dry, digesting, and scouring. It heals wounds inwardly and outwardly, and digests clotted blood.

MAIDEN-HAIR

DESCRIPTION The common maiden-hair does, from a number of black hard fibres, send forth a great many blackish shining brittle stalks, hardly a span long; in many not half so long; on each side set very thick with small round dark green leaves, spotted on the back of them like other ferns.

PLACE It grows much upon old stone walls in the western parts of England; in Wales, in Kent, and in divers other places. It is to be found, in great abundance, by the sides of springs, wells, and on the rocky, moist, and shadowy, places; and is always green.

ORDINARY WHITE MAIDEN-HAIR,
OR WALL-RUE

DESCRIPTION This has very fine pale green stalks, almost as fine as hairs, set confusedly with divers pale green leaves on very short foot-stalks, somewhat similar to the colour of garden-rue, and not much differing in form, but more diversely cut in on the edges, and thicker; smooth on the upper part, and spotted finely underneath.

PLACE It grows in many parts of the kingdom; at Dartford, and the bridge of Ashford, both in Kent; at Beaconsfield, in Buckinghamshire; on Framlingham Castle, in Suffolk; on the church walls at Mayfield, in Sussex; in Somersetshire; and divers other parts. It is green in winter as well as summer.

GOVERNMENT AND VIRTUES Both this and the former are under the dominion of Mercury. The decoction of the herb maiden-hair, being drunk, relieves those that are troubled with a cough, shortness of breath, the yellow jaundice, diseases of the spleen, stoppage of urine, and helps exceedingly to break the stone in the kidneys (in all which cases the wall-rue is also very effectual). It provokes women's menses, and stays both bleedings and fluxes of the stomach and belly, especially when the herb is dry; but, when green, it opens the body, voids choler and phlegm from the stomach and liver; it cleanses the lungs, and by rectifying the blood causes a good colour to the whole body. The herb, boiled in oil of camomile, dissolves knots, allays swellings, and dries up moist ulcers. The lye made thereof stays the falling or shedding of the hair, and causes it to grow thick, fair, and well-coloured for which purpose some boil it in wine, putting some smallage-seed thereto, and afterwards some oil. The wall-rue is as effectual as maiden-hair in all diseases of the head.

GOLDEN MAIDEN-HAIR

To the two former this may be added, which, possessing the same virtues, it is therefore needless to repeat them.

DESCRIPTION It has many small brownish-red hairs, to make up the form of leaves, growing about the ground from the root; and in the middle of them, in summer, rise small stalks of the same colour, set with very fine yellowish-green hairs on them, and bearing a small gold-yellow head, smaller than a wheat corn, standing in a great husk. The root is very small and thready.

PLACE It grows on bogs and marshy grounds, and also on dry shadowy places; at Hampstead Heath, and elsewhere.

MALLOWS AND MARSH-MALLOWS

Common mallow

Common mallows are generally so well known that they need no description.

The common marsh-mallows have divers soft, hoary, white, stalks, rising to the height of three or four feet, spreading forth many branches, the leaves, whereof are soft and hairy, somewhat smaller than the other mallow leaves, but longer pointed, cut (for the most part) into some few divisions, but deep. The flowers are many, but smaller also than the other mallows, and white, or tending

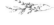

Marsh-mallow

to a blush-colour; after which come such-like round cases and seed as in the other mallows. The roots are many and long, shooting from one head, of the bigness of a thumb or finger, very pliant, tough and bending, like liquorice, of a whitish-yellow colour on the outside, and more white within, full of a slimy juice, which being laid in water, will render it as thick as jelly.

PLACE The common mallows grow in every county in the kingdom. The common marsh-mallows grow in most of the salt marshes from Woolwich down to the sea, both on the Kentish and Essex shores, and in many other places.

TIME They are in flower all the summer months, and continue till winter.

GOVERNMENT AND VIRTUES Venus owns them both. The leaves of either of the sorts before specified, and the roots also, boiled in wine or water, or broth with parsley or fennel roots, do help to open the body, and are convenient in hot agues, or other distempers of the body; if the leaves, so boiled, be applied warm to the belly, it not only voids hot choleric humours, but eases the pains and torments of the belly coming thereby; and are therefore used in all clysters conducing to those purposes. The same medicine, when used by nurses, procures them store of milk. The decoction of the seed of any of the common mallows, made in milk or wine, does exceedingly help excoriations, the phthisic, pleurisy, and other diseases of the chest and lungs that proceed from hot causes, if continued to be taken for any length of time. The leaves and root have the same effects. The juice drunk in wine, or the decoction of them therein, helps women to more speedy and easy delivery. Pliny says, that whoever takes a spoonful of any of the mallows shall that day be free from all diseases whatsoever, and that it is a good specific for the falling-sickness. The syrup also, and conserve made of the flowers, are very effectual for the same diseases, and to open the body when costive. The leaves, bruised and laid to the eyes with a little honey, takes away the impostumation of them. The leaves bruised or rubbed upon any place stung with bees, wasps, or the like, presently takes away the pains, redness, and swellings, that arise therefrom. A poultice made of the leaves, boiled and bruised, to which is added some bean or barley-flour, and oil of roses, is an especial remedy against all hard tumours, inflammations, or imposthumes; also, against the hardness of the liver or spleen, on being applied to the affected places. The juice of mallows, boiled in old oil, takes away all roughness of the skin, as also the scurf, dandruff, or dry scabs, on the head, or other parts, if anointed therewith, or washed with the decoction; and preserves the hair from falling off. It is also effectual against scaldings and burnings. The flowers boiled in oil or water (as every one is disposed), with a little honey and alum put thereto, is an excellent gargle to wash, cleanse, and heal, any sore mouth or throat, in a short space. If the feet be bathed or washed with the decoction of the leaves, roots, and flowers, it helps much the defluxions of rheum from the head. If the head be washed therewith, it prevents baldness. The green leaves (says Pliny) beaten with nitre and applied to the part, draw out thorns or pricks in the flesh; and, in short, there is no wound, external or internal, for which this is not a sovereign remedy.

The marsh-mallows are most effectual in all the diseases before mentioned. The leaves are likewise used to loosen the belly gently, and in decoctions for clysters to ease all pains of the body, opening the straight passages, and making them slippery, whereby the stone may descend the more easily, and without pain. Hippocrates used to give the decoction of the root, or the juice thereof, to drink, to those that were wounded and ready to faint through loss of blood; and applied the same, mixed with honey and rosin, to the wounds; as also the roots boiled in wine to those that had received any hurt by bruises, falls, or blows; or had any bone or member out of joint, or any swelling, pain, or ache, in the muscles, sinews, or arteries. The mucilage of the roots, and of linseed and fenugreek put together, is much used in poultices, ointments, and plasters to mollify and digest all hard swellings and the inflammation of them, and to ease pains in any part of the body. The seed, either green or dry, mixed with vinegar, cleanses the skin from morphew, and all other discolourings, being bathed therewith in the Sun.

MANDRAKE

The mandrake is male and female.

PLACE It grows in hot regions; woods, mountains, and gardens.

TIME It springs in March, flowers in April; the fruit is ripe in August.

QUALITIES AND VIRTUES It is of a cold nature. The root is phlegmatic, and may be eaten with pepper and hot pices. The apples are cold and moist; the bark of the root cold and dry, and the juice is good in all cooling ointments. The dried juice of the root, taken in a small quantity, purges phlegm and melancholy. In collyriums, it heals pains of the eyes. A suppository made of the juice, put into the fundament, causes sleep. Infused in wine, and drunk, it causes sleep, and heals pains; the apples smelt to, or the juice taken in a small quantity, also cause sleep. The seed and fruit do cleanse the womb; the leaves heal knots in the flesh, and the roots heal Saint Anthony's fire, &c. and, boiled with ivy, mollify the same. The oil of mandrakes, is very cold; yet it may be anointed upon the temples and noses of those that have a phrenzy. Also, it heals vehement pains of the head, and the tooth-ache, when applied to the cheeks and jaws, and causes sleep.

MAPLE-TREE

GOVERNMENT AND VIRTUES it is under the dominion of Jupiter. The decoction either of the leaves or bark greatly strengthens the liver; it is exceeding good to open obstructions both of the liver and spleen; and eases pains of the sides proceeding from thence.

MARIGOLDS

TIME They flower all the summer long, and sometimes in winter, if it be mild.

GOVERNMENT AND VIRTUES It is an herb of the Sun, and under Leo. They strengthen the heart exceedingly, are very expulsive, and little less effectual, in the small-pox and measles, than saffron. The juice of marigold leaves mixed with vinegar, by bathing any hot swelling therewith, instantly gives ease, and assuages the pain. The flowers, either green or dried, are much used in possets, broths, and drinks, being comfortable to the heart and spirits.

SWEET MARJORAM

Sweet marjoram is so well known, being an inhabitant in every garden, that it is needless to write any description either of this, the winter sweet marjoram, or pot-marjoram.

PLACE They grow commonly in gardens, though there are some sorts to be found growing wild, on the borders of corn-fields and pastures in various parts of the kingdom; yet it would be surperfluous to detail them, those produced in gardens being most useful.

TIME They flower in the end of summer.

GOVERNMENT AND VIRTUES It is an herb of Mercury, under Aries, and is therefore an excellent remedy for the brain, and other parts of the body and mind under the dominion of the same planet. The common sweet marjoram is warming and comfortable in cold diseases of the head, stomach, sinews, and other parts, taken inwardly or outwardly applied. The decoction thereof, being drunk, helps all diseases of the chest which hinder the freeness of breathing, and is also serviceable in obstructions of the liver and spleen. The decoction thereof made with some pellitory of Spain and long pepper, or with a little *acorus* or *origanum*, being drunk, is good for those that are begining to fall into a dropsy, for those who are troubled with a retention of water, and against pains and torments in the belly; it provokes women's menses, if it be used as a pessary. It is of great service when put into those ointments and salves that are made to warm and comfort the outward parts, as the joints and sinews; for swellings also. The powder thereof snuffed up into the nose, provokes sneezing, and thereby purges the brain; when chewed in the mouth it produces much phlegm. The oil extracted from this herb is very warm and comfortable to joints and sinews that are stiff and hard, tending to mollify and supple them. Marjoram is likewise much used in all odoriferous waters, powders, &c.

WILD MARJORAM

Called also *organe*, or *origanum*, bastard marjoram, and grove marjoram.

DESCRIPTION   Wild or field marjoram has a root which creeps much under ground, and continues a long time, sends up sundry brownish, hard, square, stalks, with small dark green leaves, very like those of sweet marjoram, but harder and somewhat broader; at the tops of the stalks stand tusts of flowers, of a deep purplish-red colour; the seed is small, and something blacker than that of sweet marjoram.

PLACE   It grows plentifully on the borders of corn-fields, and in some copses.

TIME   It flowers toward the latter end of summer.

GOVERNMENT AND VIRTUES   This is under the dominion of Mercury. It strengthens the stomach and head much; it restores lost appetite; helps the cough, and consumption of the lungs; it cleanses the body of choler, expels poison, and remedies the infirmities of the spleen; helps the bitings of venomous beasts, and such as have poisoned themselves by eating hemlock, henbane, or opium; it provokes urine, and the terms in women; helps the dropsy, scurvy, scabs, itch, and the yellow jaundice; the juice, being dropped into the ears, relieves deafness, pain, and noise in the ears.

MASTER-WORT

DESCRIPTION   common master-wort has divers stalks of winged leaves divided into sundry parts, three for the most part standing together at a small foot-stalk on both sides of the greater; and three likewise at the end of the stalk, somewhat broad, and cut in on the edges into three or more divisions, all of them dented about the brims, of a dark green colour, somewhat resembling the leaves of angelica, but that these grow lower to the ground, and on smaller stalks; among which rise up two or three short stalks, about two feet high, and slender, with leaves at the joints similar to those below, but with smaller and

PLATE 13

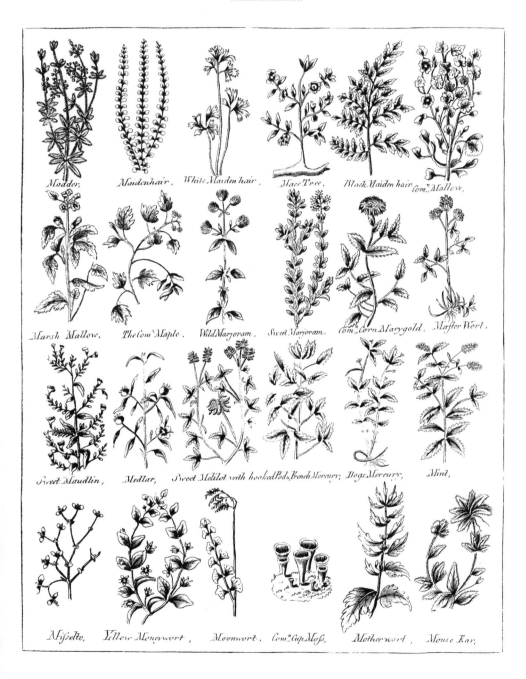

Madder,   Maidenhair,   White Maiden hair,   Mace Tree,   Black Maiden hair   Com." Mallow,

Marsh Mallow,   The Com" Maple,   Wild Marjoram,   Sweet Marjoram,   Com." Corn Marygold,   Master Worl,

Sweet Maudlin,   Medlar,   Sweet Melilot with hooked Pods, French Mercury,   Dogs Mercury,   Mint,

Miffelto,   Yellow Moneywort,   Moonwort,   Com." Cup Mofs,   Motherwort,   Mouse Ear, fewer divisions, bearing umbels of white flowers; and, after them, small thin, flat, blackish, seed, larger than dill-seeds; the root is somewhat greater, and grows slanting into the ground, shooting forth sundry heads, which taste sharp, biting the tongue, and is the hottest and sharpest part of the plant; the seed, next unto it, being somewhat blackish on the outside, and smelling well.

PLACE   It is usually grown in gardens in this kingdom.

TIME   It flowers and seeds about the end of August.

GOVERNMENT AND VIRTUES   It is an herb of Mars. The root of master-wort is hotter than pepper, and very available in all cold griefs and diseases both of the stomach and body, operation very powerfully both upwards and downwards. It is also used in a decoction, with wine, against all cold rheums, or distillations upon the lungs, and shortness of breath, if taken mornings and evenings. It also provokes urine; helps to break the stone, and expel the gravel from the kidneys; procures women's menses, and expels the dead birth. It is effectual against the dropsy, cramps, and the falling sickness. The decoction, in wine, being gargled in the mouth, extracts much water and phlegm from the brain, purging and easing it of what oppresses it. It is an excellent remedy against all sorts of cold poison; it provokes sweat: but, left the taste hereof or of the seed (which works to the like effect, though not so powerfully) should be too offensive, the best way is to take the water distilled from both the root and herb. The juice thereof, or tents dipped therein, applied to green wounds or ulcers does very soon cleanse and heal them. It is also a very good preventative against the rheumatism and gout when they originate from cold.

MASTIC-TREE

It is called in Latin *lentiscus*, and the gum or rosin, *resina lentiscina*, and *mastiche*, and *mastix*; in English, mastic.

DESCRIPTION   The mastic or lentisk-tree grows like a tree when suffered to grow up; and often it rises but as a shrub; the body and branches are of a reddish colour: tough and gentle, having their ends bending somewhat downwards, whereon do grow winged dark green leaves consisting of four couple, standing one against another, of the bigness of the large myrtle-leaf, with a reddish circle about their edges, and somewhat reddish veins on the under-side, smelling sweet, and always continuing green; the flowers grow in clusters at the joints, with the leaves, being small, and of a pale purple-green colour; after them come small blackish berries, of the size of a pepper-corn, with a hard black shell under the outer skin, and a white kernel within; it bears also certain horns, with a clear liquor in them that turns into small flies. It yields also a clear white gum, in small drops, when the stocks are cut in sundry places; which is carefully gathered and preserved.

PLACE The lentisk-tree grows in Provence, in France; and also in divers parts of Italy; in Candia, and many other places in Greece; but yields little gum there, especially in the isle of Scio.

TIME It flowers in April, and the berries are ripe in September; it is pruned and manured with as great care by the cultivators as others do their vines; the profit arising from the gum being much greater.

GOVERNMENT AND VIRTUES The lentisk-tree is under the influence of Jupiter. It is of moderately hot temperature; but the root, branches, bark, leaves, fruit, and gum, are all of a binding quality, stopping all fluxes and spitting of blood; strengthens a weak stomach, and helps falling down of the womb and fundament. The oil which is pressed out of the berries, helps the itch, leprosy, and scab, both in man and beast; gum-mastic has the like virtue of staying fluxes, taken any way in powder; or, if three or four grains of it be swallowed whole at night when going to bed, it not only eases the pains of the stomach, but binders its being affected afterwards; the powder of mastic, with amber and turpentine, is good against the running of the reins, and to check the *fluor albus* and menses in women.

SWEET MAUDLIN

DESCRIPTION common maudlin has somewhat long and narrow leaves, snipped about the edges; the stalks are two feet high, bearing at the tops many yellow flowers, set round together, and all of an equal height, in umbels, with tufts like tansy; after which flowereth small whitish seed, almost as big as wormseed. This herb is both sweet and bitter.

PLACE AND TIME It grows in gardens, and flowers in June and July.

GOVERNMENT AND VIRTUES The virtues of this herb are similar to that of costmary, or alecost; it is therefore unnecessary to repeat them.

MAY-WEED

There are three sorts of may-weed. 1. *Cotula fœtida*, stinking may-weed. 2. *Cotula non fœtida*, may-weed with no scent. Stinking mayweed grows more upright than that which has no smell, or the common camomile; neither of them creep or run on the ground as camomile does; the leaves are longer and larger than those of camomile, yet very like unto it, but of a paler green colour; the one sort has a very strong smell, the other no scent at all; the flowers are like those of camomile, but larger; there is also a sort of may-weed found in various parts of the kingdom, which has double flowers, almost as large as double camomile-flowers, which is called *cotula flore pleno*.

PLACE   The stinking may-weed grows abundantly among corn, and will blister the hands of the reapers; that which stinks not grows also very plentifully, wild, in many places, and often amongst wild camomile.

TIME   They flower all the summer months, some earlier and some later.

GOVERNMENT AND VIRTUES   May-weed is governed by Mars, yet Galen says the sophi of the Egyptians consecrated camomile to the Sun, which is much of the same temperature, but the stinking may-weed is more hot and dry, and is used for the same purposes as camomile, *viz.* to dissolve tumours, expel wind, and to ease pains and aches in the joints and other parts; it is also good for women whose matrix is fallen down, or loosened from one side to the other, by washing their feet with a decoction thereof made in water. It is likewise good to be given to smell to by such as are troubled with the rising or suffocation of the matrix.

MEALY-TREE

It is called in Latin *vibernum*; IT is also called the way-faring tree; and by Mr Parkinson, from the pliability of the twigs and branches, the pliant mealy-tree.

DESCRIPTION   This tree has (from a small body, rising to the height of a hedge-tree, or bush, covered with a dark-greyish bark) sundry, small, short but very tough and pliant branches, of a finger's thickness, whose bark is smooth and whitish, whereon grow broad leaves, like elm-leaves, but long and hoary, rough, thick, and white like meal, and a little hairy, set by couples, and finely dented about the edges; at the ends of the branches stand large tufts of white flowers, which turn into large bunches of round and flat seed, like that of the lentil, but larger; green when they are first formed, and for a considerable time afterwards, but black when they are ripe.

The branches thereof are so tough and strong, that they serve for bands to tie bundles, or any other thing; or to make fast gates leading into fields, for which purposes they are better adapted than withy, or any thing of that nature.

PLACE   It groweth as a hedge-bush, and is often cut and plashed by country people to spread on the hedges; is very frequently found in Kent, and in many other parts of this kingdom.

TIME It flowers about the end of May, and the fruit is ripe in September.

GOVERNMENT AND VIRTUES It is a plant of Saturn. The leaves thereof have a harsh binding quality, and are good to strengthen and fasten loose teeth. The decoction of the leaves thereof, and of olive-leaves together, in vinegar and water, is exceeding good to wash the mouth and throat when swelled by sharp humours falling into them; restores the uvula or palate of the mouth to its right place, when fallen down; it also stays the rheums that fall upon the jaws. The kernels of the fruit hereof, taken before they are ripe, dried and made into powder, and drunk in any liquid, stop looseness of the belly, and all sorts of fluxes. Of the roots, being steeped under ground, then boiled, and beaten a long time afterwards, bird-lime is made to catch small birds.

The leaves, boiled in lye, keep the hair from falling off the head, and change the colour into black.

MEDLAR

DESCRIPTION this tree grows near the bigness of the quince tree, with tolerably large spreading branches; longer and narrower leased than either the apple or quince, and not dented about the edges. At the end of the sprigs stand the flowers, formed of five white, great, broad-pointed leaves, marked in the middle with some white threads; after which comes the fruit, of a brownish-green colour when ripe, bearing the resemblance of a crown on the top, which was originally the five green leaves; and, being rubbed off or having fallen away, the head of the fruit appears somewhat hollow. The fruit is very harsh before it is mellow; and usually has five hard kernels within it.

There is another kind hereof, differing in nothing from the former, but that it has some thorns on it, in several places, which the other has not; and the fruit is small and not so pleasant.

PLACE AND TIME They grow in this kingdom, and flower in May generally; they bear ripe fruit in September and October.

GOVERNMENT AND VIRTUES This tree is under Saturn. A better medicine for strengthening the retentive faculties is hardly to be met with. A plaister, made of the fruit, before they are rotten, with other necessary ingredients, applied to the reins or the back, stops the miscarriage of women with child. They are very powerful in staying any fluxes of blood, or humours, in men or women. The leaves have also the same quality. The fruit, when eaten by women with child, is very effectual for those who are apt to miscarry. The decoction of them is good to gargle and wash the mouth, throat, and teeth; when there is any defluxion of blood, to stay it, or of humours which cause pains and swellings. It is a good bath for women to sit over that have their courses flow too abundantly; or for the piles when they bleed too much. The dried leaves in powder, strewed on fresh bleeding wounds, restrain the blood and close the wound quickly. The medlar stones, made into powder, and drunk in wine wherein some parsley-roots have been infused, or a little boiled, help to break and expel the stone in the kidneys.

MELILOT, OR KING'S CHAFER

DESCRIPTION This has many green stalks two or three feet high, rising from a tough, long, white, root, which dies not every year; set round about at the joints with small, and somewhat long, sweet-smelling-leaves, three together, unevenly dented about the edges. The flowers are yellow, also of a sweet scent, and formed like other trefoil, but small, standing in small spikes, one above another, for an hand's breadth long, or more, which afterwards turn into long crooked pods, wherein is contained flat seed, somewhat brown.

PLACE It grows plentifully in many parts of this kingdom; on the borders of Suffolk; in Essex, Huntingdonshire, and many other places; but most usually in corn-fields and corners of meadows.

TIME It flowers in June and July, and is ripe quickly after.

GOVERNMENT AND VIRTUES Melilot, boiled in wine, and applied to the parts, mollifies all hard tumours and inflammations that happen in the eye, or other parts of the body; and it is not unusual, in such cases, to add the yolk of a roasted egg, fine flour, poppy-seed, or endive. It heals spreading ulcers in the head, being washed with lye made thereof; being applied fresh, or boiled with any of the aforenamed articles, it relieves pains in the stomach; it also helps pains in the ears, being dropped into them; and, steeped in vinegar and rose-water, it mitigates the head-ache. The flowers of melilot and camomile are frequently mixed in clysters to expel wind and to ease pains; also in poultices, for the same purpose; and to assuage swellings or tumours in the spleen or other parts: and helps inflammations in any part of the body. The juice, dropped into the eyes, is a singular good medicine to take away any film or skin that clouds or dims the eye-sight. The head often washed with the distilled water of the herb and flowers, or a lye made therewith, is effectual to strengthen the memory, comfort the head and brain, and to preserve them from pains and the apoplexy.

DOG'S MERCURY

DESCRIPTION This is of two kinds, male and female, having many stalks, slenderer and lower than mercury, and without any branches at all upon them.

The root is set with two leaves at every joint. At the joints, with the leaves, come forth longer stalks than the former, with two hairy round seeds upon them, twice as big as those of the former mercury. From the joints come forth spikes of flowers similar to those of the French female mercury. The roots of both are numerous, and full of small fibres, which run under ground, and mat themselves very much; not perishing as the former mercury does, but remaining the whole winter, and shooting forth new branches every year, the old ones falling to the ground.

PLACE The male and female French mercury are found wild in divers parts of the kingdom: particularly at a village called Brookland, in Romney-marsh, in the county of Kent.

The dog's mercury is to be found in various parts of Kent, and elsewhere; but the female is more seldom to be met with than the male.

TIME They flourish in the summer months, and then produce their seed.

GOVERNMENT AND VIRTUES Mercury, it is said, owns this herb, but we are of opinion that it is under the dominion of Venus. The decoction of the leaves of mercury, or the juice thereof, in broth, or drunk with a little sugar put to it, purges choleric and watery humours. Hippocrates commends it wonderfully for women's diseases; when applied to the secret parts, it eases the pains of the womb; and, when used as a decoction, helps women's menses, and expels the after-birth; the decoction, mixed with myrrh or pepper, or applying the leaves externally, is effectual against the difficulty in passing urine and diseases of the bladder. It is also useful for sore and watery eyes, and for deafness and pains in the ears, by dropping the juice into them. The decoction thereof, made with water, is a safe medicine against hot fits of the ague. It also cleanses the lungs and stomach of phlegm, though rather offensive to the stomach. The juice, or distilled water, snuffed up into the nostrils, purges the head and eyes of catarrhs and rheums. Mathiolus says, that the seed, both of the male and female mercury, boiled with wormwood, and drunk, cures the yellow jaundice in a speedy manner. The leaves, or the juice, rubbed upon warts, takes them away. The juice, mixed with some vinegar, Galen says, that being applied, in the manner of a poultice, to any swelling or inflammation, it digests the swelling, and allays the inflammation.

FRENCH MERCURY

DESCRIPTION This rises up with a square green stalk, full of joints, two feet high or thereabouts, with two leaves at every joint, and branches likewise from both sides of the stalk, set with fresh green leaves, somewhat broad and long, about the bigness of the leaves of basil, finely dented about the edges.

Towards the top of the stalks and branches come forth, at every joint, in the male mercury, two small, round, green, heads, standing together upon a short foot-stalk, which, when ripe, are the seed, not bearing any flower. In the female, the stalk is longer, spike-fashion, set round about with small green husks, which are the flowers, made like small branches of grapes, which give no seed, but remain long upon the stalk without shedding. The root is composed of many small fibres, which perishes every year on the approach of winter; it rises again of its own sowing, and, where it is once suffered to sow itself, the ground will never be without it afterwards, even of both sorts, male and female.

French mercury helps conception. Costæus, in his book of the nature of plants, says, that the juice of mercury, hollyhock, and purslain, mixed together, and the hands bathed therein, defends them from burning, if they are thrust into boiling lead. This is what shew-men and merry-andrews bathe their mouths with, when they pretend to eat fire.

MINT

DESCRIPTION Of all kind of mints, the spear-mint, or hart-mint, is the most useful; the description thereof will therefore be sufficient. Spear-mint has divers round long stalks, but narrow leaves set thereon; of a dark green colour. The flowers stand in spiked heads at the tops of the branches, being of a pale-bluish colour. The smell or scent thereof is somewhat similar to that of basil; it increases by the root, under ground, as all the others do.

PLACE It is an usual inhabitant of gardens; and, though it seldom gives any good seed, yet this defect is recompensed by the plentiful increase of the root, which being once planted in a garden, is hardly to be eradicated. It flowers in August.

GOVERNMENT AND VIRTUES It is an herb of Venus. Dioscorides says, it has a heating, binding, and drying, quality; therefore the juice, taken with vinegar, stays bleeding. Two or three branches thereof, taken with the juice of sour pomegranates, stays the hiccough, vomiting, and allays choler. It dissolves imposthumes, being applied with barley-meal. If the leaves are boiled or steeped in milk before drinking, it hinders the curdling thereof on the stomach. In short, it is a very powerful stomachic. The frequent use hereof is very efficacious in stopping women's menses and the whites.

Applied to the forehead or temple, it eases pains of the head; it is good to wash the heads of young children, being a preventative against all manner of breakings out, sores, of scabs, thereon. The distilled water from mint is available for all the purposes aforesaid, yet more weakly; but the spirit thereof, when properly and chemically drawn, is much more powerful than the herb itself. Simeon Sethi says, it helps a cold liver; strengthens the belly and stomach;

causes digestion; stays vomiting and the hiccough; provokes appetite; takes away obstructions of the liver; and stirs up bodily lust; but it must not be taken in too great quantities, as it tends to make the blood thin and wheyish, and turns it into choler; therefore choleric people must abstain from it.

The powder of mint, being dried, and taken after victuals, helps digestion, and those that are splenetic. Taken in wine, it helps women in sore travail in child-bearing. It is good against the gravel and stone in the kidneys, and the difficulty in passing urine. Being smelled unto, it is comfortable for the head and memory. The decoction thereof, when used as a gargle, cures the mouth and gums, when force, and helps a stinking breath; when mixed with rue and coriander, also used as a gargle, it causes the palate of the mouth to return to its place, when down. Mint, says Pliny, exhilarates the mind, and is therefore proper for the studious. When put into any vessel containing milk, it hinders the curdling thereof, and no butter can be got therefrom.

The virtues of the wild or horse-mint, which grows in ditches, and by the sides of rivers (the description which is unnecessary, being so well known), are especially to dissolve wind in the stomach, to help the cholic, and those that are short-winded. The juice, laid on warm, helps the king's-evil, or kernels in the throat. The decoction, or distilled water, helps in a stinking breath proceeding from the corruption of the teeth; and snuffed up into the nose, purges the head. Pliny says, that eating of the leaves, and applying some of them to the face, have been found, by experience, to cure the leprosy, and, when used with vinegar, to help the scurf or dandruff of the head.

MISTLETOE

DESCRIPTION This rises up from the branch or arm of the tree whereon it grows, with a woody stem, parting itself into sundry branches, and they are again divided into many other smaller twigs, interlacing themselves one within another, very much covered with a greyish-green bark, having two leaves set at every joint, and at the end likewise, which are somewhat long and narrow, small at the bottom, but broader towards the end. At the knots or joints of the boughs and branches, grow small yellowish flowers, which turn into small, round, white, transparent, berries, three or four together, full of glutinous moisture, with a blackish seed in each of them, which was never yet known to produce any thing, though planted in gardens, and other places, for the purpose of trying it.

PLACE It grows very rarely on oak-trees in this kingdom, but upon sundry others, as well timber as fruit-trees; and is to be met with in woods, groves, &c.

TIME It flowers in the spring-time, but the berries are not ripe until October, and, remaining on the branches, serve the birds for food in severe weather.

GOVERNMENT AND VIRTUES That it is under the dominion of the Sun is without a doubt; that which grows upon the oak participates something of the nature of Jupiter, because an oak is one of his trees; as also that which grows upon pear-trees and apple-trees participates something of that nature, because he rules the trees it grows upon, having no root of its own; but why that should have more virtue that grows upon the oak is not so easily determinable, unless because it is rarest and hardest to be come at. Clusius asserts, that that which grows upon pear-trees is equally efficacious with the other sorts, provided it does not touch the ground after it is gathered; and also says, that, being hung about the neck, it remedies witchcraft. Both the leaves and berries of misletoe are of a hot and dry, nature, and of subtle parts. Bird-lime, made thereof, does mollify hard knots, tumours, and imposthumes; draws forth thick as well as thin humours from the remote parts of the body, and, being mixed with equal parts of rosin and wax, mollifies the hardness of the spleen, and heals old ulcers and sores; being mixed with sandarac and orpiment, with quick-lime and wine lees added thereto, it draws off foul nails from the flesh. Mathiolus says, that the misletoe of the oak (being the best), made into powder, and given in drink to those who have the falling sickness, does assuredly heal them; provided it be taken forty days together. Some hold it so highly in estimation, that it is termed *lignum sanctæ crucis*, or wood of the holy cross, believing it to help the falling sickness, apoplexy, and palsy, very speedily, not only when taken inwardly, but applied externally, by hanging it about the neck. Tragus says, that by bruising the green wood of any misletoe, and dropping the juice so drawn therefrom into the ears of those who are troubled with imposthumes, it heals the same in a few days.

The powder of it also cures a pleurisy, and forces the menses. Some think the misletoe that grows on the hasel-tree is better for the falling sickness, and other diseases of the head, than that which grows on the oak. Henricus ab Steers thinks it does not grow on hasel-trees till they are about an hundred years old. A young lady, having been long troubled with the falling sickness, for which she had taken every thing prescribed for her by the most famous doctors, without effect, but growing rather worse, having eight or ten dreadful fits in a day, was cured only by the powder of true misletoe, given, as much as would lie on a sixpence, early in the morning, in black cherry-water, or in beer, for some days near the full moon.

MONEY-WORT, OR HERB-TWOPENCE

DESCRIPTION The common money-wort sends forth, from a small thready root, divers long, weak, and slender, branches, lying and running upon the ground, two or three feet long or more, set with leaves two at a joint, one against another at equal distances, which are almost round, but jointed at the ends, smooth, and of a good green colour. At the joints, with the leaves from the middle forward, come forth at every joint sometimes one yellow flower, and sometimes two, standing each on a small foot-stalk, formed of five leaves, narrow and pointed at the ends, with some yellow threads in the middle; which being past, there come in their places small round heads of seed.

PLACE It grows plentifully in almost every part of the kingdom, commonly in moist grounds, by the sides of hedges, and in the middle of grassy fields.

TIME They flower in June and July, and their seed is ripe quickly after.

GOVERNMENT AND VIRTUES Venus owns it. Money-wort is singularly good to stay all fluxes in man or woman, whether they be lasks, bloody fluxes, the flowing of women's menses, bleedings inwardly or outwardly, and the weakness of the stomach that is given to casting. It is also very good for all ulcers or excorations of the lungs, or other inward parts. It is exceeding good for all wounds, whether fresh and green, or old ulcers of a spreading nature, and heals them speedily; for all which purposes, the juice of the herb; the powder drunk in water wherein hot steel has been often quenched; the decoction of the green herb in wine or water drunk; the seed, juice, or decoction, used to wash or bathe the outward places, or to have tents dipped therein and applied to the wounds; are effectual.

MOON-WORT

DESCRIPTION it rises up, usually, but with one dark green, thick, and flat, leaf, standing upon a short foot-stalk, not above two fingers breadth; but, when it flowers, bears a small slender stalk, about four or five inches high, having but one leaf set in the middle thereof, which is much divided on both sides, into sometimes five or seven parts on a side, and sometimes more, each of which parts is small next the middle rib, but broad forwards, and round-pointed, resembling a half-moon, from whence it takes its name, the uppermost parts or divisions being less than the lowest. The stalk rises above this leaf two or three inches, bearing many branches of small long tongues, every one like the spiky head of adder's tongue, of a brownish colour, which, whether they may be called the flowers or seed, is not so well certified; but, after continuing a while, resolve into a mealy dust. The root is small and fibrous. This has sometimes divers such-like leaves as are before described, with so many branches or tops rising from one stalk, each divided from the other.

PLACE It grows on hills and heaths, particularly where there is plenty of grass.

TIME It is to be found only in April and May; but in June, if hot weather comes, it generally withers and dies.

GOVERNMENT AND VIRTUES The Moon owns this herb. Moon-wort is cold and drying, in a greater degree even than adder's tongue, and is therefore serviceable in all wounds, both inward and outward. The leaves boiled in red wine, and drunk, stay the immoderate flux of women's menses, and the whites. It also stays bleeding, vomiting, and other fluxes; helps all blows and bruises, and consolidates fractures and dislocations. It is good for ruptures; but chiefly used by most, with other herbs, to make oils, or other balsams, to heal fresh or green wounds, either inward or outward, for which it is exceeding good, as is before observed.

MOSS

It would be needless to trouble the reader with a description of every kind of moss; that of the ground-moss and tree-moss, which are both well-known, being sufficient for our purpose.

PLACE The ground-moss grows in moist woods, at the bottoms of hills, in boggy grounds, shadowy ditches, and other such-like places, in all parts of the kingdom. The other grows only upon trees.

GOVERNMENT AND VIRTUES All sorts of moss are under the dominion of Saturn. The ground-moss, being boiled in wine and drunk, is held to be very efficacious in breaking the stone, and to expel and drive it forth by urine. The herb, bruised and boiled in water, and applied, eases all inflammations and pains proceeding from hot causes; and is therefore used to relieve pain arising from the gout.

The different kinds of tree-moss are cooling and binding, and partake of a digesting and mollifying quality withal, as Galen says. But each moss does partake of the nature of the tree from whence it is taken; therefore that of the oak is more binding, and is of good effect to stay fluxes in men or women; as also vomitings or bleedings, the powder thereof being taken in wine.

The oil of roses, which has had some fresh moss steeped therein for a time, and afterwards boiled and applied to the temples and forehead, does wonderfully ease the head-ache arising from a hot cause; as also the distillation of hot rheum or humours from the eyes, or other parts. The ancients used it much in their ointments and other medicines, against lassitude, and to strengthen and comfort the sinews; it may, consequently, be applied by the moderns with equal success.

MOTHER-WORT

DESCRIPTION this has a hard, square, brownish, rough, strong, stalk, rising three or four feet high at least, spreading into many branches, whereon grow leaves on each side, with long foot-stalks, two at every joint, which are somewhat broad and long, as it were rough or crumpled, with many great veins thereon, deeply dented about the edges, and almost divided. From the middle of the branches, up to the tops of them (which are very long and small), grow the flowers round about them, at distances, in sharp-pointed, rough, hard, husks, of a more red or purple colour than balm or hoarhound, but in the same manner or form as hoarhound; after which come small, round, blackish seeds, in great plenty. The root sends forth a number of long strings and small fibres, taking strong hold in the ground, of a dark yellowish or brownish colour, and remains as the hoarhound does; the smell of this being not much different from it.

PLACE It is only produced in gardens in this kingdom.

GOVERNMENT AND VIRTUES Venus owns this herb, and it is under Leo. There is no better herb to drive melancholy vapours from the heart, to strengthen it, and make the mind cheerful, blithe, and merry. It may be kept in a syrup or conserve; therefore the Latins call it *cordiaca*. The powder thereof, to the quantity of a spoonful, drunk in cold wine, is a wonderful help to women in sore travail, as also for suffocation or risings of the mother, or womb; and from these effects it most likely got the name of mother-wort. It also provokes urine, and women's menses; cleanses the chest of cold phlegm oppressing it, and kills worms in the belly. It is of good use to warm and dry up the cold humours, to digest and disperse them that are settled in the veins, joints, and sinews, of the body, and to help cramps and convulsions.

MOUSE-EAR

DESCRIPTION mouse-ear is a low herb, creeping upon the ground by small strings like the strawberry plant, from which it shoots forth small roots, whereat grow upon the ground, many small and somewhat short leaves, set in a round form together, hollowish in the middle, where they are broadest; of an hoary colour all over, and very hairy, which, being broken, produce white milk. From among these leaves spring up two or three small hoary stalks, about a span high, with a few smaller leaves thereon; at the tops whereof stands usually but one flower, consisting of many paler yellow leaves, broad at the points, and a little dented in, set in three or four rows, the largest outermost, very like a dandelion flower, and a little reddish underneath about the edges, especially if it grow in dry ground; which, after they have stood long in flower, turn into down, which, with the seed, is blown away by the wind.

PLACE It grows on the banks of ditches, and in sandy ground.

TIME It flowers in June and July, and remains green all the winter.

PLATE 14

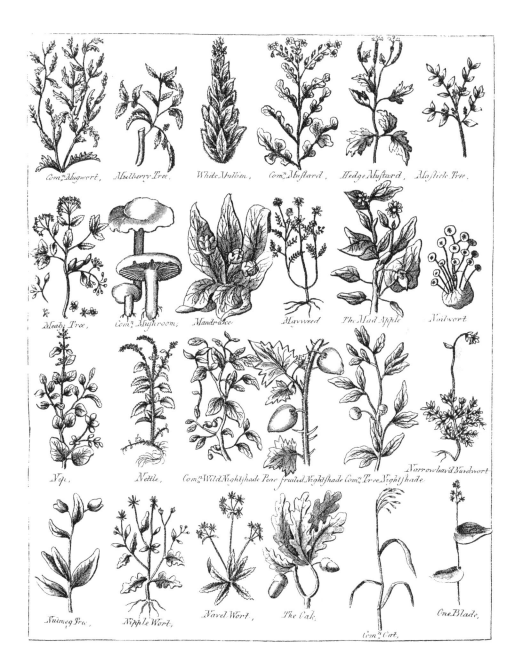

Com:ⁿ Mugwort,   Mulberry Tree.   White Mullein,   Com:ⁿ Mustard,   Hedge Mustard   Mastick Tree.

Meabi Tree,   Com:ⁿ Mushroom,   Mandrake   Mayweed   The Mad Apple   Navilwort

Nep,   Nettle,   Com:ⁿ Wild Nightshade Pear fruited Nightshade Com:ⁿ Tree Nightshade   Narrowleav'd Navelwort

Nutmeg Tree,   Nipple Wort,   Navel Wort,   The Oak,   Com:ⁿ Oat,   One Blade,

GOVERNMENT AND VIRTUES   The Moon owns this herb also. The juice thereof, taken in wine, or the decoction thereof drunk, does help the jaundice, although of long continuance; it is a special remedy against the stone, and griping pains of the bowels. The decoction thereof, with succory and centaury, is held very effectual to help the dropsy, and them that are inclining thereunto, as well as diseases of the spleen. It stays the fluxes of blood, whether at the mouth or nose, and inward bleedings also; it is very efficacious for wounds both inward and outward; it helps the bloody flux and the abundance of women's menses. There is a syrup made of the juice thereof, and sugar, by the apothecaries of Italy and other places, which is accounted very serviceable to those that are troubled with the cough or phthisic. The same is also singularly good for ruptures or burstings. The green herb, bruised, and directly applied to any fresh cut or wound, does quickly heal it; and the juice, decoction, or powder of the dried herb, is very good to stay the malignity of spreading and fretting cankers and ulcers. The distilled water of the plant is available in all the diseases aforesaid, and to wash outward wounds and sores.

MUGWORT

DESCRIPTION   common mugwort has divers leaves lying upon the ground, very much divided, or cut deeply in about the brims, somewhat like wormwood, but much larger; of a dark green colour on the upper side, and very hoary, white, underneath. The stalks rise to the height of four or five feet, having on it similar leaves to those below, but somewhat smaller, branching forth very much towards the top, whereon are set very small pale yellowish flowers like buttons, which fall away; and after them come small seed inclosed in round heads. The root is long and hard, with many small fibres growing from it, whereby it takes strong hold in the ground; but both stalk and leaf die every year, and the root shoots forth anew in the spring. The whole plant is of a tolerably good scent, and is more readily propagated by the slips than by the seed.

PLACE   It grows plentifully in many parts of this kingdom, by the road-side; also, by small water-courses; and in divers other places.

TIME   It flowers and seeds in the end of the summer.

GOVERNMENT AND VIRTUES   This is an herb of Venus; therefore maintains the parts of the body she rules, and remedies the diseases of the parts that are under her signs, Taurus and Libra. Mugwort is used with good success, among other herbs, in a hot decoction, for women to sit over, to provoke the menses, help delivery, and expel the after-birth; also, for the obstructions and inflammations of the womb. It breaks the stone, and causes one to make water when it is stopped. The juice thereof, made up with myrrh, and formed into a pessary, works the same effects; the root, being made into an ointment, with hog's-lard, takes away wens and hard knots and kernels that grow about the neck and throat, and eases pains about the neck more effectually, if some field daisies be put with it. The herb itself, being fresh, or juice thereof, taken, is a special remedy for an over-dose of opium. Three drachms of the powder of the dried leaves, taken in wine, is a speedy and the most certain cure for the sciatica. A decoction thereof, made with camomel and agrimony, takes away pains of the sinews and the cramp, if the place is bathed therewith while warm.

MULBERRY-TREE

TIME It bears fruit in the months of July and August.

GOVERNMENT AND VIRTUES Mercury rules the tree, therefore are its effects variable as his are. The mulberry partakes of different and opposite qualities; the ripe berries, by reason of their sweetness and slippery moisture, opening the body, and the unripe binding it, especially when they are dried; and then they are good to stay fluxes, lasks, and the abundance of women's menses. The bark of the root kills the broad worms in the body.

The juice, or the syrup made of the juice, of the berries, helps all inflammations or sores in the mouth or throat, and the pallet of the mouth when it is fallen down. The juice of the leaves is a remedy against the biting of serpents, and for those that have taken aconite; the leaves, beaten with vinegar, are good to lay on any place that is burnt with fire. A decoction made of the bark and leaves, is good to wash the mouth and teeth when they ache. If the root be a little slit or cut, and a small hole made in the ground next thereunto, in the harvest-time, it will give out a certain juice, which, being hardened the next day, is of good use to help the tooth-ache, to dissolve knots, and purge the belly. The leaves of mulberries are said to stay bleeding at the mouth or nose, the bleeding piles, or of any wound, being bound unto the places. A branch of the tree, taken when the Moon is at the full, and bound to the wrist of a woman whose menses overflow, stays them in a short space.

MULLEIN

DESCRIPTION common white mullein has many fair, large, woolly, white, leaves, lying next the ground, somewhat longer than broad, pointed at the ends, and dented as it were about the edges; the stalk rises up to be four or five feet high, covered over with such like leaves, but smaller, so that no stalks can be seen for the quantity of leaves thereon, up to the flowers, which come forth on all sides of the stalk, generally without any branches, and are many set together in a long spike, in some of a gold-yellow colour, in others more pale, consisting of five round pointed leaves, which afterwards have little round heads, wherein a small brownish seed is contained. The root is long, white, and woody; perishing after it has borne seed.

PLACE It grows by road-sides and lanes in many parts of the kingdom.

TIME It flowers in July, or thereabouts.

GOVERNMENT AND VIRTUES It is under the dominion of Saturn. The decoction thereof, being drunk, helps ruptures, cramps, and convulsions, and those that are troubled with an old cough; and, when used as a gargle, eases the tooth-ache. An oil, made by frequently infusing the flowers, has a very good effect on the piles. The decoction of the root, in red wine, or in water (if attended with an ague) wherein red-hot steel has been often quenched, stays the bloody flux; and also opens obstructions of the bladder and reins, when there is a stoppage of urine. A decoction of the leaves thereof, and of sage, marjoram, and camomile flowers, and the sinews being bathed therewith that are benumbed with cold, or cramps, does much ease and comfort them. Three ounces of the distilled water of the flowers, drunk morning and evening, for some days together, are said to be an excellent remedy for the gout. The juice of the leaves and flowers being laid upon rough warts, as also the powder of the dried roots, when rubbed on, does take them away; but have no effect upon smooth warts. The powder of the dried flowers is an especial remedy for those that are troubled with the cholic or belly-ache. The decoction of the root, and likewise of the leaves, is of great effect in dissolving tumours, swellings, or inflammations of the throat. The seed and leaves boiled in wine, and applied to the place, speedily draws forth thorns and splinters from the flesh, easing the pain and healing the wound. The leaves, bruised and wrapped in double papers, and covered with hot ashes and embers, in which they must be baked for some time, and then taken and laid on any blotch or boil, dissolve and heal it.

MUSHROOM

VIRTUES The Laplanders have a method of using funguses, or toadstools as we call them (which are of the same genus with the mushroom) to cure pains. They collect the largest funguses which they find on the bark of beech and other large trees, and dry them for use. Whenever they have pains in their limbs, they use some of this dry matter; pulling it to pieces with their fingers, they lay a small heap of it on the part nearest to where the pain is situated, and set it on fire. In burning away, it blisters up the part, and the water discharged thereby generally carries off the pain. It is a coarse and rough method, but generally a very successful one, especially when the patient has prudence enough to apply it in time, and resolution enough to bear the burning to a necessary degree.

MUSTARD

DESCRIPTION our common mustard has large and broad rough leaves, very much jagged with uneven and disorderly gashes, somewhat like turnip-leaves, but smaller and rougher; the stalk rises to be upwards of a foot high, and sometimes two feet high; being round, rough, and branched at the top, bearing similar leaves thereon to those below, but smaller and less divided, and divers yellow flowers one above another at the tops, after which come small rough pods, with small lank flat ends, wherein is contained round yellowish seed, sharp, hot, and biting to the tongue. The roots are small, long, and woody, when it bears stalk, and perishes every year.

PLACE This grows in gardens only, and other manured grounds.

TIME It is an annual plant, flowering in July, and the seed is ripe in August.

GOVERNMENT AND VIRTUES It is an excellent sauce for those whose blood wants clarifying, and for weak stomachs, being an herb of Mars; it is hurtful to choleric people, but highly serviceable to those who are aged, or troubled with cold diseases. Aries claims some share of dominion over this plant; it therefore strengthens the heart, and resists poison. Mustard-seed has the virtue of heating, discussing, rarefying, drawing out splinters of bones, and other things, out of the flesh; provokes the menses; is good for the falling sickness, lethargy, drowsiness, and forgetfulness, by using it both inwardly and outwardly, rubbing the nostrils, forehead, and temples, to warm and quicken the spirits, as, from its fierce sharpness, it purges the brain by sneezing, and drawing down rheums, and other viscous humours, which, by their distillation upon the lungs and chest, cause coughing; when taken inwardly, it operates more forcibly if mixed with honey. If used as a gargle, it draws up the palate of the mouth, when fallen down. It also dissolves swellings about the throat, if it be applied externally. Being chewed in the mouth, it oftentimes helps the tooth-ache. The outward application hereof upon the pained place, in cases of the sciatica, discusses the humours, and eases the pains: as also of the gout, and other joint-aches. It is frequently used to ease pains of the sides, loins, shoulders, or other parts of the body, by applying thereof as a blister, and cures the disease by drawing it to the outward part of the body; it is also used to help the falling of the hair.

HEDGE-MUSTARD

DESCRIPTION this grows up usually but with one blackish-green stalk, tough, easy to bend, but not break, branched into divers parts, and sometimes with divers stalks set full of branches, whereon grow long, rough, or hard, rugged leaves, very much torn or cut on the edges into many parts, some larger and some smaller, of a dirty green colour; the flowers are small and yellow, growing at the tops of the branches in long spikes, flowering by degrees; the stalks have small round pods at the bottom, growing upright, and close to the stalk, whilst the flowers yet shew themselves; in which are contained small yellow seed, sharp and strong, as the herb is also. The root grows down slender and woody, yet abiding, and springing again every year.

PLACE This grows generally by the roads and hedge-sides; but sometimes in the open fields.

TIME It flowers usually about July.

GOVERNMENT AND VIRTUES Mars owns this herb also. It is singularly good in all the diseases of the chest and lungs, hoarseness of voice. The juice of this herb, made into a syrup with honey or sugar, is no less effectual for the same purposes, and for coughs, wheezing, and shortness of breath. It is also serviceable to those who have the jaundice, the pleurisy, pains in the back and loins, and for torments in the belly, or the cholic; it is also used in clysters. The feed is held to be a special remedy against poison and venom, is singularly good for the sciatica, the gout, and all joint-aches, sores and cankers in the mouth, throat, or behind the ears: it is also equally serviceable in reducing the hardness and swelling of the testicles, and of women's breasts.

NAILWORT, OR WHITLOW-GRASS

DESCRIPTION this herb has no roots, save only a few strings; neither does it ever grow to be above a hand's breadth high; the leaves are very small, and something long, not much unlike those of chickweed, amongst which rise up many slender stalks, bearing numerous white flowers one above another; after which come small flat pouches containing seed.

PLACE It grows upon old stone and brick walls, and sometimes in dry gravelly grounds, especially if there be grass or moss near to shadow it.

TIME They flower very early in the year, sometimes in January and in February; before the end of April they are no longer to be found.

VIRTUES It is held to be an exceeding good remedy for those imposthumes in the joints, and under the nails, which they call whitlows, felons, adicoms, and nail-weals.

NAVEL-WORT, OR PENNY-WORT

it is called *umbilicus veneris* and *herba coxendicum*. There are seven different kinds.

DESCRIPTION AND VIRTUES
1. The small navel-wort is moist and somewhat cold and binding. It cools and repels, scours and consumes.
2. The water penny-wort is hot and ulcerating, like crowfoot; and is very dangerous to cattle who may occasionally feed thereon.
3. The bastard Italian navel-wort partakes of the true in cold and moisture.
4. The juice of the wall penny-wort heals all inflammations and hot tumours, as the erysipelas, or St Anthony's fire; it heals kibed heels, being bathed therewith and the leaves applied. The leaves and root break the stone, provoke urine, and cure the dropsy. The distilled water heals sore kidneys, pains of the bowels, piles, gout, and king's evil.
5. The common or one-summer's navel-wort is diuretic, not very hot, but exceeding dry. It provokes urine, and digests sliminess in the joints. Two drachms drunk in wine will expel much urine from dropsical persons; and, applied, will also ease the gout.
6, 7. The spotted and small red-flowered navel-wort are cold and moist, like houseleek.

PLACE The first sort grows on stone walls; the other sorts are only found on the Alps.

TIME They flower in the beginning of the spring, but flourish all the winter.

NEP, OR CATMINT

DESCRIPTION common garden nep shoots forth hard four-square stalks with a hoariness on them, a yard high or more, full of branches, bearing at every joint two broad leaves, somewhat like balm, but longer pointed, softer, whiter, and more hoary, nicked about the edges, and of a strong sweet scent. The flowers grow in large tufts at the tops of the branches and underneath them, likewise on the stalks, many together, of a whitish-purple colour. The roots are composed of many long strings or fibres, fastening themselves strongly in the ground, and retaining their leaves green all the winter.

PLACE It is only nursed up in our gardens.

TIME It flowers in July, or thereabouts.

GOVERNMENT AND VIRTUES It is an herb of Venus. It is also used for pains of the head arising from any cold cause, such as catarrhs, rheums, &c. and for swimming and giddiness thereof, and is of especial use for expelling wind from the stomach and belly. It is also effectual for the cramp or other pains occasioned by cold; and is found serviceable for colds, coughs, and shortness of breath. The juice thereof drunk in wine, helps bruises. The green herb, bruised, and applied to the part for two or three hours, eases the pain arising from the piles. The juice also, being made up into an ointment, is effectual for the same purpose. Washing the head with a decoction thereof takes away scabs; and may be used to the like effect on other parts of the body.

NETTLES

GOVERNMENT AND VIRTUES This herb Mars claims dominion over. Nettle-tops, eaten in the spring, consume the phlegmatic superfluities in the body, which the coldness and moisture of winter have left behind. The roots or leaves boiled, or the juice of either of them, or both, made into an electuary with honey or sugar, is a safe and sure medicine to open the pipes and passages of the lungs, obstruction in which is the cause of shortness of breath, and helps to expectorate tough phlegm, as also to raise the imposthumated pleurisy, and evacuate it by spitting; the juice of nettles, used as a gargle, allays the swelling of the almonds of the throat; it also effectually settles the palate of the mouth in its place, and heals and tempers the soreness and inflammation of the mouth and throat. The decoction of the leaves in wine, being drunk, is very efficacious in most of the diseases peculiarly incident to the female sex; and is equally serviceable, when applied externally, mixed with myrrh.

NIGHTSHADE

DESCRIPTION Nightshade has an upright, round, green, hollow, stalk, about a foot or half yard high, shooting forth into many branches, whereon grow numerous green leaves, somewhat broad and pointed at the ends, soft and full of juice, somewhat like unto basil, but larger, and a little unevenly dented about the edges; at the tops of the stalks and branches, come forth three or more white flowers composed of five small pointed leaves apiece, standing on a stalk together one above another, with yellow pointels in the middle, composed of four or five yellow threads set together, which afterwards turn into so many pendulous green berries of the bulk of small peas, full of green juice, and small whitish round flat seed lying within it. The root is white, and a little woody when it has given flowers and fruit, with many small fibres at it. The juice within the berries is somewhat viscous, and of a cooling and binding quality.

PLACE   It grows wild in this kingdom in the common paths and sides of hedges, in fields; and also in gardens without any planting.

TIME   It dies annually, and rises again of its own sowing; but springs not until the latter end of April at the soonest.

GOVERNMENT AND VIRTUES   It is a cold Saturnine plant. The common nightshade is wholly used to cool hot inflammations, either inwardly or outwardly, being no ways dangerous, as the other nightshades are; yet it must be used moderately; the distilled water only of the whole herb is fittest and safest to be taken inwardly; the juice, being clarified and mixed with a little vinegar, is very good to wash the mouth and throat, when inflamed. Outwardly, the juice of the herb or berries with a little vinegar and ceruse, pounded together in a leaden mortar, is very good to anoint all hot inflammations in the eyes. Pliny says, it is good for hot swellings under the throat. Care must be taken that the deadly nightshade is not mistaken for this.

DEADLY NIGHTSHADE

DESCRIPTION   the flower is bell-shaped; it has a permanent empalement of one leaf, cut into five parts; it has five stamina rising from the base of the petal; in the centre is situated an oval germen, which becomes a globular berry, having two cells sitting on the empalement, and filled with kidney-shaped seed. It is of a cold nature; in some it causes sleep; in others madness, and, shortly after, death.

WOODY NIGHTSHADE

Called also bitter sweet.

PLACE   It grows by the sides of hedges, and in moist ditches, climbing upon the bushes; with winding, woody, but brittle, stalks.

TIME   It is perennial, and flowers in June and July.

VIRTUES   The roots and stalks, on first chewing them, yield a considerable bitterness, which is soon followed by an almost honey-like sweetness; and they have been recommended in different disorders, as high resolvents and deobstruents. Their sensible operation is by sweat, urine, and stool; the dose from four to six ounces of a tincture made by digesting four to six ounces of the twigs in a quart of white wine.

NIPPLEWORT

Of this there are three kinds: 1. The ordinary nipple-wort called in Latin *lampsana vulgaris*. 2. The nipplewort of Austria, called *lampsana, papillaris*. 3. Wild or wood bastard-nipplewort, *soncho assinis lampsana sylvatica*. And in Prussia, as says Camerarius, they call it *papillaris*.

DESCRIPTION
1. The ordinary nipplewort grows with many hard upright stalks, whereon grow dark green leaves from the bottom to the top, but the higher the smaller; in some places without dents in the edges, and in others with a few uneven jags therein, somewhat like a kind of hankweed; the tops of the stalks have some small long branches, which bear many small star-like yellowish flowers on them, which turn into small-seed. The root is small and fibrous; the plant yields a bitter milk like that of the sow-thistle.
2. The Austrian nipplewort has slender, smooth, and solid, stalks, not easily broken, about two feet high, whereon stand without order, somewhat long and narrow leaves, broadest in the middle, and sharp at the ends, waved a little about the edges, and compassing them at the bottom, yielding a little milk; from the upper joints, with the leaves, grow forth small firm branches, yet a little bending, bearing each of them four or five long green husks, and in them small purplish flowers of five leaves each, notched in at the broad ends, with some small threads in the middle; which turn into down, and are blown away with the wind: the root is small and shreddy, and lasts many years.
3. The wild or wood bastard-nipplewort is like unto the first sort, but with somewhat broader leaves, and greater store of branches; but in the flowers and other parts not much different.

PLACE AND TIME   The first grows common, almost every where, upon the banks of ditches and borders of fields; the second Clusius says he found in Hungary and Saxony, and other places; the last is found near the sides of woods, and hedge-rows; they flower in summer, and the seed is ripe soon after.

GOVERNMENT AND VIRTUES   These are plants of Venus, and kindly endued with a peculiar faculty for the healing the sore nipples of women's breasts; for which reason Camerarius says that in Prussia they call it *papillaris*; it having a singular healing quality therein; and is temperate in heat and driness.

NUTMEG-TREE, AND MACE

NAMES AND DESCRIPTION   the fruit of this is called in Latin *nux mystica,* and in shops *nux moscata*. The tree grows very tall, like our pear-trees; having leaves always green, somewhat resembling the leaves of the orange-tree;

the fruit grows like our walnuts, having an outer thick husk; which, when it grows ripe, opens itself as the shell of the walnut does; shewing the nut within covered with the mace, which is of an orient crimson colour while it is fresh, but the air changes the colour to be more dead and yellowish.

GOVERNMENT AND VIRTUES The nutmegs and maces are both solar, of a temperature hot and dry in the second degree, and somewhat astringent, and are good to stay the lask; they are effectual in all cold griefs of the head or brain, for palsies, shrinking of sinews, and diseases of the womb; they cause a sweet breath, quicken the sight, and comfort the spirits; provoke urine, increase sperm, and are comfortable to the stomach; they help to procure rest and sleep, being laid to the temples, by allaying the distemper of the spirits. The mace is of the same property, but somewhat more warming and comforting, than the nutmeg; the thick oil that is drawn from both nutmegs and mace is good in pectoral complaints, to warm a cold stomach, help the cough, and to dry up distillations of rheum falling upon the lungs.

OAK

GOVERNMENT AND VIRTUES Jupiter owns the tree. The leaves and bark of the oak, and the acorn cups, do bind and dry very much; the inner bark of the tree, and the thin skin that covers the acorn, are most used to stay the spitting of blood, and the bloody flux; the decoction of the bark, and the powder of the cups, stay vomiting; lasks also, and the involuntary flux of natural seed. The acorns in powder taken in wine provoke urine, and resist the poison of venomous creatures. The decoction of acorns and the bark made in milk, and taken, resists the force of poisonous herbs and medicines, as also the virulency of cantharides, when any person, by eating them, has the bladder exulcerated, and evacuates blood. Hippocrates says, he used the fume of oak-leaves to women that were troubled with the strangling of the womb; and Galen applied them, being bruised, to cure green wounds. The distilled water of the oaken buds, before they break out into leaves, is good to be used either inwardly or outwardly to assuage inflammations, and stop all manner of fluxes in man or woman; it cools the heat of the liver, breaks the stone in the kidneys, and stays women's menses. The decoction of the leaves has the same effects. The distilled water or decoction (which last is preferable) of the leaves is one of the best remedies known for the *fluor albus*.

OATS

This grain is well known: *avena* is the Latin name; they are grown in every quarter of the globe where agriculture is carried on. They are sown in spring, and mown or reaped in September and October; but in the northern parts of this kingdom it is frequently much later before they are cut down.

NATURE AND VIRTUES They are somewhat cold and drying, and are more used for food, both for man and beast, than for physic; yet, being quilted in a bag with bay-falt, made hot in a frying-pan, and applied as warm as can be endured, they ease pains and stitches in the side, and the cholic in the belly. A poultice made of the meal of oats and oil of bays, helps the itch, leprosy, and fistulas. Oatmeal boiled in vinegar, and applied, takes away spots and freckles. It is also used in broth or milk, to bind those who have a lask, or other flux; and with sugar it is good for them that have a cough or cold.

OLIVE-TREE

Of these there are the tame and manured olive, and the wild olive-tree; the first is called in Latin *olea sativa*, and the wild kind *oleaster*, or *olea sylvestris*.

DESCRIPTION

1. It has a small tubulous impalement of one leaf, cut into four segments at the top; the former consists of one petal, which is tubulous, cut at the brim into four segments; it has two short stamina, terminated by erect summits, and a roundish germen, supporting a short single style, crowned by a thick bifid stigma; the germen afterwards turns to an oval smooth fruit, or berry, with one cell, inclosing an oblong oval nut. In Languedoc and Provence, where the olive-tree is greatly cultivated, they propagate it by truncheons split from the roots of the trees; for, as these trees are frequently hurt by hard frosts in winter, so, when the tops are killed, they send up several stalks from the root; and, when these are grown pretty strong, they separate them with an axe from the root; in the doing of which they are careful to preserve a few roots to the truncheons; these are cut off in the spring after the danger of the frost is over, and planted about two feet deep in the ground. These trees will grow in almost any soil; but, when planted in rich moist ground, they grow larger, and make a finer appearance, than in poor land; but the fruit is of less esteem, because the oil made from it is not so good as that which is produced in a leaner soil; chalky ground is esteemed best for them; and the oil, made from the trees growing in that sort of land, is much finer, and will keep longer, than the other. In England, the plants are only preserved by way of curiosity, and are placed in winter in the green-house.
2. *Oleaster*, the wild olive-tree, grows somewhat like unto the manured, but it has harder and smaller leaves, and thicker set on the branches, with sundry sharp thorns among the leaves; the blossoms and fruit come forth in the same manner as the other do, and in as great plenty, but much smaller, and scarcely coming at any time to ripeness where they naturally grow; but, where they do become ripe, they are small, with crooked points, and black. Of the olives hereof

oil is sometimes made, which is colder and more astringent than the other, and harsher in taste and greenish in colour; but the olives are much respected, and gathered to be eaten.

PLACE AND TIME   Both kinds of olives grow in the hot countries only; in any cold climate, they will never bear fruit, nor hardly endure a winter; the manured is planted where it grows, and, according to the nature of the soil or climate, produces larger or smaller olives, and in more or less plenty; and oil sweeter or more strong in taste.

GOVERNMENT AND VIRTUES   The olive-tree is a plant of Venus, and of gentle temperature. The green leaves and branches of the olive-tree, but much more of the wild olive, do cool and bind; and the juice thereof, mixed with vinegar, is peculiarly serviceable in all hot imposthumes, inflammations, swellings, St Anthony's fire, fretting or creeping ulcers, and cankers in the flesh or mouth.

Pickled olives do stir up an appetite to meat, and, although they be hard of digestion, yet are pleasing to the stomach, being apt to putrefy therein; they are not good for the eye-sight, and cause the head-ache; if they be dried, and applied to fretting and corroding ulcers, they stop their progress, and heal them. The pickled olives burned, beaten, and applied unto weals, stop their further increase, and hinder them from rising.

The water, that is taken from the green wood when heated in the fire, heals the scurf or scab in the head, or other parts; the olive-stones, being burned, are used for the same purposes.

The oil has divers virtues, according to the ripeness or unripeness of the fruit whereof it is made, and then of the time and age thereof; and of the washing it from the salt wherewith some of it is made. The oil that is made of unripe olives is more cooling and binding than that which is made of those that are ripe; which, when it is fresh and new, is moderately heating and moistening.

The green oil of unripe olives, while it is fresh, is most welcome to the stomach; it strengthens the gums, and fastens the teeth, if it be held in the mouth for any time; and, being drunk, it prevents too great a perspiration in those who are subject thereunto. The sweet oil is of most use in salads, &c. being most pleasing to the stomach and taste; but the older the oil is, the better it is for medicine. It is also a principal ingredient in almost all salves.

The soot or dregs of the oil, the older it is, is the better for various purposes, as to heal the scab in man or beast, being used with the decoction of lupines. It is very profitably used for ulcers of the fundament or privy parts, when mixed with honey, wine, and vinegar; it heals wounds, and helps the tooth-ache, being held in the mouth; if it be boiled in a copper vessel to the thickness of honey, it binds much and is effectual for all the purposes for which *lycinus* may be used; if it be boiled with the juice of unripe grapes to the thickness of honey, and applied to the teeth, it will cause them to fall out.

ONE-BLADE

DESCRIPTION This small plant never bears more than one leaf, except only when it rises up with its stalk, in which case it bears another, but seldom more, which are of a bluish-green colour, pointed with many ribs or veins therein, like plantain; at the top of the stalk grow many small white flowers, in the form of a star, smelling somewhat sweet; after which come small berries, of a reddish colour when they are ripe. The root is small, of the bigness of a rush, lying and creeping under the upper crust of the earth, shooting forth in divers places.

PLACE It grows in moist, shadowy, and grassy, places of woods, in most parts of the kingdom.

TIME It flowers about May; the berries are ripe in June; it then quickly perishes until the next year, when it springs afresh from the old root.

GOVERNMENT AND VIRTUES It is a precious herb of the Sun. Half a drachm, or at most a drachm, in powder of the roots, taken in wine and vinegar, of each equal parts, and the party laid directly down to sweat thereupon, is held to be a sovereign remedy for those that are infected with the plague, and have a sore upon them, by expelling the poison and infection, and defending the heart and spirits from danger. It is an exceeding good wound-herb, and is therefore used with others of the like nature, in making compound balms for curing wounds, either whether they are fresh and green, or old and malignant, and especially if the sinews have been burnt.

ONIONS

GOVERNMENT AND VIRTUES Mars owns them. They possess the quality of drawing corruption to them, for if you peel one and lay it upon a dunghill, you will find it rotten in half a day, by drawing putrefaction to it; it is therefore natural to suppose they would have the same attractive power if applied to a plague-sore.

Onions are flatulent, or windy; yet do they whet the appetite, increase thirst, and ease the belly and bowels; provoke the menses; and increase sperm; especially the seed of them. Being roasted under the embers, and eaten with honey or sugar and oil, they conduce much to help an inveterate cough, and expectorate the tough phlegm. The juice being snuffed up into the nostrils, purges the head, and helps the lethargy; yet the eating of them too frequently occasions the head-ache. The eating of onions, fasting, with bread and salt, is held to be a good preservative against infection. The juice of onions is reckoned good for scalds or burns. Onions, if bruised, and mixed with salt and honey, will effectually destroy warts, causing them to come out by the roots.

Onions at different stages of growh

Leeks participate of nearly the same quality as onions, though not in so great a degree. They are said to be an antidote against a surfeit occasioned by the eating of mushrooms, being first baked under the embers, and then taken when sufficiently cool to be eaten.

ORANGE-TREE

Of oranges we shall describe five kinds or sorts. These apples were called by the ancients *mala aurea Hesperidum*, the golden apples of Hesperides; and therefore Hercules made it one of his labours to kill the dragon that kept the garden where they were, and to bring them away with him. The flowers of the orange-tree are called *napha*; and the ointment that is made of them *unguentum ex napha*. Oranges are now generally called *aurantia*.

DESCRIPTION

1. The ordinary orange-tree, *mala aurantia vulgaris*, grows often to a very great height and thickness, with large spreading arms and branches, with a rougher bark below, and green on the branches; yet it is smaller in less fruitful soils; sparingly armed with sharp but short thorns; the leaves are somewhat similar to those of the lemon, but that each leaf has a piece of a leaf set under it, are not dented at all about the edges, and are full of small holes in them; the flowers are whitish, and of a strong sweet scent; the fruit hereof is round, with a thick bitter rind, of a deep yellowish-red colour, which from it takes the name of an orange colour, having a soft, thin, white, loose, substance next to the outer coloured rind; and a sour juice lying mixed amongst small skins in several parts, with seed between them in partitions; the juice of some is less sour than others, and of a taste between sour and sweet, nearly like wine.

2. The wild or crab orange-tree, *malus aurantia sylvestris*. This tree grows wild as our crab-trees do, and is fuller of branches and thicker set with thorns than the former.

3. The apple orange, called in Latin *malus aurantia, cortice dulci eduli*. The Spaniards call this orange *naranja caxel*. This differs from others not so much in the colour of the outer bark, which is of a deep gold yellowish-red, but in the whole fruit, which is throughout almost as firm as an apricot, and yet distinguished into parts, in the inside, like others; which, together with the bark and rind, is to be eaten like an apple; the rind not being rough and bitter as the others.

4. The orange without seeds, *malus aurantia, unico grano*. This only differs from that orange which has the best four juice, in having but one grain or seed in the whole juice lying within it.

5. The dwarf orange-tree, *malus aurantia pumilio*. The stock of this dwarf-tree is low, and the branches grow thick, well stored with leaves, but they are smaller and narrower than the other; the flowers also are many, and thick set on the

branches, which bear fruit more plentifully than the former, though of a smaller size, yet equally well coloured.

PLACE AND TIME   All these sorts of oranges, as well as the lemons and citrons, are brought unto us from Spain and Portugal; they hold time with the lemons, having their leaves always green, with green blossoms and ripe fruit constantly together.

GOVERNMENT AND VIRTUES   All these trees and fruits are governed by Jupiter. The fruit is of different parts and qualities; the rind of the oranges is more bitter and hot than those of the lemons or citrons, and are therefore preferable to warm a cold stomach, breaking the wind and cutting the phlegm therein; after the bitterness is taken from them, by steeping them in water for sundry days, and then preserved either wet or dry, besides their use in banquets, they are very effectual for strengthening the heart and spirits. Though the juice is inferior to those of the citron and lemon, and fitter for meat than medicine, yet four or five ounces of the juice taken at a time, in wine or ale, will drive forth putrid humours from the inward parts by sweat, and strengthen and comfort the heart. The distilled water of the flowers, besides the odoriferous scent it has as a perfume, is good against contagious diseases and pestilential fevers; by drinking thereof at sundry times, it helps also the moist and cold infirmities of the womb; the ointment that is made of the flowers is good to anoint the stomach, to help the cough, and expectorate cold raw phlegm; and to warm and comfort the other parts of the body.

ORCHIS

DESCRIPTION   To enumerate all the different sorts of it is needless; a description of the roots will be sufficient, which are to be used with some discretion. They have each of them a double root within, some of them round, others like a hand; these roots alter every year alternately; when the one rises and waxes full, the other grows lank and perishes; now it is those which are full-grown that are to be used in medicine, the other being either of no use at all, or else, according to some, thwarting the operation of the full-grown root, and undoing what otherwise it might have effected.

TIME   One or other of them may be found in flower from the beginning of April to the latter end of August.

GOVERNMENT AND VIRTUES   They are hot and moist in operation; under the dominion of Venus, and provoke lust exceedingly; which, it is said, the dry and withered roots restrain again.

ORPINE

DESCRIPTION   common orpine rises up with divers round brittle stalks thick set with fat and fleshy leaves, without any order, and very little dented about the edges, of a pale green colour; the flowers are white, or whitish, growing in tufts, after which come small chaff-like husks, with seed-like dust in them. The roots are various in their shape and size, and the plant does not grow so large in some places as in others.

PLACE   It is to be found in almost every part of this kingdom, but most commonly in gardens, where it grows to a larger size than that which is wild; it is also to be found in the shadowy sides of fields and woods.

TIME   It flowers about July, and the seed is ripe in August.

GOVERNMENT AND VIRTUES   The Moon owns this herb. Orpine is seldom used in inward medicines with us, although Tragus says, from experience in Germany, that the distilled water thereof is profitable for gnawings or excoriations in the stomach and bowels, and for ulcers in the lungs, liver, or other inward parts; as also in the matrix; being drunk for several days successively, it helps all those diseases; he also says it stays the sharpness of the humours in the bloody flux; and other fluxes of the body, or in wounds; the root thereof has also the same effect. It is used outwardly to cool any heat or inflammation upon any hurt or wound, and eases the pains of them; as also to heal scalds or burns. The juice thereof beaten with some salad-oil, and therewith anointing the parts, or the leaf bruised and laid to any green wounds in the hands and legs, does quickly heal them; and, being bound to the throat, much helps the quinsey; it is likewise found serviceable in ruptures.

The juice thereof, made into a syrup with honey or sugar, may be safely taken, a spoonful or two at a time, and with good effect, for a quinsey; and will be found more speedy in operation, as well as pleasant in taste, than some other medicines prescribed for that disorder.

PARSLEY

GOVERNMENT AND VIRTUES   It is under the dominion of Mercury, and is very comfortable to the stomach; it helps to provoke urine, women's menses, and to break wind both in the stomach and bowels; it a little opens the body, but the root possesses this last virtue in a greater degree, opening obstructions both of the liver and spleen; and is therefore accounted one of the five opening roots; Galen commends it against the falling sickness, and says it mightily provokes urine, if boiled and eaten like parsnips. The seed is also effectual to provoke urine and women's menses, expel wind, break the stone, and ease the pains and torments thereof, or of any other part of the body, occasioned by wind. The distilled water of parsley is a familiar medicine with nurses to give to children when they are troubled with wind in the stomach or belly, which they call the frets; it is also greatly useful to grown persons. The leaves of parsley, when used with bread or meal, and laid to the eyes that are inflamed with heat, or swollen, does greatly relieve them; and, being fried with butter, and applied to women's breasts that are hard through the curdling of the milk, it quickly abates the hardness; it also takes away black and blue marks arising from bruises or falls. The juice, dropped into the ears with a little wine, eases the pains thereof. Tragus recommends the following, as an excellent medicine to help the jaundice and falling sickness, the dropsy, and stone in the kidneys, *viz*. Take of the seeds of parsley, fennel, anise, and carraways, of each an ounce; of the roots of parsley, burnet, saxifrage, and carraways, of each one ounce and an half; let the seeds be bruised, and the roots washed and cut small; let them lie all night in steep in a pottle of white wine, and in the morning be boiled in a close earthen vessel until a third part or more be wasted, which, being strained and cleared, take four ounces thereof morning and evening, first and last, abstaining from drink after it for three hours. This opens obstructions of the liver and spleen, and expels the dropsy and jaundice by urine.

PARSLEY-PERT, OR PARSLEY-BREAKSTONE

DESCRIPTION the root, although it be small and thready, yet it continues many years, from whence arise many leaves lying along upon the ground, each standing upon a long small footstalk, the leaves as broad as a man's nail, very deeply indented on the edges, somewhat like a parsley leaf, but of a very dusky-green colour. The stalks are very weak and slender, about three or four fingers in length, set so full of leaves that they can hardly be seen, either having no footstalk at all, or but very short. The flowers are so small they can hardly be seen, and the seed is scarcely perceptible at all.

PLACE It is common through all parts of the kingdom, and is generally to be met with in barren, sandy, and moist, places. It may be found plentifully about Hampstead Heath, in Hyde-park, and in other places near London.

TIME It may be found all the summer through, from the beginning of April to the end of October.

GOVERNMENT AND VIRTUES Its operation is very prevalent to provoke urine and to break the stone. It is a very good salad-herb, and would pickle for winter use as well as samphire. It is a very wholesome herb. A drachm of the powder of it, taken in white wine, brings away gravel from the kidneys insensibly, and without pain. It also helps the difficulty in passing urine.

PARSNIP

DESCRIPTION The wild parsnip differs little from that of the garden, but does not grow so fair or large, nor has it so many leaves; the root is shorter, more woody, and not so fit to be eaten; therefore the more medicinable.

PLACE It grows wild in divers places, as in the marshes by Rochester, and elsewhere, and flowers in July; the seed being ripe about the beginning of August the second year after the sowing; seldom flowering the first year.

GOVERNMENT AND VIRTUES The garden parsnip is under Venus. It is exceeding good and wholesome nourishment, though rather windy; it is said to provoke venery, notwithstanding which it fattens the body much if frequently used. It is also serviceable to the stomach and reins, and provokes urine. But the wild parsnip has a cutting, attenuating, cleansing, and opening, quality therein. It eases pains and stitches in the sides, and dissolves wind both in the stomach and bowels; it also provokes urine. The root is often used, but the seed much more. The wild parsnip being preferable to that of the garden, shews nature to be the best physician.

COW-PARSNIP

DESCRIPTION this grows with three or four large, spread, winged, rough leaves, lying often on the ground, or else raised a little from it, with long, round, hairy, footstalks under them, parted usually into five divisions, the two couples standing against each other, and one at the end, and each leaf being almost round, yet somewhat deeply cut in on the edges in some leaves, and not so deep in others, of a whitish-green colour, smelling somewhat strongly; among which arises up a round crested hairy stalk, two or three feet high, with a few joints and leaves thereon, and branched at the top, where stand large umbels of white, and sometimes reddish, flowers, and, after them, flat, whitish, thin, winged seed, two always joined together. The root is long and white, with two or three long strings growing down into the ground, smelling likewise strong and unpleasant.

PLACE It grows in moist meadows, the borders and corners of fields, and near ditches, generally throughout the kingdom.

TIME It flowers in July, and seeds in August.

GOVERNMENT AND VIRTUES Mercury has the dominion over them. The seed hereof, as Galen says, is of a sharp and cutting quality, and is therefore a fit medicine for the cough and shortness of breath, the falling sickness, and the jaundice. The root is available to all the purposes aforesaid, and is also of great use to take away the hard skin that grows on a fistula, by scraping it upon the part. The seed hereof, being drunk, cleanses the belly from tough phlegmatic matter. The seed and root, being boiled in oil, and the head rubbed therewith, help not only those labouring under a phrenzy, but also the lethargy or drowsy evil. It also helps the shingles.

PEACH-TREE

DESCRIPTION the peach-tree does not grow so large as the apricot-tree, yet has it tolerable wide-spreading branches, from whence spring smaller reddish twigs, whereon are set long and narrow green leaves, dented about the edges. The blossoms are larger than those of the plum, and of a light purple. The fruit is round, and sometimes as big as a middle-sized pippin; others are smaller, and differing in colour and taste, as russet, red, or yellow, watery, or firm, with a frieze or cotton all over, a cleft therein like an apricot, and a rugged furrowed great stone within it, which contains a bitter kernel. It sooner waxes old and decays than the apricot-tree.

PLACE They are nursed up in gardens and orchards.

TIME They flower in the spring, and fructify in autumn.

GOVERNMENT AND VIRTUES Venus owns this tree, and by it opposes the ill effects of Mars. Nothing is better to purge choler in children than the leaves of this tree made into a syrup or conserve, of which two spoonfuls at a time may safely be taken. The leaves of peaches, being dried, are a safe medicine. The powder of them strewed upon fresh bleeding wounds, stays their bleeding, and closes them up. The flowers, steeped all night in a little warm wine strained forth in the morning, and drunk fasting, do gently open the belly. A syrup made of them, as the syrup of roses is made, operates more forcibly than that of roses, as it provokes vomiting. The flowers made into a conserve produce the same effect. The liquor, which drops from the tree on its being wounded, is given in the decoction of coltsfoot to those that are troubled with the cough or shortness of breath; by adding thereto some sweet wine, and putting also some saffron therein, it is good for those that are hoarse, or have lost their voice; it helps all defects of the lungs. Two drachms thereof given in the juice of lemons, or of radishes, are good for those that are troubled with the stone.

PEAR-TREE

GOVERNMENT AND VIRTUES This tree belongs to Venus, as well as the apple-tree. For their physical use, they are best discerned by their tastes. All

PLATE 15

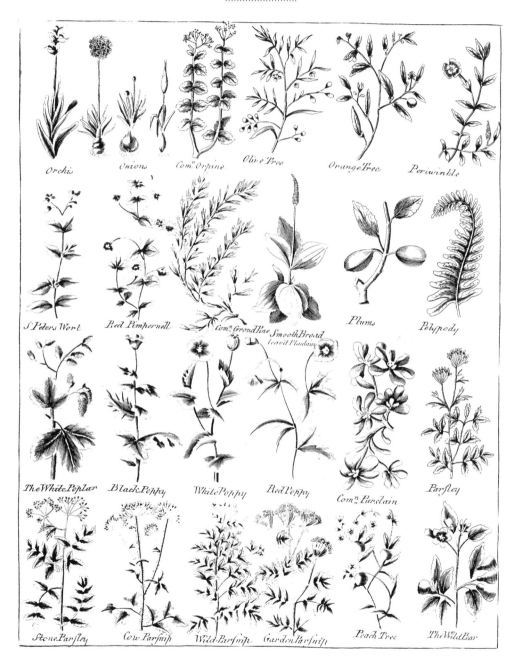

Orchis   Onions   Com.ⁿ Orpine   Olive Tree   Orange Tree   Periwinkle

S.ᵗ Peters Wort   Red Pimpernell   Com.ⁿ Ground Pine   Smooth Broad leav'd Plantain   Plums   Polypody

The White Poplar   Black Poppy   White Poppy   Red Poppy   Com.ⁿ Purslain   Parsley

Stone Parsley   Cow Parsnip   Wild Parsnip   Garden Parsnip   Peach Tree   The Wild Pear the sweet or luscious sorts, whether manured or wild, tend to open the belly more or less; those, on the contrary, that are sour and harsh, have an astringent quality; the leaves of each possess the same contrariety of properties. Those that are moist are, in some degree, of a cooling nature; but the harsh or wild sorts are much more so, and are frequently used as repelling medicines; if the wild sort be boiled with mushrooms, it makes them the less dangerous. The said pears, boiled with a little honey, help much the oppression of the stomach; but the harsher kinds are most cooling and binding. They are very useful to bind up green wounds, stopping the blood and healing the wound without further trouble or inflammation, as Galen says he has found by experience. Wild pears sooner close up the lips of green wounds than the others.

PELLITORY OF SPAIN

DESCRIPTION Pellitory is a very common plant, yet must be diligently looked after to be brought to perfection. The root goes downright into the ground, bearing leaves long and finely cut upon the stalks, lying upon the ground, much larger than the leaves of camomile are; at the top it bears one single large flower at a place, having a border of many leaves, white on the upper side, and reddish underneath, with a yellow thrum in the middle, not standing so close as that of camomile.

The other common pellitory, which grows here spontaneously, has a root of a sharp biting taste, scarcely disernible by the taste from that before described, from whence arise divers brittle stalks, more than a yard high, with narrow long leaves, finely dented about the edges, standing one above another up to the top. The flowers are many and white, standing in tufts like those of yarrow, with a small yellowish thrum in the middle. The seed is very small.

PLACE The last grows in fields, by the hedge-sides, and paths, almost every where in Britain.

TIME It flowers at the latter end of June, and in July.

GOVERNMENT AND VIRTUES It is under the government of Mercury, and is one of the best purgers of the brain that grows. Either the herb or root dried and chewed in the mouth, purges the brain of phlegmatic humours, thereby not only easing pains in the head and teeth, but also hindering the distilling of the brain upon the lungs and eyes, and preventing cough, phthisics, and consumptions, the apoplexy, and falling sickness. It is an excellent approved remedy in the lethargy. The powder of the herb or root, being snuffed up the nostrils, procures sneezing, and eases the head-ache.

PELLITORY OF THE WALL

DESCRIPTION it rises up with many brownish-red, tender, weak, clear, and almost transparent, stalks, about two feet high, upon which grow at the several joints two leaves somewhat broad and long, of a dark green colour, which afterwards turns brownish, smooth on the edges, but rough and hairy, as the stalks are also. At the joints with the leaves, from the middle of the stalks upwards, where it spreads into some branches, stand many small, pale, purplish, flowers, in hairy rough heads or husks, after which come small, black, and rough, seed, which sticks to any cloth or garment it may chance to touch. The root is somewhat long, with many small fibres thereat, of a dark reddish colour, which abides the winter, although the stalks and leaves perish, and spring afresh every year.

PLACE It generally grows wild, in most parts of the kingdom, about the borders of fields, and by the sides of walls. It prospers well when brought up in gardens, and, if once planted on the shady side, it will afterwards spring of its own sowing.

TIME It flowers in June, July, and beginning of August, and the seed is ripe soon after.

GOVERNMENT AND VIRTUES It is under the dominion of Mercury. The dried herb pellitory made up into a electuary with honey, or the juice of the herb, or the decoction thereof made up with sugar or honey, is a singular remedy for any old or dry cough, shortness of breath, and wheezing in the throat. Three ounces of the juice thereof, taken at a time, greatly helps the stoppage of urine, and expel the stone or gravel in the kidneys or bladder, and are therefore usually put among other herbs; used in clysters to mitigate pains in the back, sides, or bowels, proceeding from wind, stoppage of urine, the gravel, or stone, as aforesaid. The decoction of the herb, being drunk, eases pains of the womb, and forwards the menses; it also eases such complaints as arise from obstructions of the liver, spleen, and reins. The same decoction, with a little honey added thereto, is good to gargle a sore throat. The juice, if held a while in the mouth, eases pains in the teeth. The distilled water of the herb, drunk with some sugar, produces the same effect; it also cleanses the skin. The juice, or herb itself, bruised, with a little salt, is very effectual to cleanse fistulas and to heal them up safely; it is also of great benefit to any green wound. A poultice made hereof with mallows, and boiled in wine, mixed with wheat, bran, bean-flowers, and some oil, being applied warm to any bruised sinew, tendon, or muscle, does, in a very short time, restore it to its original strength.

The juice of pellitory of the wall, clarified and boiled into a syrup with honey, and a spoonful of it drunk every morning, is very good for the dropsy.

PENNY-ROYAL

DESCRIPTION   the common penny-royal is so well known, that it needs no description. There is another kind of penny-royal, superior to the above, which differs only in the largeness of the leaves and stalks; in rising higher, and drooping upon the ground so much. The flowers of which are purple, growing in rundles about the stalk like the other.

PLACE   The first, which is common in gardens, grows also in many moist and watery places in this kingdom. The second is found wild in Essex, and divers places on the road from London to Colchester, and parts adjacent.

TIME   They flower in the latter end of summer.

GOVERNMENT AND VIRTUES   This herb is under Venus. Dioscorides says, that penny-royal makes tough phlegm thin, warms the coldness of any part that it is applied to, and digests raw and corrupt matter: being boiled and drunk, it removes the menses, and expels the dead child and after-birth; being mixed with honey and salt, it voids phlegm out of the lungs. Applied to the nostrils, with vinegar, it is very reviving to persons fainting and swooning; being dried and burnt, it strengthens the gums, and is helpful to those that are troubled with the gout; being applied as a plaster, it takes away carbuncles and blotches from the face; applied with salt, it helps those that are splenetic, or liver-grown. The decoction does help the itch, if washed therewith; being put into baths for women to sit therein, it helps the swelling and hardness of the womb.

The green herb bruised, and boiled in wine, with honey and salt, helps the tooth-ache. It helps the cold griefs of the joints, taking away the pains and warming the cold parts, being fast bound to the place after bathing or sweating. Pliny adds, that penny-royal and mint together help faintings or swoonings, infused in vinegar, and put to the nostrils, or a little thereof put into the mouth. It easeth the head-ache, and the pains of the breast and belly, stays the gnawing of the stomach, and inward pains of the bowels; being drunk with wine, it provokes the menses, and expels the dead child and after-birth; it helps the falling-sickness: put into unwholesome or stinking water that men must drink, as at sea, and where other cannot be had, it makes it less hurtful. It helps cramps or convulsions of the sinews, being applied with honey, salt, and vinegar. It is very effectual for a cough, being boiled in milk and drunk, and for ulcers and sores in the mouth.

PEONY, MALE AND FEMALE

DESCRIPTION   The male peony rises up with many brownish stalks, whereon grow a great number of fair green, and sometimes reddish, leaves,

Male peony

Female peony

each of which is set against another upon a stalk without any particular division in the leaf. The flowers stand at the tops of the stalks, consisting of five or six broad leaves of a fair purplish-red colour, with many yellow threads in the middle, standing about the head, which after rises to be the seed-vessel, divided into two, three, or four, rough crooked pods like horns, which, being full ripe, open and turn themselves down one edge to another backward, shewing within them divers round, black, shining, seed, having also many red or crimson grains intermixed with the black, whereby it makes a very pretty show. The roots are thick and long, spreading and running down deep into the ground.

The ordinary female peony has many stalks, and more leaves than the male; the leaves not so large, but nicked on the edges, some with great and deep, others with smaller, cuts and divisions, of a dark or dead-green colour. The flowers are of a strong heady scent, most usually smaller, and of a more purple colour than the male, with yellow thrums about the head as the male has. The seed-vessels are like horns, as in the male, but smaller; the seed is black but less shining. The roots consist of many thick and short tuberous clogs, fastened at the ends of long strings, and all from the head of the root, which is thick and short, and of the like scent with the male.

PLACE AND TIME They grow in gardens, and flower usually about May.

GOVERNMENT AND VIRTUES It is an herb of the Sun, and under the lion. Physicians say, male peony roots are best; but male peony is best for men, and female peony for women. The roots are held to be of most virtue; then the seeds; next the flowers; and, last of all, the leaves. The root of the male peony, fresh gathered, has been found by experience to cure the falling sickness; but the surest way is to take the root of the male peony washed clean and stamped somewhat small, and infuse it in sack for twenty-four hours at least; afterwards strain it, and take, morning and evening, a good draught for sundry days together before and after a full moon; and this will also cure older persons, if the disease be not inveterate and past cure, especially if there be a due and orderly preparation of the body, with posset-drink made of betony, &c. .

PEPPER

KINDS AND NAMES there are several sorts of pepper, as black, white, and long, pepper; called *piper nigrum, album, et longum*. The black, and white, pepper, differ not either in manner of growing, or in form of leaf or fruit. The long pepper also grows in the same manner, but differs in the fruit. All these sorts grow on a climbing bush, in the East Indies, after one manner, that is, as hops grow with us; so that, if they be not sustained by some tree or pole, on which they may climb and spread, they will lie down on the ground, and thereon run and shoot forth small fibres at every joint. But the usual manner is

PLATE 16
....

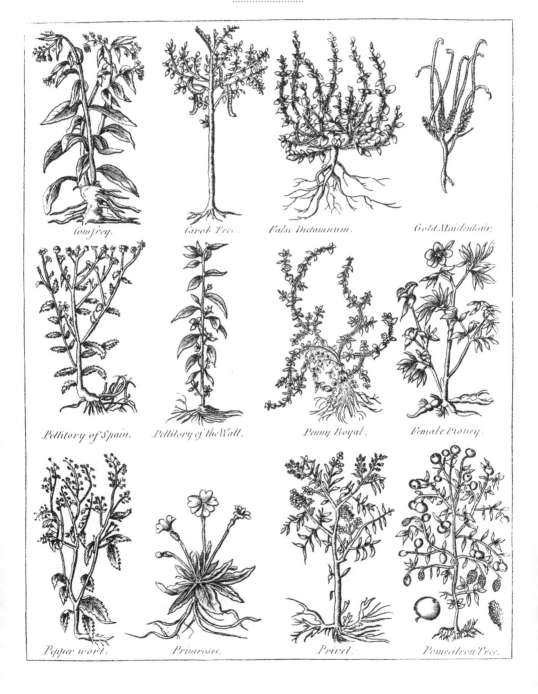

Comfrey.

Carob Tree.

False Dictamnum.

Gold Maidenhair.

Pellitory of Spain.

Pellitory of the Wall.

Penny Royal.

Female Pioney.

Pepper wort.

Primroses.

Privet.

Pomcitron Tree.

to plant a branch taken from the bush near some tall tree, great cane, or pole; and so it will quickly, by winding itself about such props, get to the top thereof; it is full of joints, and shoots forth fair, large, leaves, one at each joint, being almost round, but ending in a point, green above and paler underneath, with a great middle-rib, and four other ribs, somewhat less, spreading from it, two on each side, and smaller therein also, unto the edges, which are smooth and plain, somewhat thin, and set on a pretty long footstalk. The fruit, or pepper, whether black, white, or long, grows at the same joint, but on the contrary side, opposite to the leaf, round about a long stalk, somewhat thinly set all along thereon, or not so close as a bunch of grapes; the root has sundry joints creeping in the ground, with fibres at the joints. The white pepper is hardly distinguishable from the black, by the plants thereof, until it become ripe (for the white and black pepper grow on different bushes) but that the leaves are of a little paler green colour, and the grains or berries are white, solid, firm, without wrinkles, and more aromatic. The long pepper has leaves of very near the same form and size, but a little longer pointed, of a paler green colour, thinner also, and with a shorter foot-stalk, but four or five ribs sometimes on each side, according to the largeness of the leaf, with other smaller veins therein, and has less acrimony and hot taste than the black. The fruit of this also grows in like manner at the joints, opposite to each leaf, which are closer set together than in the black, consisting of many small grains as it were set close together in rows, and not open and separate as in the black and white pepper; of an ash colour when it is ripe.

GOVERNMENT AND VIRTUES All the peppers are under the dominion of Mars, and of temperature hot and dry almost in the fourth degree, but the white pepper is the hottest; which sort is much used by the Indians, many of whom use the leaves as Europeans do tobacco; and even the pepper itself they also chew, taking from the branch one grain after another, while they are fresh.

PEPPER-WORT, OR DITTANDER

DESCRIPTION the common pepper-wort sends forth somewhat long and broad leaves, of a light bluish-green colour, finely dented about the edges, and pointed at the ends, standing upon round hard stalks, three or four feet high, spreading many branches on all sides, and having many small white flowers at the tops of them, after which follow small seed in small heads. The root is slender, running much under ground, and shooting up again in many places; and both leaves and roots are very hot and sharp of taste, like pepper, for which cause it took the name.

PLACE It grows naturally in many parts of the kingdom, as at Clare in Essex; also near unto Exeter, Devonshire; upon Rochester Common, Kent; Lancashire, and divers other places; but is usually kept in gardens.

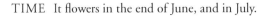
TIME It flowers in the end of June, and in July.

GOVERNMENT AND VIRTUES This herb is under the direction of Mars. Pliny and Paulus Æginetus say, that pepper-wort is very effectual for the sciatica, or any other gout, pain in the joints, or any other inveterate grief; the leaves to be bruised and mixed with hog's-lard, and applied to the place; it also amends the deformities or discolourings of the skin, and helps to take away marks, scars, and scabs, or the marks of burning with fire or iron. The juice hereof is in some places used to be given in ale to women with child, to procure them a speedy delivery.

PERIWINKLE

DESCRIPTION The common sort has many branches running upon the ground, shooting out small fibres at the joints as it runs, taking thereby hold in the ground, and roots in divers places; at the joints of these branches stand two small dark green shining leaves, somewhat like bay-leaves, but smaller, and with them come forth also flowers, one at a joint standing upon a tender footstalk, being somewhat long and hollow, parted at the brims sometimes into four, sometimes into five, leaves; the most ordinary sort are of a pale blue colour, some are pure white, and some of a dark reddish-purple colour. The root is little bigger than a rush, bushing in the ground, and creeping with its branches, and is most usually planted under hedges, where it may have room to grow.

PLACE Those with the pale blue and with the white flowers grow in woods and orchards by the hedge-sides in divers places of this land, but those with the purple flowers in gardens only.

TIME They flower in March and April.

GOVERNMENT AND VIRTUES Venus owns this herb, and says that the leaves, eaten by man and wife together, cause love between them. The periwinkle is a great binder, staying bleeding both at mouth and nose, if some of the leaves be chewed; the French use it to stay women's menses.

ST PETER'S WORT

DESCRIPTION It rises up with square upright stalks for the most part, somewhat greater and higher than St John's wort, but brown in the same manner, having two leaves at every joint, somewhat like, but larger than, St John's wort; and a little rounder pointed, with few or no holes to be seen therein, and having sometimes some smaller leaves rising from the bosom of the greater, and sometimes a little hairy also. At the tops of the stalks stand many star-like flowers, with yellow threads in the middle, very like those of St John's wort, insomuch that this is hardly to be discerned from it, but only by the largeness and height, the seed being alike in both. The root abides long, sending forth new shoots every year.

PLACE It grows in many groves and small low woods, in divers places of this land, as in Kent, Huntingdonshire, Cambridgeshire, and Northamptonshire; as also near water-courses in other places.

TIME It flowers in June and July, and the seed is ripe in August.

GOVERNMENT AND VIRTUES It is of the same property with St John's wort, but somewhat weak, and therefore more seldom used. Two drachms of the seed taken at a time, in honeyed water, purge choleric humours, as says Dioscorides, Pliny, and Galen, and thereby help those that are troubled with the sciatica. The leaves are used, as St John's wort, to help those places of the body that have been burnt with fire.

PIMPERNEL

DESCRIPTION Common pimpernel has many weak square stalks lying on the ground, beset all along with two small and almost round leaves at every joint one against another, very like chickweed; but has no footstalks, for the leaves as it were compass the stalk: the flowers stand singly, consisting of five round small pointed leaves of a fine pale red colour, with so many threads in the middle, in whose places succeed smooth round heads, wherein is contained small seed. The root is small and fibrous, perishing every year.

PLACE It grows every where almost, as well in the meadows and corn-fields as by the way-sides, and in gardens, arising of itself.

TIME It flowers from May to August, and the seed ripens in the mean time and falls.

GOVERNMENT AND VIRTUES It is a solar herb. This is of a cleansing and attractive quality, whereby it draws forth thorns or splinters, or other such-like things, from the flesh, and, put up into the nostrils, purges the head; and Galen says also, they have a drying faculty, whereby they are good to close the lips of wounds, and to cleanse ulcers. The distilled water or juice is much esteemed by the French to cleanse the skin from any roughness, deformity, or discolouring.

GROUND-PINE

DESCRIPTION   The common ground-pine grows low, seldom above a hand's breadth high, shooting forth divers small branches, set with slender small long narrow greyish or whitish leaves, somewhat hairy, and divided into three parts, many times bushing together at a joint, and sometimes some growing scatteredly upon the stalks, smelling somewhat strong like unto rosin; the flowers are somewhat small and of a pale yellow colour, growing from the joints of the stalks all along among the leaves, after which come small and round husks: the root is small and woody, perishing every year.

PLACE   It grows more plentifully in Kent than in any other county of this land; as also in many places from on this side of Dartford, along to Rochester, and upon Chatham down.

TIME   It flowers and gives seed in the summer months.

GOVERNMENT AND VIRTUES   Mars owns this herb. The decoction of ground-pine, drunk, does wonderfully prevail against the difficulty in passing urine, or any inward pains arising from the diseases of the reins and urine, and is good for all obstructions of the liver and spleen, and gently opens the body, for which purpose they were wont in former times to make pills with the powder thereof and the purple figs. It helps the diseases of the womb, used inwardly or applied outwardly, procuring the menses, and expelling the after-birth. It acts so powerfully, that it is utterly forbidden for women with child, in that it will cause abortion, or delivery before the time: it is effectual also in all pains and diseases of the joints, as gouts, cramps, palsies, sciatica, and aches; either the decoction of the herb in wine taken inwardly or applied outwardly, or both, for some time together; for which purpose the pills, made with the powder of ground-pine, and of hermodactils, with Venice turpentine, are very effectual. These pills also are good for the dropsy, to be continued for some time. The same is a good help for the jaundice, and for griping pains in the joints, belly, or inward parts; it helps also all diseases of the brain, proceeding of cold and phlegmatic humours and distillations, as also the falling-sickness. It is a good remedy for a cold cough, especially in the beginning.

PITCH AND TAR

KINDS AND NAMES   There are two sorts of pitch: the one moist, called liquid pitch, the other is hard and dry: they do both run out of the pine and pitch tree, and out of certain other trees, as the cedar, turpentine, and larch, trees, by burning of the wood and timber of them. Pitch is called in Latin *pix*, in French *poix*, in Dutch *peck*. The liquid pitch is called in Latin *pix liquida*, in

Brabant *teer*, and in English tar. The dry pitch is called in Latin *pix arida*, and *navalis*; in English ship-pitch or stone-pitch; in Dutch *steen-peck*.

GOVERNMENT AND VIRTUES The pitch and tar are both solar, hot and dry in the second degree, and of subtle parts, but the stone-pitch is the driest; the liquid pitch or tar is the hottest and of more subtle parts. Liquid-pitch, taken with honey, does cleanse the breast, and is good to be licked in by those that are troubled with shortness of breath, whose inside is clogged with corrupt matter. It mollifies and brings to perfection all hard swellings, and is good to anoint the neck against the squinancy or swelling of the throat; it is good to be put into mollifying plasters, anodyne to take away pains, and maturative or ripening medicines; being applied with barley-meal, it softens the hardness of the matrix and fundament.

The stone-pitch, being pounded very small, with the fine powder of frankincense, heals hollow ulcers and fistulas, filling them up with flesh: the stone-pitch is not so strong as the liquid pitch, but is much better, it being more apt to close up the lips of wounds.

PITCH-TREE

This tree is called in latin *picea* and *pitis*.

DESCRIPTION The pitch-tree is of an indifferent bigness, and tall stature, but not so great as the pine-tree, and always green, like the pine and fir tree. The timber is fat, and does yield an abundance of rosin of divers sorts; the branches are hard, and parted into other sprays, most commonly cross-wise, upon which grow small green leaves, not round about the branches, but by every side, one right over against another, like little feathers: the fruit is smaller than the fruit of the pine-tree. In burning of this tree, there does issue out pitch, as does also out of the pine-tree.

PLACE AND TIME The pitch-tree grows in many places of Greece, Italy, France, and Germany; and the fruit thereof is ripe in September.

GOVERNMENT AND VIRTUES The leaves, bark, fruit, kernels, or nuts, of this tree, are almost of the same nature, virtues, and operations, as the leaves, bark, fruit, and kernels, of the pine-tree. Out of the pine and pitch-trees come three sorts of rosin, besides the pitch and tar.
1. The one flows out by force of the heat of the Sun in summer, from the wood or timber where it is broken or cut.
2. The other is found both upon and between the bark of the pine and pitch-tree, and most commonly in such parts thereof as are cut or any other way impaired.

3. The third kind grows betwixt the scales of the fruit.

All the rosins are solar, and of an hot and dry temperature, and of a scouring and cleansing nature. Rosin does cleanse and heal fresh wounds, and therefore is a principal ingredient in all ointments and plasters that serve for that purpose. It softens hard swellings, and is comfortable to bruised parts or members, being applied or laid to, with oils, ointments, or plasters, appropriated to that use.

PLANTAIN

TIME It is in its beauty about June, and the seed ripens shortly after.

GOVERNMENT AND VIRTUES It is under the command of Venus, and cures the head by antipathy to Mars, and the privities by sympathy to Venus; neither is there hardly a martial disease but it cures. The juice of plaintain, clarified and drunk for divers days together, either by itself or in other drink, prevails wonderfully against all torments or excoriations in the bowels, helps the distillations of rheum from the head, and stays all manner of fluxes, even women's menses when they flow too abundantly.

It is good to stay spitting of blood, and other bleeding at the mouth, or the making of foul or bloody water by reason of any ulcer in the reins or bladder; and also stays the too free bleeding of wounds. It is held an especial remedy for those that are troubled with the phthisic, or consumption of the lungs, or ulcers in the lungs, or coughs that come of heat. The decoction or powder of the roots or seed is much more binding for all the purposes aforesaid than the leaves. The roots of plantain and pellitory of Spain beaten to powder, and put into hollow teeth, take away the pains of them: the clarified juice or distilled water dropped into the eyes cools the inflammations in them, and takes away the pin and web; and, dropped into the ears, eases pains in them, and helps and restores the hearing: the same also, with juice of houseleek, is profitable against all inflammations and breakings out of the skin, and against burnings and scaldings by fire or water. The plantains are singular good wound-herbs, to heal fresh or old wounds or sores, either inward or outward.

PLUMS

GOVERNMENT AND VIRTUES All plums are under Venus. The dried fruit, sold by the grocers under the name of damask prunes, do somewhat loosen the belly, and, being stewed, are often used, both in health and sickness, to procure appetite, and gently open the belly, allay choler, and cool the stomach. The juice of plum-tree leaves, boiled in wine, is good to wash and gargle the mouth and throat, to dry the flux of rheum coming to the palate, gums, or almonds of the ears.

The gum of the tree is good to break the stone. The gum, or leaves, boiled in vinegar, and applied, will kill tetters and ringworms. Mathiolus says, the oil pressed out of the stones, as oil of almonds is made, is good against the inflamed piles, the tumours or swellings of ulcers, hoarseness of the voice, roughness of the tongue and throat, and likewise pains in the ears. Five ounces of the said oil, taken with one ounce of muscadine, will expel the stone, and help the cholic.

POLYPODY OF THE OAK

DESCRIPTION   This is a small herb, consisting of nothing but roots and leaves, bearing neither stalk, flower, nor seed, as it is thought. It has three or four leaves rising from the root, every one singly by itself, of about a hand's length, which are winged, consisting of many small narrow leaves, cut into the middle rib, standing on each side of the stalk, large below, and smaller up to the top, not dented or notched on the edges at all like the male fern; of a sad-green colour, and smooth on the upper side, but on the under side somewhat rough, by reason of some yellowish spots thereon. The root is smaller than one's little finger, lying sloping, or creeping along under the upper crust of the earth, brownish on the outside, greenish within, of a sweet harshness in taste, set with certain rough knobs on each side thereof, having also much moss or yellow hair upon it, and some fibres underneath, whereby it is nourished.

PLACE   It grows as well upon old rotten stumps or trunks of trees, as oak, beech, hasel, willow, or any other, as in the woods under them, and upon old mud walls; also in mossy, stony, and gravelly, places, near unto the woods. That which grows upon oak is accounted the best, but the quantity thereof is scarcely sufficient for common use.

TIME   Being always green, it may be gathered for use at any time.

GOVERNMENT AND VIRTUES   It is an herb of Saturn. Polypodium of the oak is dearest; but that which grows upon the ground is best to purge melancholy; if the humour proceed from other causes, choose your polypodium accordingly. Mesue says, that it dries up thin humours, digests thick and tough and purges burnt choler, and especially thick and tough phlegm, and thin phlegm also, even from the joints; and is therefore good for those that are troubled with melancholy, or quartan agues, especially if it be taken in whey or honeyed water, in barley water, or the broth of a chicken, with epythimum, or with beets and mallows. It is also good for the hardness of the spleen, and for prickings or stitches in the sides, as also for the cholic; some choose to put to it some fennel, aniseed, or ginger, and an ounce of it may be given at a time in a decoction, if there be not sena or some other strong purger mixed with it. A drachm or two of the powder of the dried roots, taken fasting in a cup of honeyed water, works gently and for the purposes aforesaid. The distilled water, both from the roots and leaves, is much commended for the quartan ague, if taken for several days together; as also against the cough, shortness of breath, and wheezings, and those distillations of thin rheum upon the lungs which cause phthisics, and oftentimes consumptions. The fresh roots beaten small, or the powder of the dried roots mixed with honey, and applied to any of the limbs out of joint, does much help them.

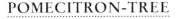

POMECITRON-TREE

There are three kinds of pomecitrons. The tree is generally called *malus medica, vel citria.*

DESCRIPTION
1. The greater pomecitron-tree, or *malus citra major*. This tree does not grow very high in some places, but rather with a short crooked body, and in others not much lower than the lemon-tree, spreading out into sundry great long arms and branches; set with long and sharp thorns, and fair, large, and broad, fresh green leaves, a little dented about the edges, with a shew of almost invisible holes in them, but less than the orange-leaves have; of a very sweet scent, the flowers green at the leaves, all along the branches, being somewhat longer than those of the orange; made of five thick, whitish, purple, or bluish, leaves, with some threads in the middle, after which follows fruit all the year, being seldom seen without ripe fruit, and half-ripe, and some young and green, and blossoms, all at once. This kind bears great and large fruit, some the size of a musk melon, others less, but all of them with a rugged, bunched out, and uneven, yellow bark, thicker than in any of the other sorts, with a sour juice in the middle, and somewhat great, pale, whitish, or yellow, seed, with a bitter kernel lying in it; the smell of this fruit is very strong and comfortable to the senses.
2. The smaller pomecitron-tree, *citra malus minor, five limonera*; this tree grows very like the former, but the leaves are somewhat smaller and shorter, and so are the thorns; the flowers are of a deep-bluish colour, and the fruit less and longer than they, but no larger than the small fruit of the former; the rind is also thick and yellow, but not so rugged, having more sour juice and fewer seeds.
3. *Citria malus, sive limonera pregnans*. This differs very little from the foregoing tree described.

PLACE AND TIME All these sorts of citrons are cultivated in Spain, by the curious, but were transported thither from sundry places abroad. The great pomecitron was brought first from Media and Persia, and was therefore called *malum Medicum* and *malum Persicum*. The last was brought for the Fortunate Islands. They are continually in flower, and bear fruit throughout the year.

GOVERNMENT AND VIRTUES These are solar plants, yet they are of different qualities; all the parts of the fruit hereof, both the outer and inner rind, as well as the juice and seed, are of excellent use, though of contrary effects one to another; some being hot and dry, whilst others are cold and dry.

The outer yellow rind is very sweet in smell, highly aromatic and bitter in taste; and, dried, it warms and comforts a cold and windy stomach, and disperses cold, raw, and undigested, humours therein, or in the bowels, and mightily expels wind.

Being chewed in the mouth, it helps a stinking breath; it also helps digestion, and is good against melancholy. The outer rinds are often used in cordial electuaries, and preservatives against infection and melancholy.

The inner white rind of this fruit is rather unsavoury, almost without taste, and is not used in physic. The sour juice in the middle is cold, and far surpasses that of lemons in its effects, although not so sharp in taste. It is singularly good to suppress the choler and hot distemper of the blood, and to quench thirst; and corrects the bad disposition of the liver. It stirs up an appetite, and refreshes the over-spent and fainting spirits. The seed not only equals the rind in its virtues, but in many instances surpasses it.

POMEGRANATE-TREE

KINDS AND NAMES The pomegrante-tree is distinguished into three kinds; that is, the manured pomegranate bearing fruit, and the greater and less wild kind: that first is called *malus punicum* and *malus granata*, and the fruit *malum punicum* and *malum granatum*, because it is supposed that they were brought over, from that part of Africa where old Carthage stood, into that part of Spain which is now called Granada, and from thence called Granatum. The flowers of the manured kind are called *citin*; but Pliny calls the flowers of the wild kind *citinus*, and the flowers of both kinds, *balaustium*; but *citinus* is more properly the cup wherein stand the flowers of both kinds; *balaustium* is with us generally taken for the double flowers of the wild kind only.

DESCRIPTION The pomegranate-tree bearing fruit, *malus punica sativa*. This tree grows not great in the warm countries, and where it is natural, not above seven or eight feet high, spreading into many slender branches, here and there set with thorns, and with many very fair, green, shining, leaves, like the leaves of large myrtle, every one upon a small and reddish footstalk. Among the leaves come forth here and there the flowers, which are like bell-flowers, broad at the brims, and smaller at the bottom, being one whole leaf divided at the top into five parts, of an orient-crimson colour naturally, but much paler with us, and many veins running through it, with divers threads in the middle, and standing in a brownish hollow cup, or long hard husk; the fruit is great and round, with a hard, smooth, brownish-red, rind; not very thick, but yellowish on the inside, and a crown at the top, stored plentifully with a fine clear liquor or juice, like wine, full of seeds inclosed in skins, and the liquor among them. Sometimes this breaks the rind as it grows, which will cause it to rot very soon.

PLACE AND TIME The manured kinds grow in Spain, Italy, Portugal, and other warm countries; but here in England they are preserved and housed with great care (yet come not to perfection) and the wild kind with much more; they seldom flower with us.

GOVERNMENT AND VIRTUES The Sun governs these plants and fruits. Pomegranates are hot and moist, but yet moderate; all the sorts breed good blood, yet do they yield but slender nourishment; they are very helpful to the stomach: those that are sweet are most pleasant, yet they somewhat heat, and breed wind and choler, and therefore they are forbidden in agues; and those that are sour are fit for a hot fainting stomach, stay vomiting, and provoke urine, but are somewhat offensive to the teeth and gums in the eating. The seed within the fruit, and the rind thereof, do bind very forcibly, whether the powder or the decoction be taken, and stay casting, the bloody flux, women's menses, and are said to be good for the dropsy: the flowers work the same effects.

POPLAR-TREE

DESCRIPTION There are two sorts of poplars which are very familiar with us, *viz.* the white and the black: The white sort grows large, and tolerably high, covered with a smooth, thick, white, bark, especially the branches, having large leaves cut into several divisions, almost like a vine leaf, but not of so deep a green on the upper side, and hoary white underneath, of a good scent, the whole representing the form of colts foot. The catkins, which it brings forth before the leaves, are long, of a faint reddish colour, which fall away, and but seldom bear good seed with them. The wood hereof is smooth, soft, and white, very finely waved, whereby it is much esteemed.

The black poplar grows higher and straighter than the white, with a greyish bark, bearing broad and green leaves somewhat like ivy-leaves, not cut in on the edges like the white, but whole and dented, ending in a point, and not white underneath, hanging by slender long foot-stalks, which, with the air, are continually shaken as the aspen-leaves are. The catkins hereof are greater than of the white, composed of many round green berries, as it were set together in a long cluster, containing much downy matter, which, on being ripe, is blown away with the wind. The clammy buds hereof, before they are spread into leaves, are gathered to make the *unguentum populeon*, and are of a yellowish-green colour, and small, somewhat sweet, but strong. The wood is smooth, tough, and white, and easy to be cloven. On both these trees grows a sweet kind of musk, which formerly used to be put into sweet ointments.

PLATE 17

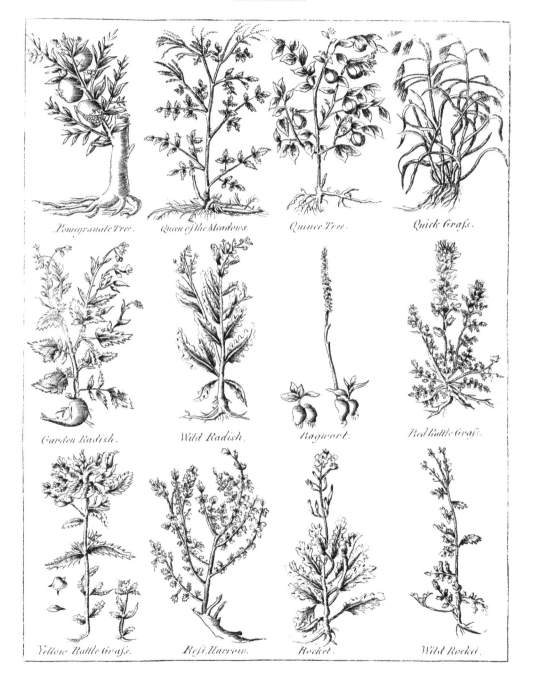

Pomegranate Tree.   Queen of the Meadows.   Quince Tree.   Quick Grass.

Garden Radish.   Wild Radish.   Ragwort.   Red Rattle Grass.

Yellow Rattle Grass.   Rest Harrow.   Rocket.   Wild Rocket.

PLACE They grow in moist woods, and by the water-side, in all parts of the kingdom; but the white sort is not so frequently to be met with as the other.

TIME They are in leaf at the end of summer, but the catkins come before the leaves, as above-mentioned.

GOVERNMENT AND VIRTUES Saturn has dominion over both. The white poplar, says Galen, possesses a cleansing property; one ounce in powder of the bark thereof being drunk, says Dioscorides, is a remedy for those that are troubled with the sciatica, or the difficulty in passing urine. The juice of the leaves, dropped warm into the ears, eases the pains thereof. The young clammy buds or eyes, before they break out into leaves, bruised, and a little honey put to them, are a good medicine for a dull sight. The black poplar is held to be more cooling than the white, and therefore the leaves bruised with vinegar, and applied, help the gout. The seed, drunk in vinegar, is held good against the falling sickness. The water, that drops from the hollow places of this tree, takes away warts, pushes, weals, and other out-breakings in the body. The young black poplar buds, says Mathiolus, are much used by women to beautify their hair, bruising them with fresh butter, and straining them after they have been kept for some time in the Sun. The ointment called *populeon*, which is made of this poplar, is singularly good for all heat and inflammation in any part of the body, and tempers the heat of wounds. It is much used to dry up the milk in women's breasts, when they have weaned their children.

POPPY

Of these there are three kinds, *viz.* the white and black of the garden, and the erratic wild poppy, or corn-rose.

White poppy

DESCRIPTION The white poppy has at first four or five whitish-green leaves lying upon the ground, which rise with the stalk, compassing it at the bottom of them, and are very large, much cut or torn in on the edges, and dented also. The stalk, which is usually four or five feet high, has sometimes no branches at the top, and usually but two or three at most, bearing but one head, each wrapped in a thin skin, which bows down before it be ready to blow, and then, rising and being broken, the flower within it spreads itself open, and consists of four very large round white leaves, with many whitish round threads in the middle, set about a small round green head, having a crown, or star-like cover, at the head thereof, which, growing ripe, becomes as large as a great apple, wherein are contained a great number of small round seed, in several partitions or divisions next unto the shell, the middle thereof remaining hollow and empty. All the whole plant, leaves, stalks, and heads, while they are fresh, young, and green, yield a milk, when they are broken, of an unpleasant bitter taste, almost ready to

Black poppy

Red poppy

provoke puking, and of a strong heady smell, which, being condensed, is called opium. The root is white and woody, perishing as soon as it has given ripe seed.

The black poppy differs but little from the former, until it bears its flower, which is somewhat less, and of a black-purplish colour, but without any purple spots in the bottom of the leaf. The head of the seed is much less than the former, and opens itself a little round about the top, under the crown, so that the seed, which is very black, will fall out, if the head is turned downwards.

The wild poppy, or corn-rose, has long and narrow leaves, very much cut in on the edges into many divisions, of a light green colour, and sometimes hairy withal: The stalk is blackish and hairy also, but not so tall as the garden kinds, having some such like leaves thereon as grow below, parted into three or four branches sometimes, whereon grow small hairy heads, bowing down before the skin breaks wherein the flower is inclosed, which, when it is full blown, is of a fair yellowish-red or crimson colour, and in some much paler, without any spot in the bottom of the leaves, having many black soft spots in the middle, compassing a small green head, which, when it is ripe, is no larger than one's little finger end, wherein is contained much black seed, smaller by half than that of the garden. The root perishes every year, and springs again of its own sowing. Of this kind there is one smaller in all the parts thereof, but differing in nothing else.

PLACE   The garden kinds naturally grow wild in any place, but are all sown in gardens, where they grow. The wild poppy, or corn-rose, is plentiful enough, and many times too much so, in the corn-fields in all parts of the kingdom, also upon the banks of ditches and by hedge-sides. The smaller wild kind is also to be met with in those places, though not so plentifully as the former.

TIME   The garden kinds are usually sown in the spring, which then flower about the end of May, and somewhat earlier, if they are of their own sowing. The wild kinds usually flower from May until July, and the seed of them is ripe soon after their flowering.

GOVERNMENT AND VIRTUES   The herb is lunar, and the juice of it is made into opium. The garden poppy-heads, with the seed, made into a syrup, are frequently, and to good effect, used to procure rest and sleep to the sick and weak, and to stay catarrhs and defluxions of hot thin rheums from the head into the stomach, and upon the lungs, causing a continual cough, the fore-runner of a consumption; it helps also hoarseness of the throat, and when a person has lost the power of articulation; for all which complaints the oil of the seed is also a good remedy. The black seed, boiled in wine and drunk, is also said to stay the flux of the belly, and the menses.

The empty shells of the poppy-heads are usually boiled in water, and given to procure sleep; the leaves likewise, when so boiled, possess the same virtue. If the head and temples be bathed with the decoction warm, the oil of poppies, the green leaves or heads bruised and applied with a little vinegar, or made into a poultice with barley-meal, or hog's grease, it cools and tempers all inflammations, as also the disease called St Anthony's fire. It is generally used in treacle and mithridate, and in all other medicines that are used to procure rest and sleep, and to ease pains in the head, as well as in other parts. It is also used to cool inflammations, agues, or phrensies, and to stay defluxions which cause a cough or consumption, and also other fluxes of the belly: it is frequently put into hollow teeth to ease the pain thereof, and has been found by experience to help gouty pains.

The wild poppy, or corn-rose, Mathiolus says, is good to prevent the falling sickness. The syrup made with the flowers is given with good effect to those that have the pleurisy; and the dried flowers also, either boiled in water, or made into powder, and drunk, either in the distilled water of them, or in some other drink, work the like effect. Galen says, the seed is dangerous to be used inwardly.

PRIMROSES

These are so well known, that they need no description. Of the leaves of primroses is made an excellent salve to heal green wounds.

PRIVET

DESCRIPTION The common privet runs up with many slender branches, to a tolerable height and breadth, and is frequently used in forming arbours, bowers, and banqueting-houses, and shaped sometimes into the forms of men, horses, birds, &c. which, though at first requiring support, grow afterwards strong enough of themselves. It bears long and narrow green leaves by couples, and sweet-smelling white flowers in tufts at the ends of the branches, which turn into small black berries that have a purplish juice within them, and some seeds that are flat on the one side, with a hole or dent therein.

PLACE It grows in divers woods in Great Britain.

TIME The privet flowers in June and July, and the berries become ripe in August and September.

GOVERNMENT AND VIRTUES It is under the influence of the Moon, and is but little used in physic in these times, except in lotions to wash sores and sore mouths, and to cool inflammations and dry up fluxes. There is a sweet water also distilled from the flowers, which is good for all those diseases that require cooling and drying, and therefore helps all fluxes of the belly or stomach, bloody fluxes, and women's menses, being either drunk, or otherwise applied; as also for those that void blood at their mouth or at any other place; likewise for distillations of rheums in the eyes.

PURSLAIN

Garden purslain, being used as a salad-herb, is so well known that it needs no description.

GOVERNMENT AND VIRTUES This is an herb of the Moon. It is good to cool any heat in the liver, blood, reins, and stomach, and, in hot agues, nothing better can be administered; it stays hot and choleric fluxes of the belly, the menses, *flour albus*, gonorrhea, and running of the reins.

The seed is more effectual than the herb, and is singularly useful in cooling the heat and sharpness of the urine, lust, venerous dreams, and the like, insomuch that the over frequent use of it extinguisheth the heat and virtue of natural procreation. The juice of the herb is held equally effectual for all the purposes aforesaid; as also to stay vomitings; taken with some sugar or honey, it helps an old dry cough, shortness of breath, and the phthisic, and stays immoderate thirst. The distilled water of the herb is used by many, being more palatable, with a little sugar, to produce the same effects. The juice also is good in ulcers and inflammations of the secret parts, likewise of the bowels, and hæmorrhoids when they are ulcerous, or have excoriations in them.

The juice is also used with oil of roses for the above purposes, for women's sore breasts, and to allay heat in all other sores or hurts. It is likewise good for sore mouths, and gums that are swelled, as well as to fasten loose teeth. Camerarius says, that the distilled water cured the tooth-ache when all other remedies failed, and that the thickened juice, made into pills with the powders of gum tragacanth and arabic, being taken, greatly relieves those that make bloody water. Applied to the gout, it eases pains thereof, and helps hardness of the sinews, if not arising from the cramp, or a cold cause. The herb, if placed under the tongue, assuages thirst.

QUEEN OF THE MEADOWS, OR MEADOW-SWEET

DESCRIPTION The stalks of this are reddish, rising to be three feet high, sometimes four or five feet, having at the joints thereof large winged leaves set on each side of a middle-rib, being hard, rough, or rugged, crumpled like elm-leaves, having also some smaller leaves with them (as agrimony has), somewhat deeply dented about the edges, of a sad-green colour on the upper side, and greyish underneath, of a pretty sharp scent and taste, somewhat like unto burnet; and a leaf thereof, put into a cup of claret, gives it a fine relish: at the top of the stalks and branches stand many tusts of small white leaves thick together,

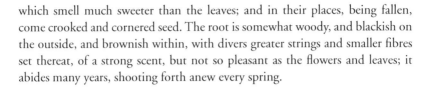

which smell much sweeter than the leaves; and in their places, being fallen, come crooked and cornered seed. The root is somewhat woody, and blackish on the outside, and brownish within, with divers greater strings and smaller fibres set thereat, of a strong scent, but not so pleasant as the flowers and leaves; it abides many years, shooting forth anew every spring.

PLACE It grows in moist meadows, or near the courses of water.

TIME It flowers in some place or other all the three summer months, *viz.* June, July, and August; and the seed is ripe quickly after.

GOVERNMENT AND VIRTUES Venus claims dominion over this herb. It is used to stay all manner of bleedings, fluxes, vomitings, and women's menses, as also their whites; it is said to take away the fits of quartan agues, and to make a merry heart, for which purpose some use the flowers, and some the leaves. It speedily helps those that are troubled with the cholic, being boiled in wine; and, with a little honey, taken warm, it opens the belly: but, boiled in red wine, and drunk, it stays the flux of the belly. Being outwardly applied, it heals ulcers. The leaves, when they are full grown, being laid upon the skin, will, in a short time, raise blisters thereon. The water thereof helps the heat and inflammation of the eyes.

QUICK-GRASS

KINDS AND NAMES There are several sorts of these grasses, some growing in the fields and other places of the upland ground, and others near the sea: it is also called dog-grass, and *gramen caninum*; the other several names shall follow in the descriptions.

DESCRIPTION
1. Common quick-grass, *gramen caninum vulgare*. This grass creeps far about under ground, with long white jointed roots, and small fibres almost at every joint, very sweet in taste, as the rest of the herb is, and interlacing one another; from whence shoot forth many fair and long grass leaves, small at the ends, and cutting or sharp on the edges; the stalks are jointed like corn with the like leaves on them, and a long spiked head, with long husks on them, and hard rough seed in them.
2. Quick-grass with a more spreading panicle, *gramen caninum longius, radicatum, et paniculatum*. This differs very little from the former, but in the tuft, or panicle, which is more spread into branches, with shorter and broader husks; and in the root, which is fuller, greater, and farther spread.
3. The smaller quick-grass with a sparsed tuft, *gramen caninum, latiore panicula minus*. This small quick-grass has slender stalks, about half a foot high, with

many very narrow leaves, both below and on the stalks; the tuft, or panicle, at the top, is small according to the plant, and spreads into sundry parts, or branches: the root is small and jointed, but creeps not so much, and has many more fibres than the others have, and is a little browner, but more sweet.

4. Low-bending quick-grass, *gramen caninum, arvense*. This creeps much under ground, but in a different manner, the stalk taking root in divers places, and scarcely rising a foot high; with such-like green leaves as the ordinary, but shorter; the spiked head is bright, and spreads abroad somewhat like the field-grass.

5. *Gramen caninum supinum monspeliense.* This differs very little from the last, in any other part thereof than in the panicle, or spiked head: which is longer, and not spread or branched into parts as that is.

6. A small sweet grass like quick-grass, *gramen exile tenuifolium, canariæ simile, sive gramen dulce*. This small grass has many low creeping branches, rooting at the joints, like the two last, having a number of small and narrow leaves on them, much less than they; and a small sparsed panicle, somewhat like the red dwarf grass.

7. Wall-grass with a creeping root, *gramen murorum radice repente*. This wall-grass, from a blackish creeping root, springs forth with many stalks a foot high, bending or crooking with a few narrow short leaves on them, at whose tops stand small white panicles, of an inch and a half long, made of many small chaffy husks.

PLACE AND TIME   The first is usual and common in divers plowed grounds and gardens, where it is often more bold than welcome, troubling the husbandmen as much, after the plowing up of some of them (as to pull up the rest after the springing, and, being raked together, to burn them) as it does the gardeners, where it happens, to weed it out from amongst their trees and herbs; the second and third are more scarce, and delight in sandy and chalky grounds; the three next are likewise found in fields that have been plowed and do lie fallow; and the last is often found on old decayed walls in divers places; they flourish in the beginning of summer.

GOVERNMENT AND VIRTUES   These are plants of Mercury. The root is of temperature cold and dry, and has a little mordacity in it, and some tenuity of parts; the herb is cold in the first degree, and moderate in moisture and dryness; but the seed is much more cold and drying. This quick-grass is most medicinal of all other sorts of grasses: it is effectual to open obstructions of the liver and spleen, and the stoppings of urine, the decoction thereof being drunk; and to ease the griping pains in the belly, and inflammations; and to waste the excrementitious matter of the stone in the bladder, and the ulcers thereof; also the root, being bruised and applied, does knit together and consolidate wounds: the seed does most powerfully expel urine, binds the belly, and stays vomiting.

QUINCE-TREE

DESCRIPTION The ordinary quince-tree grows often to the height and bigness of an apple-tree, but more usually lower, and crooked, with a rough bark, and branches spreading far abroad. The leaves are somewhat like those of the apple-tree, but thicker, broader, and fuller of veins, and whiter on the under-side, not dented at all about the edges. The flowers are large and white, sometimes dashed over with a blush. The fruit, when ripe, is yellow, and covered with a white frieze or cotton, thick set on the younger, and growing less as they become thoroughly ripe, bunched out oftentimes in some places, some being like an apple, and some a pear, of a strong heady scent, nor durable to keep, and of a sour, harsh, and unpleasant, taste, to eat fresh; but, being scalded, roasted, baked, or preserved, it becomes more pleasant.

PLACE AND TIME It thrives and grows best near the water-side, and is common throughout Great Britain; it flowers not until the leaves come forth. The fruit is ripe in September or October.

GOVERNMENT AND VIRTUES Old Saturn owns the tree. Quinces, when they are green, help all sorts of fluxes in man or woman, and choleric lasks, castings, and whatsoever needs astriction; yet the syrup of the juice, or the conserve, is rather opening, and, if a little vinegar be added, it stirs up the languishing appetite, and strengthens the stomach; some spices being added, it comforts and cheers the decayed and fainting spirits, helps the liver when oppressed, so that it cannot perfect the digestion, and corrects choler and phlegm. If you would have them purging, put honey to them instead of sugar; and, if more laxative, for choler, rhubarb; for phlegm, turbith; for watery humours, scammony: but, if more forcibly to bind, use the unripe quinces, with roses, acacia, or hypocistis, and some torrified rhubarb. If there be need of any outward binding and cooling of any hot fluxes, the oil of quinces, or any medicine that may be made thereof, is very available to anoint the belly or other parts. It likewise strengthens the stomach and belly, and the sinews that are loosened by sharp humours falling on them. The mucilage, taken from the seeds of quinces, and boiled in a little water, is very good to cool the heat, and heal the sore breasts of women. The same with a little sugar is good to lenify the harshness and soreness of the throat and roughness of the tongue.

RADISH AND HORSE-RADISH

Garden radish

DESCRIPTION The horse-radish has its first leaves rising before winter, about a foot and a half long, very much cut in or torn on the edges into many parts, of a dark green colour, with a great rib in the middle; after those have been up a while, others follow, greater, rougher, broader, and longer, whole, and

Wild radish

not divided as the first, but only somewhat roundly dented about the edges. The stalk, when it bears flowers (which is but seldom) is great, rising up with some few smaller leaves thereon to three or four feet high, spreading at the top many small branches of white flowers, of four leaves each; after which come small pods, like those of shepherd's purse, but seldom with any seed in them. The root is large, long, white, and rugged, shooting up divers heads of leaves; but it does not creep within ground, nor run above ground; and is of a strong, sharp, and bitter, taste, almost like mustard.

PLACE It is found wild in some places in England, but is chiefly planted in gardens, where it thrives in moist and shadowy places.

TIME It flowers but seldom, but, when it does, it is in July.

GOVERNMENT AND VIRTUES They are both under Mars. The juice of horse-radish, given to drink, is held to be very effectual for the scurvy. The root bruised and laid to the place grieved with the sciatica, joint-ache, or hard swellings of the liver and spleen, does wonderfully help them all. The distilled water of the herb and roots is more commonly taken with a little sugar for all the purposes aforesaid. Garden radishes are eaten as salad; for such as are troubled with the gravel, stone, or stoppage of urine, they are good physic; the juice of the roots may be made into a syrup for that use.

RAGWORT

It is called St James's wort, stagger-wort, stammer-wort, and seggrum.

DESCRIPTION The greater common ragwort has many large and long dark green leaves lying on the ground, very much rent and torn on the sides into many pieces; from among which rise up sometimes one and sometimes two or three square or crested blackish stalks three or four feet high, sometimes branched, bearing divers such-like leaves upon them at several distances unto the tops, where it branches forth into many stalks bearing yellow flowers, consisting of a number of leaves set as a pale, or border, with a dark yellow thrum in the middle, which at last turns into down, and, with the small blackish grey seed, are carried away with the wind. The root is made of many fibres, whereby it is firmly fastened into the ground, and abides many years.

There is another sort hereof different from the former only in this, that it rises not so high; the leaves are not so finely jagged, nor of so dark a green colour, but rather whitish, soft, and woolly, and the flowers usually paler.

PLACE They both grow wild in pastures and untilled grounds in many places, and oftentimes both of them in one field.

TIME They flower in June and July, and the seed is ripe in August.

GOVERNMENT AND VIRTUES Ragwort is under the command of Venus. The decoction of this herb is good for ulcers in the mouth or throat, and for swellings, hardness, or imposthumations, for it thoroughly cleanses and heals them; as also the quinsey and the king's evil. It helps to stay catarrhs, thin rheum, and defluxions from the head into the eyes, nose, or lungs.

The juice is found by experience to be good to heal green wounds. It is also much commended to help aches and pains, either in the fleshy parts or in the nerves and sinews; as also the sciatica, or pain of the hips. Bathe the places with the decoction of the herb, or anoint them with an ointment made of the herb bruised and boiled in hogs'-lard, with mastic and olibanum in powder added to it after it is strained. In Sussex this herb is called rag-wood. Externally it has been praised with good reason against swellings, and in inflammations: they are to be boiled to softness, and applied as a warm poultice with bread and oil.

RATTLE-GRASS

Of this there are two kinds, the red and the yellow.

Red rattle-grass

DESCRIPTION The common red rattle grass has sundry reddish hollow stalks, and sometimes green, rising from the root, lying for the most part on the ground, yet some growing more upright, with many small reddish or greenish leaves set on both sides of a middle-rib finely dented about the edges: the flowers stand at the tops of the stalks and branches, of a fine purplish-red colour; after which come flat blackish seed in small husks, which, lying loose therein, will rattle with shaking. The root consists of two or three small whitish strings, with some fibres thereat.

Yellow rattle-grass

The common yellow rattle has seldom above one round green stalk, rising from the root, about half a yard or two feet high, and but few branches thereon, having two long and somewhat broad leaves set at a joint, deeply cut in on the edges, resembling the comb of a cock, broadest next the stalk. The flowers grow at the tops of the stalks, with some shorter leaves with them, hooded after the same manner as the others, but many of a fair yellow colour, in some paler, in some whiter. The seed is contained in large husks; the root is smaller and slender, perishing every year.

PLACE They grow in meadows and woods generally throughout England.

TIME They are in flower from midsummer till August.

GOVERNMENT AND VIRTUES They are both under the dominion of the Moon. The red rattle is reckoned good to heal fistulas and hollow ulcers, and to stay the flux of humours to them, or any other flux of blood, being boiled in red or white wine and drunk. The yellow rattle, or cock's comb, is held to be good for those that are troubled with a cough.

SWEET, OR **AROMATICAL REED**

KINDS AND NAMES There is one sort called *calamus aromaticus mathioli*, Mathiolus's aromatical reed; a second called *calamus aromaticus Syriacus vel Arabicus suppositivus*, the supposed Syrian or Arabian aromatical reed; and the third, the true *acorus* of Dioscorides, or sweet-smelling reed, called in shops *calamus aromaticus*, and likewise a*corus verus, sive calamus officinarum*.

DESCRIPTION
1. Mathiolus's aromatical reed. This grows with an upright tall stalk, set full of joints at certain spaces up to the top (not hollow, but stuffed full of a white spongeous pith, of a gummy taste, somewhat bitter, and of the bigness of a man's finger) and at every one of them a long narrow leaf, of a dark green colour, smelling very sweet, differing therein from all other kinds of reeds; on the tops whereof grows a bushy or feather-like panicle, resembling those of the common reed. The root is knobby, with divers heads thereat, whereby it increases and shoots forth new heads of leaves, smelling also very sweet, having a little binding taste, and sharp withal.
2. The supposed Syrian or Arabian aromatical reed, rises up from a thick root three or four inches long, big at the head and small at the bottom, with one stalk, sometimes more, two cubits high, being straight, round, smooth, and easy to break into splinters; full of joints, and about a finger's thickness, hollow and spongy within, of a whitish-yellow colour; the stalk is divided into other branches, and they again into other smaller ones, two usually set together at a joint, with two leaves under them likewise, very like unto the leaves of lysimachia, the willow-herb or loosestrife, but less, being an inch an half long; compassing the stalk at the bottom, with sundry veins running all the length of them; from the joints rise long stalks, bearing sundry yellow small flowers, made of leaves like also unto lysimachia, with a small pointel in the middle, after which follow small, blackish, long heads or seed-vessels, pointed at the end, and having in them small blackish seed: the stalk has little or no scent, yet not unpleasant, as Alpinus says, being bitter, with a little acrimony therein; but Bauhinus says, it is of an aromatical taste, and very bitter.
3. The sweet-smelling reed, or *calamus officinarum*, or *acorus verus*, has many flags, long and narrow fresh green leaves, two feet long, or more; yet oftentimes somewhat brownish at the bottom, the one rising or growing out of the side of the other, in the same manner that other flags or flower-de-luces grow, which are thin on both sides, and ridged or thickest in the middle; the longest, for the most part, standing in the midst, and some of them as it were curled or plaited

towards the ends or tops of them; smelling very sweet, as well when they are green and fresh as when they are dried and kept a long time; which do so abide in a garden a long time, as though it never did nor never would bear flower; the leaves every year drying down to the ground, and shooting out fresh every spring; but, after three or four years abiding in a place, it shoots forth a narrow long leaf by itself, flat like-unto the other leaves, especially from the middle upwards; but from the bottom to the middle it is flat, at which place comes forth one long round head, very seldom two; in form and bigness like unto the catking or aglet of the hasel-nut tree, growing upright, and of the length and thickness of one's finger, or rather bigger; set with several small lines or divisions, like unto a green pine-apple; of a purplish-green colour for the most part; out of which bunches shoot forth small pale-whitish flowers, consisting of four small leaves apiece, without so good a scent as the leaves, falling quickly away, and not yielding any seed. The root is thick and long, lying under the surface of the ground, shooting forward, and with small roots or suckers, on all sides like unto the garden valerian, whitish on the outside, or greenish if it lie above the ground, and more pale or whitish on the inside, with many joints thereabouts, and whereat it has or does shoot forth long thick fibres underneath, whereby it takes strong hold in the ground.

PLACE AND TIME The first is said by Mathiolus, and others, to grow in India, Syria, and Judæa; the dry stalks of the second are said to grow at the foot of Mount Libanus, in Syria, not far from Tripoli, in the wet grounds there; the third in sundry moist places in Egypt, and by the lake Gennesareth in Judæa, and in divers places of Syria and Arabia.

The other *calamus* of the shops, or true *acorus*, grows in many places of Turkey, in moist grounds, whence the largest roots, the firmest, whitest, and sweetest, are brought unto us; it grows also in Russia and thereabouts, in great plenty. It is sometimes found in moist grounds in Yorkshire, and the northern parts of England.

GOVERNMENT AND VIRTUES These reeds are under the dominion of Venus, of a temperate quality. The *calamus* of Dioscorides, he says, has these properties: It provokes urine, and, boiled with grass-roots and smallage, it helps those that have the dropsy; it fortifies the reins, and is good against the difficulty in passing urine, and is also profitable for those that have the rupture; the fumes of it, taken through a tobacco-pipe, either by itself or with some dried turpentine, cure a cough; it is put into baths for women to sit in.

It is used in mollifying oils and plasters, that serve to ripen hard imposthumes, as also for the sweet scent thereof. Galen says, it being of a temperature moderate, between heat and cold, and somewhat astringent, and having a very little acrimony, it is profitably used among other things that help the liver and stomach, does provoke urine, is used with other things in fomentations for inflammations, and gently to move the menses.

The root is of much use in all antidotes against poison or infection. The hot fumes of the decoction made in water, and taken in at the mouth through a funnel, are good to help those that are troubled with a cough. A drachm of the powder of the roots, with as much cinnamon, taken in a draught of wormwood wine, is good against convulsions or cramps. An oxymel or syrup made hereof in this manner is effectual for all cold spleens and livers: Take of the roots of acorus one pound; wash and pick them clean, then bruise them, and steep them for three days in vinegar, after which time let them be boiled together to the consumption of the one half of the vinegar, which, being strained, set to the fire again, putting thereto as much honey as is sufficient to make it into a syrup; an ounce of this syrup in the morning, in a small draught of the decoction of the same roots, is sufficient for a dose; the whole roots, preserved either in honey or sugar, are effectual for the same purposes; but the green roots, preserved, are better than the dried roots, which are first steeped and then preserved. It likewise mollifies hard tumours in any part of the body.

REST-HARROW, OR CAMMOAK

DESCRIPTION   Common rest-harrow rises up with divers rough woody twigs, two or three feet high, set at the joints without order, with little-roundish leaves, sometimes more than two or three at a place, of a dark green colour, without thorns while they are young, but afterwards armed in sundry places with short and sharp thorns. The flowers come at the tops of the twigs and branches, whereof it is full, fashioned like pease, or bloom blossoms, but smaller, flatter, and somewhat close, of a faint purplish colour: after which come small pods, containing small, flat, and round, seed. The root is blackish on the outside, and whitish within: very rough and hard to break when it is fresh and green, and as hard as an horn when it is dried, thrusting down deep into the ground, and spreading likewise, every piece being likely to grow again if it be left in the ground.

PLACE   It grows in many places of Great Britain, as well in arable as in waste ground.

TIME   It flowers in general about the beginning or middle of July, and the seed is ripe in August.

GOVERNMENT AND VIRTUES   It is under the dominion of Mars. It is good to provoke urine and to break and expel the stone, which the powder of the bark of the root taken in wine performs effectually. Mathiolus says, the same helps the disease called *hernia carnosa*, the fleshy rupture, by taking the said powder for some months together constantly, and that it has cured some which seemed incurable by any other means than by cutting or burning. The decoction thereof, made with some vinegar, and gargled in the mouth, eases the tooth-ache, especially when it comes of rheum; and is very powerful to open obstructions of the liver and spleen, and other parts. A distilled water, made in *balneo mariæ* with four pounds of the roots hereof, first sliced small, and afterwards steeped in a gallon of Canary wine, is very good for all the purposes aforesaid, and to cleanse the passages of the urine. The powder of the said root, made into an electuary or lozenges with sugar, as also the bark of the fresh roots boiled tender, and afterwards beaten into a conserve with sugar, works the like effect. The powder of the roots, strewed upon the brims of ulcers, or mixed with any other convenient thing and applied, consumes the hardness, and causes them to heal the better.

RHUBARB, OR RHAPONTIC

Though the name may speak it foreign, yet it grows with us in England, and that frequently enough, in our gardens; and is nothing inferior to that which is brought us out of China; take therefore a description at large of it, as follows.

DESCRIPTION At the first appearing out of the ground, when the winter is past, it has a great round brownish head, rising from the middle or sides of the root, which opens itself into sundry leaves one after another, very much crumpled or folded together at the first, and brownish; but afterwards it spreads itself, and becomes smooth, very large, and almost round, every one standing on a brownish stalk, of the thickness of a man's thumb when they are grown to their fulness, and most of them two feet and more in length, especially when they grow in any moist or good ground; and the stalk of the leaf also, from the bottom thereof to the leaf itself, is also two feet; the breadth thereof from edge to edge, in the broadest place, is also two feet; of a sad or dark green colour, of a fine tart or sourish taste, much more pleasant than the garden or wood sorrel. From among these rises up sometimes, but not every year, a strong thick stalk, not growing so high as the patience, or garden-dock, with such round leaves as grow below, but smaller at every joint up to the top, and among the flowers, which are white, spreading forth into many branches, and consisting of five or six small white leaves each, after which come brownish three-square seed, like unto other docks, but larger. The root grows in time to be very great, with divers great spreading branches from it, of a dark brownish or reddish colour on the outside, with a pale yellow skin under it, which covers the inner substance or root; which rind and skin being pared away, the root appears of so fresh and lively a colour, with fresh-coloured veins running through it, that the choicest of that rhubarb that is brought us from beyond the seas cannot excel it: which root, if it be dried carefully, and as it ought (which must be in our country by the gentle heat of a fire, in regard the Sun is not hot enough here to do it) and every piece kept from touching one another, will hold its colour almost as well as when it is fresh; and has been approved of, and commended, by those who have oftentimes used it.

PLACE AND TIME It grows in gardens, and flowers about the beginning or middle of June, and the seed is ripe in July. The roots, that are to be dried and kept all the year following, are not to be taken up before the stalk and leaves be quite withered and gone, and that is not until the middle or end of October; and, if they be taken a little before the leaves do spring, or when they are sprung up, the roots will not have so good a colour in them.

MONK'S RHUBARB, OR GARDEN PATIENCE

DESCRIPTION This is a dock, bearing the name of rhubarb for some purging quality therein, and grows up with large tall stalks, set with somewhat broad and long fair green leaves, not dented. The tops of the stalks, being divided into many small branches, bear reddish or purplish flowers, and three-square seed, like unto other docks. The root is long, great, and yellow, like unto the wild docks, but a little redder, and, if it be a little dried, shews less discoloured veins than the next does when it is dry.

BASTARD-RHUBARB, OR GREAT ROUND-LEAVED DOCK

DESCRIPTION This has divers large, round, thin, yellowish-green leaves, rising from the root, a little waved above the edges, every one standing on a thick and long brownish foot-stalk; from among which rises up a pretty big stalk, about two feet high, with some such-like leaves growing thereon, but smaller; at the top whereof stand, in a long spike, many small brownish flowers, which turn into hard three-square shining brown seed, like the garden patience before described. This root grows larger, with many branches of great fibres, yellow on the outside, and somewhat pale yellow within, with some discoloured veins, like the rhubarb first described, but much less, especially when it is dry.

PLACE AND TIME These also grow in gardens; they flower in June, and the seed is ripe in July.

GOVERNMENT AND VIRTUES Mars claims predominancy over all the wholesome herbs: a drachm of the dried root of monk's rhubarb, with a scruple of ginger, made into powder and taken fasting in a draught or mess of warm broth, purges choler and phlegm downwards, very gently and safely, without danger: the seed thereof, contrarily, does bind the belly, and helps to stay any sort of lask or bloody flux. The distilled water thereof is very profitably used

PLATE 18

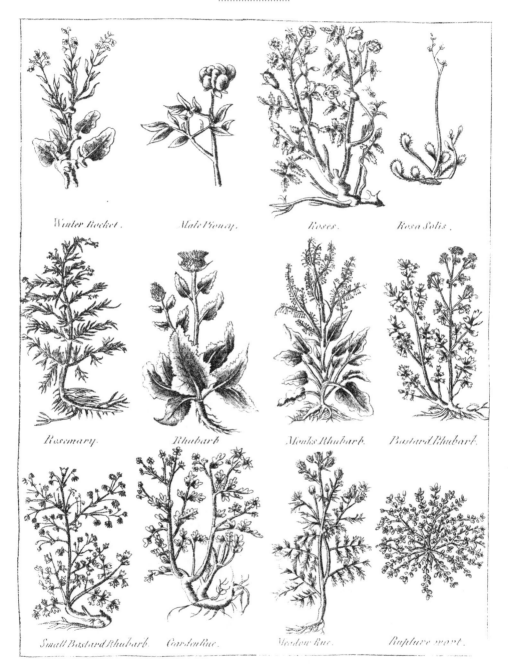

Winter Rocket.   Male Piony.   Roses.   Rosa Solis.

Rosemary.   Rhubarb   Monks Rhubarb.   Bastard Rhubarb.

Small Bastard Rhubarb.   Garden Rue.   Meadow Rue.   Rupture wort.

238

to heal scabs, and to allay the inflammation of them; the juice of the leaves or roots, or the decoction of them in vinegar, is used as a most effectual remedy to heal scabs and running sores.

The properties of that which is called the English rhubarb are the same with the former, but much more effectual, and has all the properties of the true Indian rhubarb, except the force of purging, wherein it is but of half the strength thereof, and therefore a double quantity must be used; it likewise has not that bitterness and astriction; in other things it works almost in an equal quality, which are these, it purges the body of choler and phlegm, being either taken of itself, made into powder and drunk in a draught of white wine, or steeped therein all night, and taken fasting, or put among other purges, as shall be thought convenient, cleansing the stomach, liver, and blood, opening obstructions, and helping those griefs that come thereof; as the jaundice, dropsy, swelling of the spleen, tertian and day agues, and pricking pain in the sides; and also it stays spitting of blood. The powder, taken with cassia dissolved, and a little Venice turpentine, cleanses the reins, and strengthens them, and is very effectual to stay the running of the reins. It is also given for the pains and swellings in the head, for those that are troubled with melancholy, and helps the gout and the cramp. The powder of rhubarb, taken with a little mumia and madder-roots, in some red wine, dissolves clotted blood in the body, happening by any fall or bruise, and heals burstings and broken parts as well inward as outward: the oil, likewise, wherein it has been boiled, works the like effects; it is used to heal those ulcers that happen in the eyes and eye-lids, being steeped and strained; as also to assuage swellings and inflammations. Whey or white wine are the best liquors to steep it in, and thereby it works more effectually in opening obstructions, and purging the stomach and liver.

RICE

DESCRIPTION   This grain, or corn, rises up with a stronger stalk than wheat, about a yard high, with sundry joints, and a large thick leaf at each of them, like the reed; at the top it bears a spiked tuft spread into branches, whose blooming is said to be purplish, with the seed standing severally on them inclosed in hard brown straked husk, and an arm at the head of every one of them; which, being hulled, is very white, of the bigness almost of wheat-corns, blunt at both ends.

NAMES   Rice is called in Latin *oriza*, and the Italians call it *rizo*, the French *ris*.

PLACE AND TIME This grain originally was brought out of the East Indies, where in many places it yields two crops in a year, being the chiefest corn they live upon, and not with them only, but through all Ethiopia and Africa; and thence has been brought into Syria, Egypt, Italy, &c. It delights to grow in moist grounds, and is ripe about the middle of autumn.

GOVERNMENT AND VIRTUES It is a solar grain, chiefly to stay the lasks and fluxes of the stomach and belly, especially if it be a little parched before it be used, and steel quenched in the milk wherein it is boiled, being somewhat binding and drying. The flower of rice is of the same property, and is sometimes applied to women's breasts, to stay inflammations therein.

ROCKET

DESCRIPTION The common wild rocket has longer and narrower leaves much more divided into slender cuts and jags on both sides of the middle-rib than the garden kinds have, of a sad-green colour, from among which rises up divers stiff stalks, two or three feet high, sometimes set with the like leaves, but smaller, and much less upwards, branched from the middle into sundry stalks, bearing yellow flowers of four leaves each, as the others are, which afterwards yield small reddish seed, in small long pods, of a more bitter and hot biting taste than the garden kinds, as are the leaves likewise.

Rocket

Wild rocket

PLACE It is found wild in most places of Great Britain.

TIME It flowers about June and July, and the seed is ripe in August.

GOVERNMENT AND VIRTUES Mars rules them. The wild rocket is more strong than the garden kinds; it serves to help digestion, and provokes urine exceedingly. The herb, boiled or stewed, and some sugar put thereto, helps the cough in children, being taken often. The seed also, taken in drink, increases milk in nurses, and wastes the spleen.

WINTER ROCKET, OR CRESSES

DESCRIPTION Winter rocket, or winter cresses, has divers somewhat like turnip-leaves, with smaller pieces next the bottom, and broad at the ends, which so abide all winter (if it spring up in autumn, when it is used to be eaten) from among which rises up divers small round stalks full of branches, bearing many small yellow flowers of four leaves each, after which come small long pods with reddish seed in them. The root is rather stringy, and perishes every year after the seed is ripe.

PLACE It grows of its own accord in gardens, and fields, by the way-sides, in divers places.

PLATE 19

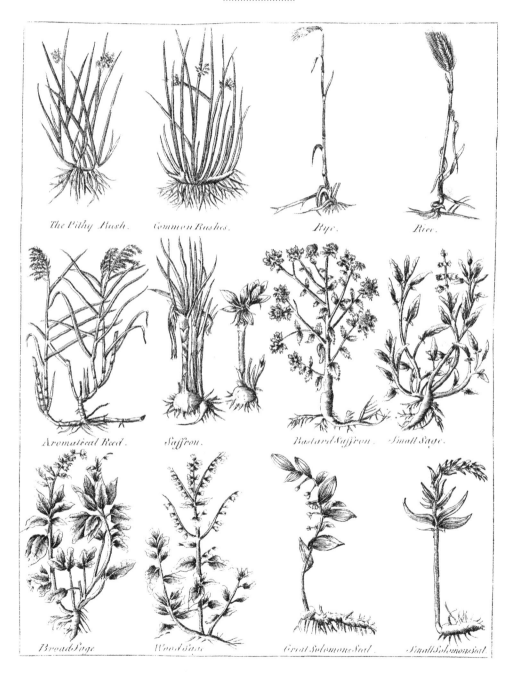

The Pithy Rush. Common Rushes. Rye. Rice.

Aromatical Reed. Saffron. Bastard Saffron. Small Sage.

Broad Sage Wood Sage Great Solomons Seal. Small Solomons Seal.

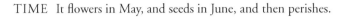

TIME It flowers in May, and seeds in June, and then perishes.

GOVERNMENT AND VIRTUES This is profitable to provoke urine, to help the difficulty in passing urine, and to expel gravel and the stone; it is also of good effect in the scurvy. It is found by experience to be a good herb to cleanse inward wounds; the juice or decoction, being drunk, or outwardly applied to wash ulcers and sores cleanses them by sharpness, and hinders the dead flesh from growing therein, and heals them by the drying quality.

ROSA SOLIS, OR SUN-DEW

DESCRIPTION it has divers small round hollow leaves, somewhat greenish, but full of certain red hairs, which makes them seem red, every one standing upon his own footstalks, reddish hairy likewise. The leaves are continually moist in the hottest day, for the hotter the sun shines on them the moister they are, with a certain sliminess, the small hairs always holding this moisture. Among these leaves rise up small slender stalks, reddish also, three or four fingers high, bearing divers small white knobs one above another, which are the flowers; after which, in the heads, are contained small seeds: the root is a few small hairs.

PLACE It grows usually in bogs and in wet places, and sometimes in moist woods and meadows.

TIME It flowers in June, and then the leaves are fittest to be gathered.

GOVERNMENT AND VIRTUES The Sun rules it, and it is under the sign of Cancer. Rosa solis is accounted good to help those that have salt rheum distilling on their lungs, which breeds a consumption, and therefore the distilled water thereof in wine is held fit and profitable for such to drink, which water will be of a gold-yellow colour: the same water is held to be good for all other diseases of the lungs, as phthisics, wheezing, shortness of breath, or the cough; as also to heal the ulcers that happen in the lungs; the leaves outwardly applied to the skin will raise blisters, which has caused some to think it dangerous to be taken inwardly.

ROSEMARY

TIME It flowers in April and May with us, and sometimes again in August.

GOVERNMENT AND VIRTUES The Sun claims privilege in it, and it is under the cœlestial Ram. It is very comfortable to the stomach in all the cold griefs thereof, helping digestion, the decoction or powder being taken in wine. It is a remedy for wind in the stomach or bowels, and expels it powerfully, as also wind in the spleen. It helps those that are liver-grown, by opening the obstructions thereof. Both Dioscorides and Galen say, that, if a decoction be made thereof with water, and they that have the yellow jaundice do exercise their bodies presently after the taking thereof, it will certainly cure them. The flowers, and the conserve made of them, are good to comfort the heart, and to expel the contagion of the pestilence; to burn the herb in houses and chambers corrects the air in them. The dried leaves, smoked, help those that have a cough, phthisic, or consumption, by warming and drying the thin distillations which cause those diseases.

The leaves are much used in bathings, and, made into ointments or oils, are good to help cold benumbed joints, sinews, or members. The chemical oil, drawn from the leaves and flowers, is a sovereign help for all the diseases of the head and brain spoken of before; as also to take a drop, two, or three, as the cause requires, for the inward griefs; yet must it be done with discretion, for it is very quick and piercing, and therefore but a very little must be taken at a time. There is also another oil made in this manner: Take what quantity you will of the flowers, and put them into a strong glass close stopped, tie a fine linen cloth over the mouth, and turn the mouth down into another strong glass, which being set in the Sun, an oil will distil down into the lower glass, to be preserved as precious for divers uses, both inward and outward.

ROSES

I hold it needless to trouble the reader with a description of these, since both the garden roses and the wild roses of the briers are well enough known; take therefore the virtues of them as follows; and first I shall begin with the garden kinds.

GOVERNMENT AND VIRTUES   Red roses are under Jupiter, damask under Venus, and white under the Moon. The white and the red roses are cooling and drying, and yet the white is taken to exceed the red in both those properties, but is seldom used inwardly in medicine. The decoction of red roses, made with wine, and used, is very good for the head-ache, and pains in the eyes, ears, throat, and gums, as also for the fundament, the lower bowels, and the matrix. The same decoction, with the roses remaining in it, is profitably applied to the region of the heart to ease the inflammation therein; as also St Anthony's fire, and other diseases of the stomach. Being dried and beaten to powder, and taken into steeled wine or water, it helps to stay women's menses.

The yellow threads in the middle of the red roses (which are erroneously called the rose seed), being powdered, and drunk, in the distilled water of quinces, stays the defluxion of rheum upon the gums and teeth, preserving them from corruption, and fastens them if they be loose, being washed and gargled therewith, and some vinegar of squills added thereto. The heads, with seed, being used in powder, or in a decoction, stay the lask and spitting of blood.

Red roses do strengthen the heart, stomach, and liver, and the retentive faculty; they mitigate the pains that arise from heat, assuage inflammations, procure rest and sleep, stay running of the reins and fluxes of the belly; the juice of them does purge and cleanse the body from choler and phlegm. The husks of the roses with the beards and nails, are binding and cooling, and the distilled water of either of them is good for heat and redness in the eyes, and to stay and dry up the rheums and watering of them. Of the red roses are usually made many compositions, all serving to sundry good uses, viz. electuary of roses; conserve, both moist and dry, which is more usually called sugar of roses; syrup of dried roses, and honey of roses; the cordial powder called *diarrhodon abbatis* and a*romatica rosarum*; the distilled water of roses, vinegar of roses, ointment and oil of roses, and the rose-leaves dried, which, although no composition, is yet of very great use and effect.

The electuary is purging, whereof two or three drachms taken by itself in some convenient liquor is a purge sufficient for a weak constitution; but may be increased to six drachms, according to the strength of the patient. It purges choler without trouble, and is good in hot fevers, and pains of the head arising from hot choleric humours and heat in the eyes, the jaundice also, and joint-aches proceeding of hot humours. The moist conserve is of much use, both binding and cordial; for, until it be about two years old, it is more binding than cordial, and after that more cordial than binding; some of the younger conserve, taken with mithridatum, mixed together, is good for those that are troubled with distillations of rheum from the brain to the nose, and defluxions of rheum into the eyes, as also for fluxes and lasks of the belly; and, being mixed with the powder of mastic, is very good for the running of the reins. The old conserve, mixed with *aromaticum rosarum*, is a very good cordial against faintings, swoonings, weakness, and tremblings of the heart, strengthening both it and a weak stomach, helps digestion, stays casting, and is a very good preservative in the time of infection. The dry conserve, which is called sugar of roses, is a very good cordial to strengthen the heart and spirits, as also to stay defluxions. The syrup of dried red roses strengthens a stomach given to casting; cools an over-heated liver, comforts the heart, resists putrefaction and infection, and helps to stay lasks and fluxes. Honey of roses is much used in gargles and lotions, to wash sores, either in the mouth, throat, or other parts, both to heal them and to stay the fluxes of humours falling upon them; it is also used in clysters. The cordial powders, called *diarrhodon abbatis* and *aromaticus rosarum*, do comfort and strengthen the heart and stomach, procure an appetite, help digestion, stop vomiting, and are very good for those that have slippery bowels, to strengthen them and to dry up their moisture.

Red-rose water is of well-known and familiar use in all occasions (and better than damask-rose water) being cooling and cordial, quickening the weak and faint spirits, used either in meats or broths, to wash the temples, to smell at the nose, or to smell the sweet vapours thereof out of a perfuming pot, or cast on a hot fire-shovel; it is also of good use against the redness and inflammations of the eyes, to bathe them therewith, and the temples of the head also against pain and ache, and to procure rest and sleep. The ointment of roses is much used against heat and inflammations in the head, to anoint the forehead and temples, and, being mixed with *unguentum populeon*, to procure rest; it is also used for the heat of the liver, of the back and reins, and to cool and heal pushes, weals, and other red pimples rising in the face or other parts. Oil of roses is not only used by itself to cool any hot swellings or inflammations, and to bind and stay fluxes of humours unto sores, but is also put into ointments and plasters that are cooling and binding, to restrain the flux of humours. The dried leaves of the red roses are used both inwardly and outwardly, being cooling, binding, and cordial; for with them are made both *aromaticum rosarum*, *diarrhodon abbatis*, and *saccharum rosarum*, each of whose properties are before declared.

Rose-leaves and mint, heated and applied outwardly to the stomach, stay castings, and very much strengthen a weak stomach; and, applied as a fomentation to the region of the liver and heart, do much cool and temper them, and also serve instead of a rose-cake, to quiet the over-hot spirits and cause rest and sleep. The syrup of damask roses is both simple and compound, and made with agaric. The simple solutive syrup is a familiar, safe, gentle, and easy, medicine, purging choler, taken from one ounce to three or four; yet this is remarkable herein, that the distilled water of this syrup should notably bind the belly. The syrup with agaric is more strong and effectual, for one ounce thereof by itself will open the body more than the other, and works as much on phlegm as choler. The compound syrup is more forcible in working on melancholy humours, and against the leprosy, itch, tetters, &c. and the French disease. Also honey of roses solutive is made of the same infusions that the syrup is made of, and therefore works the same effect both opening and purging, but is oftener given to phlegmatic than choleric persons, and is more used in clysters than in potions, as the syrup made with sugar is. The conserve and preserved leaves of these roses are also operative in gently opening the belly.

The simple water of the damask roses is chiefly used for fumes to sweeten things, as the dried leaves thereof to make sweet powders and fill sweet bags. The wild roses are few or none of them used in physic, but yet are generally held to come near the nature of the manured roses. The fruit of the wild brier, which are called hops, being thoroughly ripe, and made into a conserve with sugar, besides the pleasantness of the taste, does gently bind the belly and helps digestion. The brier-ball is often used, being made into powder and drunk, to break the stone, provoke urine when it is stopped, and to ease and help the cholic.

GARDEN RUE

GOVERNMENT AND VIRTUES It is an herb of the Sun, and under Leo. Being boiled or infused in oil, it is good to help the wind-cholic. It helps the gout or pains in the joints of hands, feet, or knees, applied thereunto: and with figs it helps the dropsy, being bathed therewith; being bruised, and put into the nostrils, it stays the bleeding thereof. It takes away weals and pimples, if, being bruised with a few myrtle leaves, it be made up with wax and applied. It cures the morphew, and takes away all sorts of warts, if boiled in wine with some pepper and nitre, and the places rubbed therewith; and, with alum and honey, helps the dry scab, or any tetter or ringworm.

MEADOW RUE

DESCRIPTION Meadow rue rises up with a yellow stringy root, much spreading in the ground, and shooting forth new sprouts round about, with many herby-green stalks, two feet high, crested, set with joints here and there, and many large leaves on them below, being divided into smaller leaves, nicked or dented in the forepart, of a sad-green colour on the upper side, and pale green underneath. Toward the top of the stalk there shoots forth divers short branches, on every one whereof there stand two, three, or four, small round heads or buttons, which breaking the skin that incloses them shew forth a tuft of pale greenish-yellow threads, which falling away, there come in their places small three-cornered cods, wherein is contained small, long, and round, seed. The plant has a strong unpleasant smell.

PLACE It grows in many places in England, in the borders of moist meadows, and by ditch-sides. Pliny writes, that there is such friendship between it and the fig-tree, that it prospers no where so well as under that tree, and delights to grow in sunny places.

TIME It flowers about July, or the beginning of August.

GOVERNMENT AND VIRTUES Dioscorides says, that this herb, bruised and applied, perfectly heals old sores: and the distilled water of the herb and flowers does the like. It is used by some, among other pot-herbs, to open the body; but the roots, washed clean, boiled in ale, and drunk, are more opening than the leaves. The root, boiled in water, and the places of the body most troubled with vermin or lice washed therewith, while it is warm, destroys them utterly. In Italy it is used against the plague, and in Saxony against the jaundice. It is an enemy to the toad, as being a great enemy to poison. The ancient astrologers declare this herb has a property of making a man chaste; but a woman it fills with lust.

RUPTURE-WORT

DESCRIPTION   This spreads very many small branches round about upon the ground, about a span long, divided into many parts, full of small joints set very thick together, whereat come forth two very small leaves of a yellowish-green colour, branches and all, where grows forth also a number of exceeding small yellowish flowers, scarcely to be discerned from the stalks and leaves, which turn into seeds as small as the very dust. The root is very long and small, thrusting down deep into the ground. This has no smell nor taste at first, but afterward has a little astringent taste, without any manifest heat, yet a little bitter and sharp.

PLACE   It grows in dry, sandy, rocky, places.

TIME   It is fresh and green all the summer.

GOVERNMENT AND VIRTUES   This herb is under the dominion of Saturn. Rupture-wort has not its name in vain, for it is found by experience to cure the rupture, not only in children, but also in grown persons, if the disease be not too inveterate, by taking a drachm of the powder of the dried herb every day in wine, or the decoction made in wine and drunk, or the juice or distilled water of the green herb taken in the same manner; and helps all other fluxes either in men or women; vomitings also, and the gonorrhea, or running of the reins, being taken any of the ways aforesaid. It does also most assuredly help those that have the difficulty in passing urine, or are troubled with the stone or gravel. The same also much helps all stitches in the side, all griping pains in the stomach or belly, the obstructions of the liver, and cures the yellow jaundice likewise. It heals wounds, and helps defluxions of rheum from the head to the eyes, nose, and teeth, being bruised green and bound thereto.

RUSHES

Although there are many kinds of rushes, yet I shall confine myself to those which are best known, and most medicinal, as the bull-rushes, and other of the soft and smooth kinds; which grow so commonly in almost every place in Great Britain, and are so generally noted, that it is needless to write any description of them. Briefly then take the virtues of them, as follows:

Common rushes

GOVERNMENT AND VIRTUES   The seeds of these soft rushes, say Dioscorides and Galen, toasted, and drunk in wine and water, stay the lask and the menses, when they come down too abundantly; but it causes the head-ache. They likewise provoke sleep, but must be given with caution. Pliny says, the root, boiled in water to the consumption of one-third, helps the cough.

The pithy rush

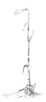

RYE

GOVERNMENT AND VIRTUES Rye is more digesting than wheat; the bread and the leaven thereof ripens and breaks imposthumes, biles, and other swellings; the meal of rye, put between a double cloth, moistened with a little vinegar, and heated in a pewter dish, and bound fast to the head while it is hot, does much ease the continual pains of the head. Mathiolus says, that the ashes of rye-straw, put into water, and suffered therein a day and a night, will heal the chaps of the hands or feet.

SAFFRON

PLACE It grows frequently at Walden in Essex, and in Cambridgeshire.

GOVERNMENT AND VIRTUES It is an herb of the Sun, and under the Lion, and therefore strengthens the heart exceedingly. Let not above ten grains be given at one time, for, being taken in an immoderate quantity, it may hurt the heart instead of helping it. It quickens the brain, for the Sun is exalted in Aries; it helps the consumption of the lungs and difficulty of breathing: it is an excellent thing in epidemical diseases, as pestilence, small-pox, and measles. It is a notable expulsive medicine, and remedy for the yellow jaundice. My own opinion is, that hermodactils are nothing else but the roots of saffron dried; and my reason is, that the roots of all crocus, both white and yellow, purge phlegm as hermodactils do; and, if you dry the roots of any crocus, neither your eyes nor your taste shall distinguish them from hermodactils.

SAGE

TIME It flowers in or about June, July, and August.

Broad sage

Small sage

GOVERNMENT AND VIRTUES Jupiter claims this, and it is good for the liver, and to breed good blood. The juice of sage, taken in warm water, helps a hoarseness and cough. The leaves sodden in wine, and laid upon the place affected with the palsy, helps much, if the decoction be drunk also. Sage taken with wormwood is good for the bloody flux. Sage is of excellent use to help the memory, warming and quickening the senses; and the conserve made of the flowers is used to the same purpose. Gargles likewise are made with sage, rosemary, honey-suckles, and plantane, boiled in wine or water, with some honey or alum put thereto, to wash sore mouths and throats. With other hot and comfortable herbs, sage is boiled to bathe the body and legs in the summer-time, especially to warm cold joints or sinews troubled with the palsy or cramp, and to comfort or strengthen the parts.

WOOD-SAGE

DESCRIPTION Wood-sage rises up with square hoary stalks two feet high at the least, with two leaves at every joint, somewhat like other sage leaves, but smaller, softer, whiter, and rounder, and a little dented about the edges, and smelling somewhat stronger; at the tops of the stalks and branches stand the flowers on a slender long spike, turning themselves all one way when they blow, and are of a pale and whitish colour, smaller than sage, but hooded and gaping like it; the seed is blackish and round, four usually seen in a husk together; the root is long and stringy, with divers fibres thereat; and it abides many years.

PLACE It grows in woods, and by wood-sides, as also in divers fields and by-lanes in Great Britain.

TIME It flowers in June, July, and August.

GOVERNMENT AND VIRTUES The herb is under Venus. The juice of the herb, or the powder thereof dried, is good for moist ulcers and sores in the legs or other parts, to dry them, and causes them to heal more speedily. It also cures green wounds.

SAMPHIRE

*First
samphire*

DESCRIPTION Rock-samphire grows with a tender green stalk, about half a yard or two feet at the most, branching forth almost from the very bottom, and stored with sundry thick, and almost round, somewhat long, leaves, of a deep green colour, sometimes three together, and sometimes more, on a stalk, and are sappy, and of a pleasant, hot, or spicy, taste. At the tops of the stalks and branches stand umbles of white flowers, and after them come large seed bigger than fennel-seed, yet somewhat like. The root is great, white, and long, continuing many years, and is of an hot spicy taste.

*Second
samphire*

PLACE It grows on the rocks that are often moistened by the sea.

TIME It flowers and seeds in the end of July and August.

*Third
samphire*

GOVERNMENT AND VIRTUES It is an herb of Jupiter, and was in former times wont to be used more than it now is. It is a safe herb, very pleasant both to the taste and stomach, helping digestion, and in some sort opening the obstructions of the liver and spleen, provoking urine, and helping thereby to wash away the gravel and stone.

Sanicle

*Great
sanicle*

SANICLE

DESCRIPTION The ordinary sanicle sends forth many great round leaves, standing upon long brownish stalks, every one cut or divided into five or fix parts, and some of those also cut in, somewhat like the leaf of a crow-foot or dove's foot, finely dented about the edges, smooth, and a dark green shining colour, and sometimes reddish about the brims, from among which rise up small round green stalks, without any joint or leaf thereon, expect at the top, where it branches forth into flowers, having a leaf divided into three or four parts at that joint with the flowers, which are small and white, starting out of small round greenish-yellow heads, many standing together in a tuft; in which afterwards are the seeds contained, which are small round rough burs, somewhat like the seeds of clover, and stick in the same manner upon any thing that they touch. The root is composed of many black strings of fibres set together at a little long head, which abides with the green leaves all the winter.

PLACE It is found in many shadowy woods, and other places, in England.

TIME It flowers in June, and the seed is ripe shortly after.

GOVERNMENT AND VIRTUES This is one of Venus's herbs. It is exceeding good to heal green wounds, or any ulcers, imposthumes, or bleedings, inwardly. It helps to stay fluxes of blood either by the mouth, urine, or stool, and lasks of the belly, the ulceration of the kidneys also, and the pains in the bowels, and the running of the reins, being boiled in wine or water, and drunk.

SARACEN'S CONSOUND, OR SARACEN'S WOUND-WORT

DESCRIPTION This grows very high, sometimes with brownish stalks, and other times with green and hollow, to a man's height, having many long and narrow green leaves snipped about the edges, somewhat like those of the peach-tree, or willow leaves, but not of such a white-green colour: the tops of the stalks are furnished with many pale yellow star-like flowers standing in green heads, which, when they are fallen, and the seed ripe (which is somewhat long, small, and of a yellowish-brown colour wrapped in down) is therewith carried away by the wind. The root is composed of many strings or fibres, set together at a head, which perish not in winter, though the stalks dry away. The taste of this herb is strong and unpleasant, and so is the smell. Wonders are related of the virtues of this herb against hurts and bruises; and it is a great ingredient in the Swiss arquebusade-water. It is balsamic and diuretic; and all its occult powers are judiciously combined in Dr Sibly's Solar Tincture: which medicine no family should ever be without, particularly such as live remote from medical assistance.

PLATE 20

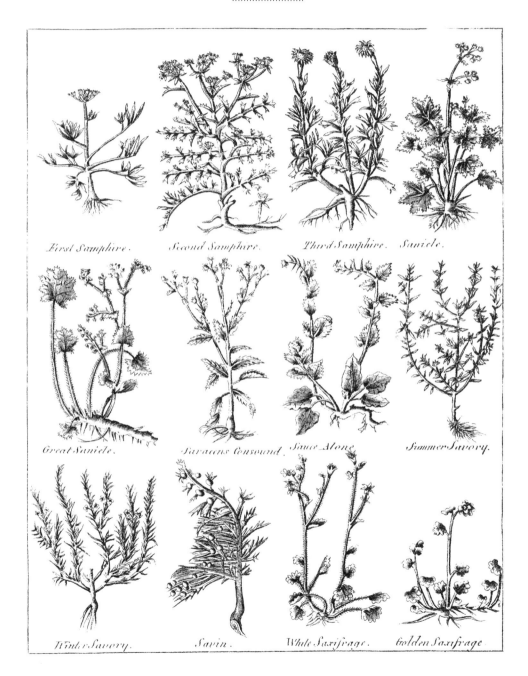

First Samphire.   Second Samphire.   Third Samphire.   Sanicle.

Great Sanicle.   Saracens Consound.   Sauce Alone.   Summer Savory.

Winter Savory.   Savin.   White Saxifrage.   Golden Saxifrage.

PLACE It grows in moist and wet grounds by the side of woods, and sometimes in moist places of the shady groves, as also by the water-side.

TIME It flowers generally about the middle of July, and the seed is soon ripe, and carried away by the wind.

GOVERNMENT AND VIRTUES Saturn owns this herb. Among the Germans, this wound-herb is preferred before all others of the same quality. Being boiled in water, it helps continual agues; and this said water, or the simple water of the herb distilled, or the juice or decoction, are very effectual to heal any green wound. It is no less effectual for the ulcers in the mouth or throat, by washing and gargling them therewith. Briefly, whatsoever has been said of bugle or sanicle may be found herein.

SARSAPARILLA

This is reckoned amongst the sorts of prickly bindweeds, of which there are two sorts, and this sarsaparilla brought from the West Indies makes the third kind. Their names with their descriptions severally follow.

DESCRIPTION
1. Prickly bindweed with red berries, called in Latin *smilax aspera sructu rubro*. This grows up with many branches, wherewith it winds about trees and other things, set with many crooked pricks or thorns like a bramble, all the whole length, binding this way and that in a seemly proportion; at every joint it bows or bends itself, having a somewhat broad and long leaf thereat, standing upon a long foot-stalk, and is broad at the bottom, with two forked round ends, and then grows narrower unto the point; the middle-rib on the backside of most of them having many small thorns or pricks, and also about the edges; the lowest being the largest, and growing smaller up to the top, smooth and of a fair green colour, and sometimes spotted with white spots. At the joints with the leaves also come forth tendrils, like a vine, whereby it winds itself; the flowers stand at the tops of the branches at three or four joints, many breaking forth into a cluster, which are white, composed of six leaves each, star-fashion, and sweet in scent, after which come the fruit, which are red berries when they are ripe, of the bigness of asparagus-berries or small grapes; and in some less, wherein are contained sometimes two or three hard black stones, like those of asparagus. The root is slender, white, and long, in hard dry grounds not spreading far, but in the looser and moister places running down into the ground a pretty way, with divers knots and joints.
2. Prickly bindweed with black berries, *smilax aspera fructu nigro*. This other prickly bindweed grows like the former, the branches being joined in like manner with thorns on them, but not climbing like the former; the leaves are

somewhat like it, not having those forked ends at the bottom of every leaf, but almost wholly round, and broad at the bottom, of a darker-green colour also, seldom having any thorns or pricks, either on the back or edges of the leaves, with tendrils like a vine also: the flowers come forth in the same manner, and are star-fashion, consisting of six leaves like the other, of an incarnate or blush colour, with a round red umbone in the middle of every one, which is the beginning of the berry, which when it is ripe will be black, being more sappy or fleshy than the other, with stones or kernels within them like unto it: the roots hereof are bigger and fuller than the former for the most part, and spread further under the ground.

3. Sarsaparilla of America, s*milax aspera Peruviana*. The sarsaparilla that comes from America into Spain has been seen fresh, even the whole plant, and has been verified in all things to resemble the prickly bindweed, and in nothing different from it. But certainly the plant of sarsaparilla that grows in Peru and the West Indies is a peculiar kind of itself, differing from the *smilax aspera* as mechoacan does from our briony: this does wind itself about poles or any thing else it can lay hold on to climb on; the branches have crooked prickles growing on them as the *smilax aspera* has, but fewer and not so sharp; it has very green leaves like those of bindweed, but longer, and cornered like ivy-leaves, ending in a long point: the flowers are said to be very great and white, every one as big as a middle-sized dish, which, opening in the morning, fades at night; which occasioned the Spaniards to call the whole plant *buenos noches*, that is, good night. Gerrard describes the sarsaparilla to be the roots of a shrub, having leaves like ivy; but says nothing of the flowers or fruit, which it may be believed were not then discovered.

PLACE AND TIME   The two first grow in Italy, Spain, and other warm countries, whether continent or isles, throughout Europe and Asia. The third is found only in the West Indies; the best is said to come from the Honduras, others not so good from other places, as the fertility or barrenness of the ground, and the temperature of the climate, afford it; and it has ripe berries early in hot countries.

GOVERNMENT AND VIRTUES   These are all plants of Mars, of an healing quality, howsoever used. The true sarsaparilla is held generally not to heat, but rather to dry, the humours; yet it is easily perceived, that it does not only dry the humours, but wastes them away, by a secret and hidden property therein. It is much used in many kinds of diseases; as in all cold fluxes from the head and brain, rheums, and catarrhs, as also in all cold griefs of the stomach, and expels wind very powerfully. It helps not only the French disease, but all manner of aches in the sinews or joints.

SAUCE-ALONE, OR JACK-BY-THE-HEDGE

DESCRIPTION   The lower leaves of this are rounder than those that grow towards the tops of the stalks, and are set singly, one at a joint, being somewhat round and broad, and pointed at the ends, dented also, about the edges, somewhat resembling nettle-leaves for the form, but of a more fresh-green colour, and not rough or pricking; the flowers are very small, and white, growing at the tops of the stalks one above another; which being past, there follow small and long round pods, wherein are contained small round seeds, somewhat blackish. The root is stringy and thready, perishing every year after it has given seed, and raises itself again of its own sowing. The plant, or any part thereof, being bruised, smells of garlic, but is much more pleasant, and tastes somewhat hot, sharp, and biting, almost like rocket.

PLACE   It grows under walls, and by hedge-sides, and pathways in fields in many places.

TIME   It flowers in June, July, and August.

GOVERNMENT AND VIRTUES   It is an herb of Mercury. This is eaten by many country people as sauce to their salt fish; it warms the stomach, and causes digestion. The juice thereof, boiled with honey, is reckoned to be as good as hedge-mustard for the cough, to cut and expectorate the tough phlegm. The seed, bruised and boiled in wine, is a good remedy for the wind-cholic, or the stone, being drunk warm. The leaves also, or the seed boiled, are good to be used in clysters to ease the pains of the stone. The green leaves are held to be good to heal ulcers in the legs.

SAUNDERS

KINDS AND DESCRIPTION   In our shops, for physical use we have three sorts of saunders, whereof the white and yellow are sweet woods, but the yellow is the sweetest; the red has no scent. The saunders-tree grows to be as big as a walnut-tree, having fresh-green leaves like the mastic-tree, and darkish-blue flowers, the fruit being like cherries for the size, but without any taste; black when they are ripe, and quickly falling away. The wood itself is without scent, as it is said, while it is living and fresh, and smells sweet only when it is dry. The white and the yellow woods are so hard to be distinguished before that time, that none but those Indians that usually fell those trees do know their difference before-hand; and can tell which will prove better than others: the chiefest part, and smelling sweetest, is the heart of the wood. They are distinguished by these names, *santalum album citrinum, et rubrum.*

GOVERNMENT AND VIRTUES All the saunders are under the solar regimen, they are cooling and cordial, and used together in sundry cordial medicines; but the white and the yellow are the more cordial and comfortable, by reason of their sweetness; and the red more cooling and binding; which quality neither of the other are without, though in a lesser proportion. The red is often used to stay thin rheum falling from the head, and to cool hot inflammations, hot gouts, and in hot agues to cool and temper the heat; but the white and yellow are both cordial and cephalic, applied with rose-water to the temples, procuring ease in the head-ache, and are singular good for weak and fainting stomachs through heat, and in the hot fits of agues. They are very profitably applied in fomentations for the stomach, spirits, and palpitations of the heart, which also do comfort and strengthen them, and temperate the melancholy humour, and procure alacrity and mirth, which quality is attributed to the yellow more than the white.

SAVIN

To describe a plant so well known is needless, it being almost in every garden, and remaining green all the winter.

GOVERNMENT AND VIRTUES It is under the dominion of Mars, being hot and dry in the third degree; and being of exceeding clean parts, is of a very digesting quality: if you dry the herb into powder, and mix it with honey, it is an excellent remedy to cleanse ulcers, and fistulas; but it hinders them from healing. The same is good to break carbuncles and plague-sores; it also helps the king's-evil, being applied to the place: being spread upon a piece of leather, and applied to the navel, it kills the worms in the belly; helps scabs and the itch, running sores, cankers, tetters, and ringworms; and, being applied to the place, may happily cure venereal sores. This I thought proper to mention, as it may safely be used outwardly; but inwardly it cannot be taken without manifest danger, particularly to pregnant women, or those who are subject to flooding.

WINTER AND SUMMER SAVOURY

Winter savoury

GOVERNMENT AND VIRTUES Mercury claims the dominion over this herb. They are both of them hot and dry, especially the summer kind, which is both sharp and quick in taste. It cuts tough phlegm in the chest and lungs, and helps to expectorate it the more easily; quickens the dull spirits in the lethargy, the juice thereof being snuffed or cast up into the nostrils.

Summer savoury

BURNET-SAXIFRAGE

DESCRIPTION The greater sort of our English burnet-saxifrage grows up with divers long stalks of winged leaves, set directly opposite one to another on both sides, each being somewhat broad, and a little pointed and dented about the edges, of a sad-green colour. At the tops of the stalks stand umbels of white flowers, after which comes small and blackish seed: the root is long and whitish, abiding long. Our smaller burnet-saxifrage has much finer leaves than the former, very small, and set one against another, deeply jagged about the edges, and of the same colour as the former. The umbels of the flowers are white, and the seed very small; and so is the root, being also somewhat hot to the taste.

PLACE These grow in most meadows in England, and are to be found concealed in the grass scarcely to be discerned.

TIME They flower about July, and the seed is ripe in August.

GOVERNMENT AND VIRTUES These herbs are both of the Moon. These saxifrages are as hot as pepper; and Tragus says, by his experience, they are more wholesome. They have the same properties that the parsleys have. The roots or seed, being used either in powder, or in decoction, or any other way, help to break and void the stone in the kidneys. Being boiled in the distilled water hereof, it is good to be given to those that are troubled with cramps and convulsions. Some make the seed into comfits (as they do carraway-seed). The juice of the herb, dropped into the most grievous wounds of the head, dries up their moisture and heals them quickly.

COMMON WHITE-SAXIFRAGE

DESCRIPTION This has a few small reddish kernels, covered with some skins lying among divers small blackish fibres, which send forth several round, faint or yellowish-green leaves, greyish underneath, lying above the ground, unevenly dented about the edges, and somewhat hairy, green, stalks, two or three feet high, with a few such round leaves as grow below, but smaller, and somewhat branched at the top, whereon stand pretty large white flowers of five leaves each, with some yellow threads in the middle, standing in a long-crested brownish-green husk. After the flowers are past, there arises sometimes a round hard head, sorked at the top, wherein is contained small blackish seed; but usually they fall away without any seed; and it is the kernels or grains of the root which are usually called the white saxifrage-seed, and so used.

PLACE It grows in many parts of Great Britain; in meadows and grassy sandy places: it used to grow near Lamb's Conduit, on the back-side of Gray's Inn.

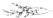

TIME It flowers in May, and is then gathered, as well for that which is called the seed as to distil; for it quickly perishes down to the ground in hot weather.

GOVERNMENT AND VIRTUES It is very effectual to cleanse the reins and bladder, and to dissolve the stone ingendered in them, and to expel it and the gravel by urine; to help the difficulty in passing urine; for which purposes the decoction of the herb or roots in white wine is most usual. The distilled water of the whole herb, roots, and flowers, is most commonly taken. It frees and cleanses the stomach and lungs from thick and tough phlegm. There are not many better medicines to break the stone than this.

SCABIOUS

Great scabious

Sheep's scabious

Third scabious

DESCRIPTION The common field-scabious grows up with many hairy, soft, whitish-green, leaves, some whereof are but very little if at all jagged on the edges, others very much rent and torn on the sides, and have threads in them, which, upon the breaking, may be plainly seen; from among which rise up divers hairy green stalks, three or four feet high, with such-like hairy green leaves on them, but more deeply and finely divided, branched forth a little. At the tops, which are naked and bare of leaves for a good space, stand round heads of flowers, of a pale-bluish colour, set together in a head, the outermost whereof are larger than the inward, with many threads also in the middle, somewhat flat at the top, as the head with seed is likewise. The root is great, white and thick, growing down deep in the ground, and abides many years.

There is another sort of field-scabious, different in nothing from the former, but only that it is smaller.

The corn-scabious differs little from the first, but that it is greater, and the flowers more inclining to purple; and the root creeps under the surface of the earth, and runs not deep in the ground as the first does.

PLACE The first grows most usually in meadows, especially about London, every where. The second in some of the dry fields near London, but not so plentiful as in the former. The third in the standing corn, or fallow fields, and the borders of such-like fields.

TIME They flower in June and July, and some abide flowering until it be late in August, and the seed ripens in the mean time.

There are many other sorts of scabious, but those here described are most familiar with us; the virtues both of these and the red being much alike, you will take them as follows.

GOVERNMENT AND VIRTUES Mercury owns the plant. Scabious is very effectual for all sorts of coughs, shortness of breath, and all other diseases of the breast and lungs. The decoction of the herb and roots, outwardly applied, does wonderfully help all sorts of hard or cold swellings in any part of the body, and is as effectual for any shrunk sinew or vein. The juice of scabious made up with the powder of borax and camphire, cleanses the skin. The head being washed with the same decoction, it cleanses it from dandruff, scurf, sores, itches, and the like, being used warm. Tents, dipped in the juice or water thereof, heal green wounds. The herb bruised, and applied, does in a short time loosen and draw forth any splinter, or other thing, lying in the flesh.

SCAMMONY

DESCRIPTION The true scammony has a long root of a dark ash-colour on the outside, and white within, and of the bigness of an arm, with a pith in the middle thereof, and many fibres thereat, from whence arise many long, round, green, branches, winding themselves like a bindweed about stakes and trees, or any other thing that stands next it, unto a good height, without any clasping tendrils, like the true or wild vine: from the joints of the branches come forth the leaves, every one by itself upon short footstalks, somewhat broad at the bottom, with two corners next thereto, and some also round; and then growing long and narrow to the end, being of a fair-green colour, and smooth, somewhat shining. Towards the tops of the branches, at the joints with the leaves, come forth large whitish bell-flowers, with wide open brims and narrow bottoms, after which come round heads, wherein is contained three or four black seeds; if any part of this plant be broken, it yields forth a milk, not hot, nor burning, nor bitter, yet somewhat unpleasant, provoking loathing, and almost casting.

NAMES It is called scammonia both in Greek and Latin. The dried juice, which is most in use, is called also scammoniacum in the druggists and apothecaries shops, as also with most writers, and some call the plant so too. When it is prepared, that is, baked in a quince under the embers, or in an oven, or any other way, it is called diagridium.

PLACE AND TIME Scammony grows in Syria, and the farther eastern parts, where no frosts come in the winter; for where any frost comes it quickly perishes, consequently it flourishes in hot climates only.

GOVERNMENT AND VIRTUES This is a martial plant. It purges both phlegm, yellow choler, and watery humours, very strongly; but, if it be indiscreetly given, it will not only trouble the stomach more than any other medicine, but will also scour the guts, in working too powerfully, and therefore is not fit to be given to any gentle or tender body.

Dioscorides says, if the juice be applied to the womb, it destroys the birth, being mixed with honey and ox-gall; and, rubbed on weals, pimples, and

PLATE 21

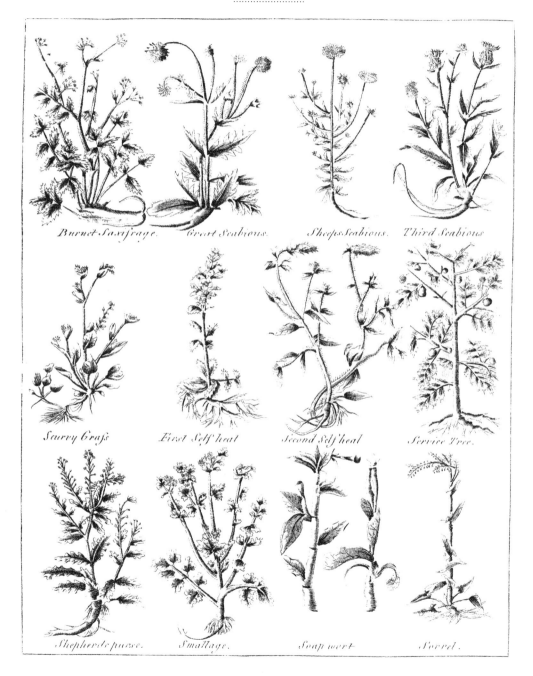

Burnet Saxifrage.   Great Scabious.   Sheeps Scabious.   Third Scabious

Scurvy Grass   First Self heal   Second Self heal   Service Tree.

Shepherds purse.   Smallage.   Soap wort   Sorrel.

pushes, takes them all away; being dissolved in rose-water and vinegar, and the head moistened therewith, it eases the continual pains thereof. A drachm or two of the roots of scammony purge in the same manner as the juice does, if some of the things that are appointed therewith be given in it. The roots boiled in water, and made into a poultice, with barley-meal, eases the sciatica, being laid thereon; it takes away scurfs and scabs if they be washed with the vinegar wherein the roots have been boiled, and also heals imposthumes.

SCURVY-GRASS

DESCRIPTION Our ordinary English scurvy-grass has many thick leaves, more long than broad, and sometimes longer and narrower; sometimes smooth on the edges, and sometimes a little waved; sometimes plain, smooth, and pointed, sometimes a little hollow in the middle, and round pointed, of a sad green, and sometimes a bluish colour, every one standing by itself upon a long footstalk, which is brownish or greenish also, from among which rise small slender stalks, bearing a few leaves thereon like the other, but longer and less for the most part; at the tops whereof grow many whitish flowers with yellow threads in the middle, standing about a green head which becomes the seed-vessel. The seed is reddish, tasting somewhat hot: the root is composed of many white strings, which stick deeply in the mud, wherein it chiefly delights; yet it will grow in upland and dry grounds; and tastes a little brackish, or salt, even there, but not so much as where it has salt water to feed upon.

PLACE It grows all along the Thames side, on the Essex and Kentish shores, from Woolwich round about the sea coasts to Dover, Portsmouth, and even to Bristol, where it is in plenty; the other, with round leaves, grows in the marshes in Holland in Lincolnshire, and other places of Lincolnshire by the sea-side.

Dutch scurvy-grass is most known and frequent in gardens, and has divers fresh, green, and almost round, leaves, rising from the root, not so thick as the former, yet in some rich ground very large, not dented about the edges, nor hollow in the middle, every one standing on a long footstalk; from among these rise up divers long slender weak stalks, higher than the former, and with more white flowers, which turn into smaller pods, and smaller brownish seed, than the former: the root is white, small, and thready: the taste of this is not salt at all, but hot, aromatical, and spicy.

TIME It flowers in April or May, and the seed is ripe soon after.

GOVERNMENT AND VIRTUES It is an herb of Jupiter. The English scurvy-grass is more used for its salt taste, which does somewhat open and cleanse; but the Dutch scurvy-grass is of better effect, and chiefly used by those that have the scurvy, especially to purge and cleanse the blood, the liver, and the spleen, for all which diseases it is of singular good effect, by taking the juice in the spring every morning fasting in a cup of drink.

SEBESTEN, OR ASSYRIAN PLUM

DESCRIPTION AND NAMES The sebesten-tree grows not so high as the plum-tree. It is covered with a whitish bark; the branches are green, whereon grow rounder, thicker, and harder, leaves. The blossoms are white, and consist of five leaves each, growing together on a long stalk, which afterwards turn into small berries, rather than plums, of blackish-green colour when they are ripe, every one standing in a little cup, of a sweet taste, and glutinous or clammy substance, and a very thick skin; within which lies a three-square hard stone, with a thick shell and a small kernel; these are gathered and laid in the Sun, whereby they grow wrinkled: and so they are kept and brought to us in boxes.

WILD SEBESTEN

The wild sebesten is in all things like the other, but that it grows lower, much like unto a hedge-bush, and with smaller and thinner leaves. The flowers and fruit are like, but less.

In shops they have only the name of sebesten, but in Latin the tree is called *myxos*, *myxa*, and *mixaria*.

PLACE AND TIME The first grows in Syria, and is but planted in Egypt, whence they were brought into Italy in Pliny's time, and grafted on the service-tree, and do now grow in many places in their orchards. It is so tender, that it will not endure the cold with us. The wild kind, as Alpinus says, is natural in Egypt: they flower in May, and the fruit is ripe in September.

GOVERNMENT AND VIRTUES This is a plant of Venus: the Arabians and Greeks hold that they open the body as much, or rather more, by reason of the mucilage in them, than the damask prunes: more however while they are green, and less when they are dry: yet the decoction of them, or the infusion of them in broth, although dried and taken whole, works effectually; which Fuschius denies, and affirms that they are rather binding. They serve to cool any intemperate heat of the stomach or liver, and therefore are good in hot agues, and to purge choler, whereof they come. There is a kind of bird-lime made of these fruits by boiling them a little in water to take away the skins and stones, and afterwards boiling them more to a consistence; the which (as says Mathiolus) was used at Venice to catch birds; but Alpinus says they use it in Egypt as a plaster to dissolve hard tumours or swellings.

SELF-HEAL

First self-heal

It is called prunel, carpenter's herb, hook-heal, and sickle-wort.

DESCRIPTION The common self-heal is a small, low, creeping, herb, having many small roundish pointed leaves, somewhat like the leaves of wild mints, of a dark green colour, without any dents on the edges, from among which rise divers small leaves up to the tops, where stand brownish spiked heads, of many small brownish leaves like scales and flowers set together, almost like the head of cassidony, which flowers are gaping, and of a bluish-purple, or more pale below, in some places sweet, but not so in others. The root consists of many strings or fibres downward, and spreads strings also, whereby it increases. The small stalks, with the leaves, creeping upon the ground, shoot forth fibres taking hold of the ground, whereby it is made a great tuft in short time.

Second self-heal

PLACE It is found in woods and fields every where.

TIME It flowers in May, and sometimes in April.

GOVERNMENT AND VIRTUES This is an herb of Venus. It is a special herb for inward and outward wounds: take it inwardly in syrups for inward wounds: outwardly, in unguents and plasters. As self-heal is like bugle in its form, so also in the qualities and virtues, serving with good success. If it be accompanied with bugle, sanicle, and other the like wound-herbs, it will be the more effectual. It is a good remedy for green wounds, to close the lips of them.

SENA

DESCRIPTION The true sena is said to grow in Arabia and Syria, and is transported from Alexandria to us. There is a bastard sena which is kept in many gardens with us, commonly called colutea, which is its Latin name.

GOVERNMENT AND VIRTUES It is under the dominion of Mercury. The leaves of sena (which only are used) are hot near the first degree, and dry in the third; it is of a purging faculty, but leaves a binding quality after the purging; it opens obstructions, and cleanses and comforts the stomach, being corrected with some anise-seed, carraway-seed, or ginger. It cleanses and purifies the blood, and causes a fresh and lively habit of the body,

The bastard sena works very violently both upwards and downwards, offending the stomach and bowels.

SERVICE-TREE

TIME It flowers before the end of May, and the fruit is ripe in October.

GOVERNMENT AND VIRTUES Services, when they are mellow, are fit to be taken to stay the fluxes, scowering, and castings, yet less than medlars; if they be dried before they be mellow, and kept all the year, they may be used in decoction for the said purpose, either to drink, or to bathe the parts requiring it; and are profitably used in that manner to stay the bleeding of wounds. The service-tree is under the dominion of Saturn.

SHEPHERD'S PURSE

It is also called shepherd's scrip, shepherd's pouch, toy-wort, pick-purse, and case-weed.

DESCRIPTION The root is small, white, and perishes every year. The leaves are small and long, of a pale green colour, and deeply cut on both sides: amongst which springs up a stalk which is small and round, containing small leaves upon it even to the top. The flowers are white, and very small; after which come the little cases which hold the seed, which are flat, almost in the form of a heart.

PLACE They are frequent in Great Britain, commonly by the paths-side.

TIME They flower all the summer, some of them so fruitful, that they flower twice a year.

GOVERNMENT AND VIRTUES It is under the dominion of Saturn, and of a cold, dry, and binding, nature. The herb, being made into a poultice, helps inflammations. A good ointment may be made of it for all wounds, especially wounds in the head.

SMALLAGE

PLACE It grows naturally in wet and marshy grounds; but, if it be sown in gardens, it there prospers very well.

TIME It abides green all the winter, and seeds in August.

GOVERNMENT AND VIRTUES It is an herb of Mercury. Smallage is hotter, drier, and much more medicinable than parsley, for it much more opens obstructions of the liver and spleen, rarefies thick phlegm, and cleanses it and the blood withal. The juice, put to honey of roses, and barley water, is very good to gargle the mouth and throat of those that have sores and ulcers in them, and will quickly heal them: the same lotion also cleanses and heals ulcers elsewhere.

SOLOMON'S SEAL

Great solomon's seal

Small solomon's seal

DESCRIPTION   The common solomon's seal rises up with a round stalk about half a yard high, bowing or bending down, set with single leaves one above another, somewhat large, and like the leaves of the lily-convalley, or May-lily, with an eye of bluish upon the green, with some ribs therein, and more yellowish underneath. At the foot of every leaf, almost from the bottom up to the top of the stalk, come forth small, long, white, and hollow, pendulous flowers, somewhat like the flowers of May-lily, but ending in five long points, for the most part two together at the end of a long foot-stalk, and sometimes but one, and sometimes also two stalks with flowers at the foot of a leaf, which are without any scent at all, and stand all on one side of the stalk. After they are past, come in their places small round berries, green at first, and blackish green, tending to blueness, when they are ripe, wherein lie small, white, hard, and stony, seed. The root is of the thickness of one's finger or thumb, white and knobbed in some places, with a flat circle representing a seal, whence it took the name, lying along under the surface of the earth, and not running very low, but with many fibres underneath.

PLACE   It is frequent in divers places of Kent, Essex, and other counties.

TIME   It flowers about May, or the beginning of June; and the root abides and shoots anew every year.

GOVERNMENT AND VIRTUES   Saturn owns the plant. The root of Solomon's seal is found by experience to be available in wounds, hurts, and outward sores, to heal and close up the lips of those that are green, and to dry up and restrain the flux of humours to those that are cold: it is good to stay vomitings and bleedings wheresoever, as likewise all fluxes in man or woman

SOPE-WORT, OR BRUISE-WORT

DESCRIPTION   the root creeps under ground far and near, with many joints therein, of a brown colour on the outside, and yellowish within, shooting forth in divers places many weak round stalks, full of joints, set with two leaves apiece at every one of them on the contrary side, which are ribbed somewhat like that of plantain, and fashioned like the common field white campion leaves, seldom having any branches from the sides of the stalks, but set with divers flowers at the top standing in long husks like the wild campions, made of five leaves each, round at the ends, and a little dented in the middle, of a pale rose colour, almost white, sometimes deeper, sometimes paler.

PLACE It grows wild in low and wet grounds in many parts of England, by the brooks and sides of running waters.

TIME It flowers usually in July, and so continues all August and part of September.

GOVERNMENT AND VIRTUES Venus owns it. The country people in many places do use to bruise the leaves of sope-wort, and lay it to their fingers, hands, or legs, when they are cut, to heal them. Some say it is diuretic, and expels gravel and stone in the kidneys, and is also good to void hydropical waters, thereby to cure the dropsy.

SORREL

GOVERNMENT AND VIRTUES It is under the dominion of Venus. Sorrel is prevalent in all hot diseases, to cool any inflammation and heat of blood, and is a cordial to the heart, for which the seed is more effectual, being more drying and binding. The roots also, in a decoction, or in powder, are effectual for all the said purposes. The decoction of the roots is taken to expel the gravel and stone. A syrup made with the juice of sorrel and fumitory is a sovereign help to kill those sharp humours that cause the itch. The leaves wrapped up in a colewort leaf, and roasted under the embers, and applied to a hard imposthume, or sore, both ripen and break it. The distilled water of the herb is of much good use for all the purposes aforesaid; and the leaves eaten in a salad are excellent for the blood.

WOOD-SORREL

DESCRIPTION This grows low upon the ground, having a number of leaves coming from the root, made of three leaves like trefoil, but broad at the ends, and cut in the middle, of a faint yellowish-green colour, every one standing on a long footstalk, which at their first coming up are close folded together to the stalk; but, opening afterwards, are of a fine sour relish, and yield a juice which will turn red when it is clarified, and makes a most dainty clear syrup. Among these leaves rises up divers slender weak footstalks, with every one of them a flower at the top, consisting of five small pointed leaves, star-fashion, of a white colour in most places, and in some dashed over with a small show of bluish on the back-side only. After the flowers are past, follow small round heads, with small yellowish seed in them. The roots are nothing but small strings fastened to the end of a small long piece, all of them being of a yellowish colour.

PLACE It grows in many places of England, in woods and other places not too much open to the Sun.

TIME It flowers in April and May.

GOVERNMENT AND VIRTUES Venus owns it. Wood-sorrel serves to all the purposes that the other sorrels do, and is more effectual in cooling and tempering heats and inflammations, to quench thirst, to strengthen a weak stomach, to procure an appetite, to stay vomiting, and is very excellent in any contagious sickness.

The syrup made of the juice is effectual in all the cases aforesaid, and so is the distilled water of the herb. Sponges or linen cloths wet in the juice, and applied outwardly to any hot swellings or inflammations, do much cool and help them. The same juice taken, and gargled in the mouth, for some time, and frequently repeated, does wonderfully help ulcers therein. It is of singular service for wounds in any part of the body, to stay the bleeding and to cleanse and heal the wounds; and helps to stay any hot defluxions into the throat or lungs and cleanses the viscera.

Great
southernwood

SOUTHERNWOOD

TIME It flowers for the most part in July and August.

Small
southernwood

GOVERNMENT AND VIRTUES It is a Mercurial plant, worthy of more esteem than it has. Dioscorides says, that the seed bruised, heated in warm water, and drunk, helps those that are troubled with the cramps, or convulsions of the sinews, the sciatica, or difficulty in making water. The same taken in wine is an antidote, or counter-poison, and drives away serpents and other venomous creatures; as also the smell of the herb, being burnt, does the same.

The oil thereof, anointed on the back-bone before the fits of agues come, prevents them; it takes away inflammations in the eyes, if it be put with some part of a roasted quince, and boiled with a few crumbs of bread and applied. Boiled with barley-meal, it takes away pimples, pushes, or weals, that rise in the face or other part of the body. The seed as well as the dried herb is often given to kill worms in children. The herb bruised helps to draw forth splinters and thorns out of the flesh.

PLATE 22

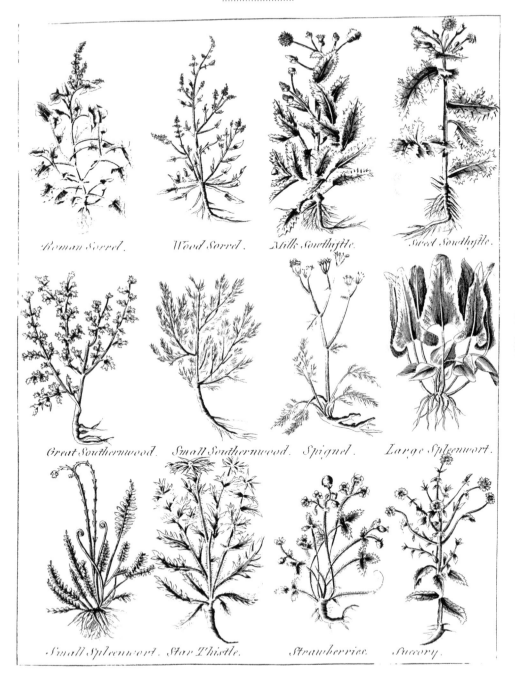

Roman Sorrel.   Wood Sorrel.   Milk Sowthistle.   Sweet Sowthistle.

Great Southernwood.   Small Southernwood.   Spignel.   Large Spleenwort.

Small Spleenwort. Star Thistle.   Strawberries.   Succory.

SOW-THISTLES

PLACE They grow in our gardens and manured grounds, and sometimes by old walls, the path-sides of fields and highways.

GOVERNMENT AND VIRTUES This and the former are under the influence of Venus. Sow-thistles are cooling, and somewhat binding, and are very fit to cool an hot stomach, and to ease the gnawing pains thereof. The decoction of the leaves and stalks causes abundance of milk in nurses, and is good for those whose milk curdles in their breasts.

The herb bruised, or the juice, is profitably applied to all hot inflammations in the eyes, or wheresoever else, and for weals, blisters, or other the like eruptions, or heat, in the skin; also for the heat and itching of the hæmorrhoids, and the heat and sharpness of humours in the secret parts of man or woman. The distilled water of the herb is not only effectual for all the diseases aforesaid, to be taken inwardly with a little sugar but outwardly, by applying cloths or sponges wetted therein. It is good for women to wash their faces therewith, to clear the skin, and to give a lustre thereto. The virtue of this plant lies in its milky juice, which is of great value in difficulty of hearing.

SPIGNEL

DESCRIPTION The roots of common spignel do spread much and deep in the ground, many strings or branches growing from one head, which is hairy at the top, of a blackish-brown colour on the outside, and white within, of a pleasant smell and aromatic taste, whence rise sundry long stalks of fine cut leaves like hairs, smaller than dill, set thick on both sides of the stalk, and of a good scent. Among these leaves rise up round stiff stalks, with a few joints and leaves, and at the tops an umbel of fine pure white flowers, at the edges whereof sometimes will be seen a show of reddish-blue colour, especially before they be full blown, and are succeeded by small somewhat round seed, bigger than the ordinary fennel, and of a browner colour, divided into two parts, and crested on the back, as most of the umbelliferous seeds are.

PLACE It grows wild in Lancashire, Yorkshire, and other northern counties; and is also planted in gardens.

GOVERNMENT AND VIRTUES It is an herb of Venus. The roots boiled in wine or water, and drunk, help the wind, swellings, and pains, in the stomach, and all joint-aches. If the powder of the roots be mixed with honey, and the same taken as a licking medicine, it breaks tough phlegm, and dries up the rheum that falls on the lungs.

SPIKENARD

Spikenard

It is naturally an Indian plant, called *nardus Indica*; therefore I shall proceed to declare its virtues, not troubling you at all with its description.

VIRTUES Spikenard is of a heating drying faculty, and eases pains of the stone in the reins and kidneys, being drunk in cold water; to women with child it is forbidden to be taken inwardly.

English spikenard

The oil of spikenard purges the brain of rheum, being snuffed up the nostrils; being infused certain days in wine, and then distilled in a hot bath, the water is good inwardly and outwardly to be used for any coldness of the members. It comforts the brain, and helps cold pains of the head, and the shaking palsy.

SPLEEN-WORT, OR CETRACH

Large spleen-wort

DESCRIPTION The smooth spleen-wort, growing from a black, thready, and bushy root, sends forth many long single leaves, cut in on both sides into round dents, almost to the middle, which is not so hard as that of polypody, each division being not always set opposite unto the other, but between each, smooth, and of a light green on the upper side, and a dark-yellowish roughness on the back, folding or rolling itself inward at the first springing up.

Small spleen-wort

PLACE It grows as well upon stone walls as moist and shadowy places about Bristol and the other the west parts plentifully; as also on Framingham Castle, on Beckonsfield church in Berkshire, at Stroud, in Kent, and elsewhere, and abides green all the winter.

GOVERNMENT AND VIRTUES Saturn owns it. It is generally used against infirmities of the spleen: it helps with the difficulty in passing urine, and wastes the stone in the bladder, but the use of it in women hinders conception.

STAR-THISTLE

DESCRIPTION The common star-thistle has divers long and narrow leaves lying next the ground, cut or torn on the edges, somewhat deeply, into many almost even parts, soft or a little woolly all over the green, among which rise up divers weak stalks parted into many branches, all lying or leaning down to the ground, so that it seems a pretty bush, set with many divided leaves up to the tops, where severally stand long and small whitish-green heads, set with sharp and long white pricks (no part of the plant being else prickly) which are somewhat yellowish: out of the middle whereof rises the flower, composed of many small reddish-purple threads; and in the heads, after the flowers are past,

PLATE 23

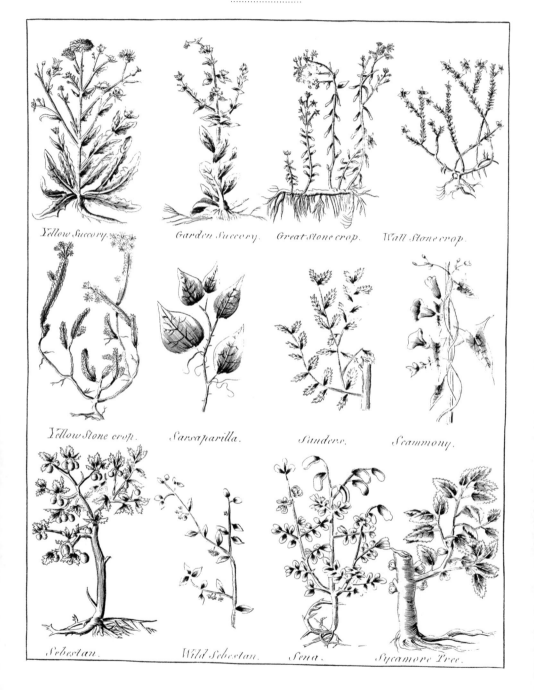

Yellow Succory.   Garden Succory.   Great Stone crop.   Wall Stone crop.

Yellow Stone crop.   Sarsaparilla.   Sanders.   Scammony.

Sebestan.   Wild Sebestan.   Sena.   Sycamore Tree.

come small whitish round seed, lying down as the others do. The root is small, long, and woody, perishing every year, and rising again of its own sowing.

PLACE It grows wild in the fields about London in many places.

TIME It flowers early, and seeds in July, and sometimes in August.

GOVERNMENT AND VIRTUES This, like almost all thistles, is under Mars. The seed of this star-thistle made into powder, and drunk in wine, helps to break the stone, and expel it. Baptista Sardus does much commend the distilled water, to help the French disease, to open obstructions of the liver, and cleanse the blood from corrupted humours: and it is profitably given against quotidian or tertian agues.

STONECROP, OR SMALL HOUSELEEK

Great stonecrop

DESCRIPTION It grows with divers trailing branches upon the ground, set with many thick, fat, roundish, whitish, leaves, pointed at the ends; the flowers stand many of them together, somewhat loosely; the roots are small, and run creeping under the ground.

Yellow stonecrop

PLACE It grows upon the stone walls and mud walls, upon the tiles of houses and penthouses, and amongst rubbish, and in most gravelly places.

TIME It flowers in June and July, and the leaves are green all the winter.

Wall stonecrop

GOVERNMENT AND VIRTUES It is under the dominion of the Moon, cold in quality, and something binding, and therefore very good to stay defluxions, especially such as fall upon the eyes. It is so harmless an herb, you can scarce use it amiss.

STORAX-TREE

KINDS There are accounted three sorts of the storax-tree, whose names shall follow with their descriptions.

DESCRIPTION

1. The usual storax-tree is called in Latin *styrax arbor vulgaris*. This storax-tree grows very like the quince-tree, both for form and bigness, the leaves also are long and round, and somewhat like, but far less: whitish underneath, and stiff, the flowers stand both at the joints with the leaves, and at the ends of the branches, consisting of five or six large whitish leaves, like those of the orange-

tree, with some threads in the middle, after which come round berries, set in the cups that the flowers were in before, of the bigness of hasel-nuts, pointed at the ends, and hoary all over; each standing on a long foot-stalk, containing within them certain kernels in small shells. This yields most fragrant sweet gum, and clear, of the colour of brown honey.

2. Storax with maple-leaves, *styrax folio aceris*. From a round root, covered with a crested or as it were a jointed bark, come forth, out of knots, three or five broad leaves, like those of the maple or plane-tree, standing on small blackish long stalks, and are divided in three or five parts, full of veins, dented about the edges, and pointed at the ends.

3. Red storax, called in Latin *styrax rubra*. This has formerly by some been thought to be the bark of some kind of tree that went under the name of storax. But Serapio and Avicen divide storax into *liquida* and *sicca*: by *liquida* meaning the pure gum flowing from the tree; and by the *sicca* the fæces of the expressed oil from the fruit.

PLACE AND TIME The first grows in Provence of France, in Italy, Candy, Greece, and some other parts of Turkey, where it yields no gum; but in Syria, Silicia, Pamphylia, Cyprus, and those hotter countries, it grows much. It flowers in the spring, yielding fruit in September.

GOVERNMENT AND VIRTUES This is a solar plant: there is no part of this tree in use with us, but the gum that issues out of it is of temperature hot in the second degree, and dry in the first; it heats, mollifies, and digests; and is good for coughs, catarrhs, and hoarseness. Pills made with it and a little turpentine, and taken, gently loosen the belly. It is good to be put into baths, for lameness of the joints. It is also good to be put with white frankincense to perfume those that have catarrhs, rheums, and defluxions from the head to the nose, eyes, or other parts, by casting it on quick coals, and holding the head over the smoke. It dissolves hard tumours in any part, and is good for the king's evil.

STRAWBERRIES

TIME They flower in May ordinarily, and the fruit is ripe shortly after.

GOVERNMENT AND VIRTUES Venus owns the herb. Strawberries, when they are green, are cold and dry; but when they are ripe they are cold and moist. The berries are excellent good to cool the liver, the blood, and the spleen, or a hot choleric stomach; to refresh and comfort the fainting spirits, and to quench thirst. They are good also for other inflammations, yet it is not amiss to refrain from them in a fever, less by their putrifying in the stomach they increase the fits. The water of the berries, carefully distilled, is a sovereign remedy and cordial in the pacification of the heart.

PLATE 24

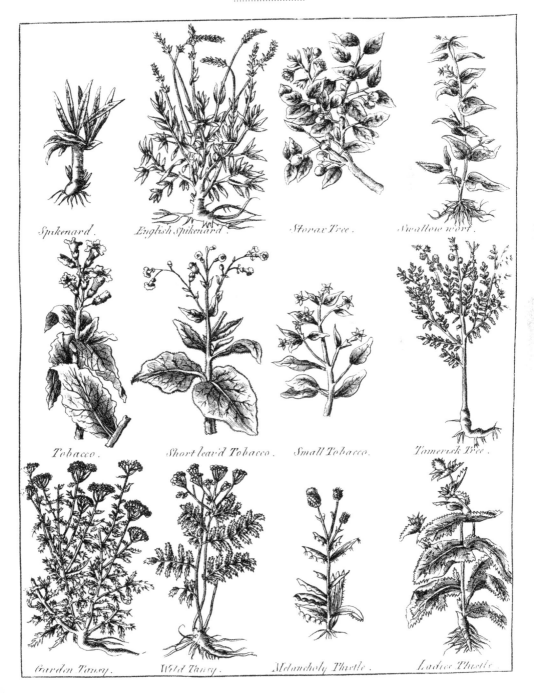

Spikenard.   English Spikenard.   Storax Tree.   Swallow wort.

Tobacco.   Short leav'd Tobacco.   Small Tobacco.   Tamerisk Tree.

Garden Tansy.   Wild Tansy.   Melancholy Thistle.   Ladies Thistle.

SUCCORY

DESCRIPTION The garden-succory has longer and narrower leaves than endive, and more cut in and torn at the edges, and the root abides many years; it bears also many blue flowers like endive, and the seed is hardly distinguishable from the seed of the smooth or ordinary endive.

GOVERNMENT AND VIRTUES It is an herb of Jupiter. Garden-succory, as it is more dry and less cold than endive, so it opens more. A handful of the leaves or roots boiled in wine or water, and a draught thereof drunk fasting, drives forth choleric and phlegmatic humours; opens obstructions of the liver, gall, and spleen; helps the yellow-jaundice, the heat of the reins, and of the urine. A decoction thereof made with wine, and drunk, is very effectual against long lingering agues; and a drachm of the seed in powder drunk in wine before the fit of an ague helps to drive it away.

SWALLOW-WORT

KINDS Of this there are three kinds; the usual Latin name of swallow-wort is *asclepias* or *Venice toxicum*; their distinct names follow in their descriptions.

DESCRIPTION
1. Swallow-wort with white flowers, *asclepias flore albo*. This swallow-wort rises up with divers slender weak stalks to be two or three feet long, not easy to break, scarcely able to stand upright, and therefore for the most part leans or lies upon the ground, if it find not any thing to sustain it; whereon are set two leaves at the joints, being somewhat broad and long pointed at the end; of a dark green colour, and smooth at the edges. At the joints with the leaves, towards the tops of the stalks, and at the tops themselves, come forth divers small white flowers, consisting of five pointed leaves apiece, of a sweet scent; after which come small long pods, thick above, in a great deal of white silken down, which when the pod is ripe opens of itself, and sheds both seed and cotton upon the ground, if it be not carefully gathered. The roots are a great bush, of many strings fastened together at the head, smelling somewhat strong while they are fresh and green, but more pleasant when they are dried; both leaves and stalks perish every winter, and arise anew in the spring of the year, when the stalks, at their first springing, are of a blackish brown.
2. Swallow-wort with black flowers, called in Latin *asclepias flore nigro*. This grows in the same manner that the former does, having long slender rough branches, rising out to a greater height than the other, and twining about whatsoever stands next unto them; having such-like dark green leaves set by couples, but somewhat smaller, and of a dark-purplish colour; after which come more plentifully such-like cods, with a white silver down and seeds in them

as the former. The roots hereof are not so bushy as the other, neither smell so strong; neither does it give any milky but a watery juice when broken.

3. Swallow-wort of Candy, *asclepias Cretica*. This rises up in the same fashion as the former do, with many slender flexible green branches, with leaves set at the joints on either side, as the white kind has, and are very like them, but somewhat of a paler white colour. The flowers stand in the same manner, three or four together upon a stalk, but are somewhat of a paler white colour; to whom succeed sometimes but one pod, and sometimes two together, thicker and shorter than those of the white kind; streaked all along and double-forked at the ends, wherein lie silk and seeds as in the former; the roots have not so strong a smell as the last, and have, as well as the rest of the plant, a scent like Box-leaves.

PLACE AND TIME The two first grow in rough and untilled ground; upon divers mountains in France, about Narbonne, Marseille, and Montpelier, and in Italy also; the last in Candy. They flower in the months of June and July, and sometimes not until August; and their cods are ripe about a month after; the empty hulks abide on the dry branches when the seed and silk are fallen out.

GOVERNMENT AND VIRTUES These are solar plants. The powder of the roots, taken with peony-seeds, is good against the falling-sickness; or, with basil-seed, or the rind of pomecitron-seeds, is good against melancholy. The leaves and flowers boiled, and made into a poultice, and applied to the hard tumours or swellings of women's breasts, cure them speedily.

SYCAMORE-TREE

KINDS There are two sorts of this tree, the one bearing fruit out of the body and greater arms of the tree only, the other upon stalks without leaves. The first is called in Latin, *sycomorus* and *sicus Egyptia*, the Egyptian fig-tree, and is the true sycamore-tree; those trees which are vulgarly called sycamores in England, are a kind of maple.

DESCRIPTION

1. This sycamore grows to be a very great tree, bigger than the mulberry-tree, with large arms and branches, full of round and somewhat long leaves, pointed at the ends, and dented about the edges, very like the leaves of the mulberry-tree; but harder and rougher, like fig-leaves; this bears small figs, or fruit, and no flower, differing in that from all other trees; for it brings forth the fruit out of the very body or trunk of the tree only, and the elder branches next to the body, and no where else; and are very like unto white or wild figs, and of the same bigness; but much sweeter, and without any kernels. The whole tree, and every part, abounds with milk, if the bark be but gently wounded; but if it be cut too deep, it yields no milk at all; which makes it to bear three or four times a year, new

rising out of the places where the old grew. The root is solid, hard, and black, and will abide fresh long after it is felled.

2. The other sycamore is called *sycomorus altera, seu ficus Cypria*, the sycamore of Cyprus. This grows to be as big as a plum-tree, or white poplar-tree, the arms and branches bearing broad and somewhat round leaves, like unto the elm, but very like unto the former; this bears such-like fruit as figs, but smaller, which rise both from the body and the greater arms, but not as the former, but on certain stalks in branches, which rise by themselves without any leaves with them; and are as sweet as figs. They bear four times every year, but not unless they be slit, that the milk in them may come forth.

PLACE AND TIME The first grows chiefly in Egypt, Syria, and Arabia, and other places adjacent; the other in Cyprus, Caria, and Rhodes.

GOVERNMENT AND VIRTUES These are under the particular influence of Venus. The fruit makes the belly soluble, but by its overmuch moisture it troubles the stomach, and gives but little nourishment. The milk that is taken from the tree, by gently piercing the bark, and afterwards dried and made into trouches, and kept in an earthen pot, has a property to soften humours, and dissolve them, and to solder and close together the lips of green wounds. The fruit itself, being applied as a plaster, works the same effect.

TAMARISK-TREE

TIME It flowers about the end of May, or in June, and the seed is ripe and blown away in the beginning of September.

GOVERNMENT AND VIRTUES It is under the dominion of Saturn. If the root, leaves, or young branches, be boiled in wine, and drunk, and applied outwardly, it is very powerful against the hardness of the spleen. The bark is as effectual, if not more, to all the purposes aforesaid; and both it and the leaves boiled in wine, and the mouth and the teeth washed therewith, help the tooth-ache, the ear-ache, and the redness and watering of the eyes. The said decoction, with some honey put thereto, is good to stay gangrenes and fretting ulcers. The wood is very effectual to consume the spleen, and therefore to drink out of cups and cans made thereof is good for splenetic persons. The ashes of the wood are used for all the purposes aforesaid; and, besides, do quickly help the blisters raised by burnings or scaldings by fire or water.

GARDEN TANSEY

TIME It flowers in June and July.

GOVERNMENT AND VIRTUES Venus governs this herb. The herb bruised, and applied to the navel, stays miscarriages; also it consumes those phlegmatic humours which the cold and moist constitution of winter usually infects the body with, and that was the first reason of eating tansey in the spring. The decoction of the common tansey, or the juice drunk in wine, is a singular remedy for all the griefs that come by stopping of the urine, helps the difficulty in passing urine, and those that have weak reins and kidneys. It is very profitable to dissolve and expel wind in the stomach, belly, or bowels. If it be bruised, and often smelled to, as also applied to the lower part of the belly, it is very profitable for such women as are given to miscarry in child-bearing, to cause them to go out their full time; it is used also against the stone in the reins, especially to men. The herb fried with eggs, which is called a tansey, helps to digest, and carry downward, those bad humours that trouble the stomach. Being boiled in oil, it is good for the sinews shrunk by cramps, or pained with cold. The seed is very profitably given to children for worms, and the juice in drink is as effectual; and it is in this last capacity that it is principally to be regarded.

WILD TANSEY, OR SILVER-WEED

PLACE It grows almost in every place.

TIME It flowers in June and July.

GOVERNMENT AND VIRTUES This is likewise an herb of Venus. Wild tansey stays the lask, and all the fluxes of blood, in men or women, which some say it will do if the green herb be worn in the shoes, so it be next the skin; it stays also spitting or vomiting of blood. Being boiled in wine and drunk, it eases the griping pains of the bowels, and is good for the sciatica and joint-aches. The same boiled in vinegar with honey and alum, and gargled in the mouth, eases the pains of the tooth-ache, fastens loose teeth, helps the gums that are sore, and settles the palate of the mouth in its place when it is fallen down. Being bruised and applied to the soles of the feet, and the wrists, it wonderfully cools the hot fits of agues, be they never so violent. The distilled water cleanses the skin; and dropped into the eyes, or cloths wet therein and applied, takes away the heat and inflammations in them.

THISTLES

PLACE Some grow in fields, some in meadows, and some among the corn; others on heaths, greens, and waste grounds, in many places.

TIME They all flower in July and August, and their seed is ripe quickly after.

GOVERNMENT AND VIRTUES Mars rules them. Thistles are good to strengthen the stomach. Pliny says, that the juice bathed on the place that wants hair, it being fallen off, will cause it to grow again speedily.

FULLER'S THISTLE, OR TEASEL

It is so well known, that it needs no description, being used by the cloth-workers.

The wild teasel is in all things like the former, but that the prickles are small, soft, and upright, not hooked or stiff: and the flowers of this are of a fine-bluish or pale-carnation colour, but of the manured kind whitish.

PLACE The first grows, being sown, in gardens or fields, for the use of cloth-workers. The other near ditches in many places of Great Britain.

TIME They flower in July, and are ripe near the end of August.

GOVERNMENT AND VIRTUES It is an herb of Venus. Dioscorides says, that the root bruised and boiled in wine until it be thick, and kept in a brazen vessel or pot, and afterwards spread as a salve and applied, does heal fistulas, and also takes away warts and wens. The juice of the leaves, dropped into the ears, kills worms in them. The distilled water of the leaves, dropped into the eyes, takes away redness and mists in them that hinder the sight, and is often used by women to preserve their beauty, and to take away redness and inflammations, and all other discolourings.

MELANCHOLY THISTLE

DESCRIPTION it rises up with a tender single hoary-green stalk, bearing thereon four or five long hoary-green leaves, dented about the edges, the points whereof are little or nothing prickly, and at the top usually but one head, yet sometimes from the bosom of the uppermost leaf there shoots forth another smaller head, scaly and somewhat prickly, with many reddish-purple thrums in the middle, which, being gathered fresh, will keep the colour a great while, and fade not from the stalk in a long time, while it perfects the seed. The root has many long strings fastened to the head, or upper parts, which is blackish, and perishes not.

There is another sort, little differing from the former, but that the leaves are more green above and more hoary underneath, and the stalk, being about two feet high, bearing but one large scaly head, with threads and seeds as the former.

PLACE They grow in many moist meadows of this land, as well in the southern as in the northern parts.

PLATE 25

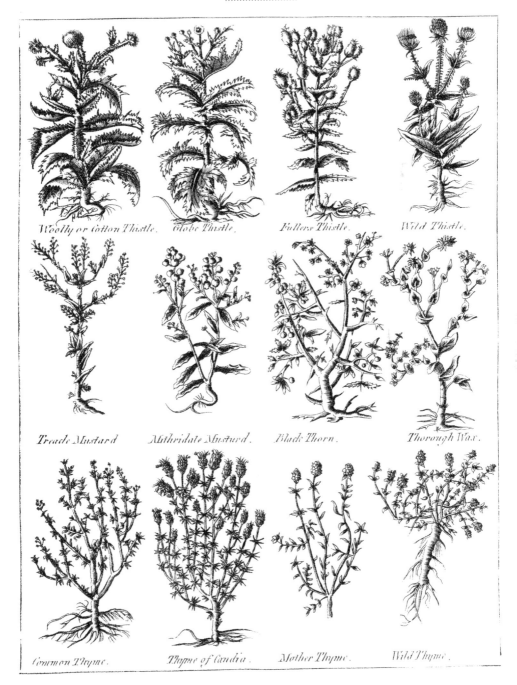

Woolly or Cotton Thistle.   Globe Thistle.   Fullers Thistle.   Wild Thistle.

Treacle Mustard.   Mithridate Mustard.   Black Thorn.   Thorough Wax.

Common Thyme.   Thyme of Candia.   Mother Thyme.   Wild Thyme.

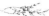
TIME They flower about July or August, and their seed ripens quickly after.

GOVERNMENT AND VIRTUES It is under Capricorn, and therefore under both Saturn and Mars. Their virtues are but few, but those not to be despised; for the decoction of the thistle in wine, being drunk, expels superfluous melancholy out of the body, and makes a man merry.

OUR LADY'S THISTLE

DESCRIPTION our lady's thistle has divers large and broad leaves, lying on the ground, cut in and as it were crumpled, but rather hairy on the edges; of a white-green shining colour, wherein are many lines and strakes of a milky white colour running all over, and set about with many sharp and stiff prickles, among which rises up one or more strong, round, and prickly, stalks, set full of the like leaves up to the top, where, at the end of every branch, comes forth a great, prickly, thistle-like, head, strongly armed with pricks, and with bright purple thrums rising out of the middle of them; after they are past, the seed grows in the said heads, lying in a great deal of soft white down, which is somewhat flattish and shining, large and brown. The root is great, spreading in the ground, with many strings and small fibres fastened thereto. All the whole plant is bitter in taste.

PLACE It is frequent on the bank of almost every ditch.

TIME It flowers and seeds in June, July, and August.

GOVERNMENT AND VIRTUES Our lady's thistle is under Jupiter, and thought to be as good as *carduus benedictus* for agues, as also to open obstructions of the liver and spleen, and thereby is good against the jaundice. It provokes urine, breaks and expels the stone, and is good for the dropsy. The seed and distilled water are held powerful to all the purposes aforesaid: and, besides, it is often applied both inwardly to drink, and outwardly with cloths or sponges to the region of the liver, to cool the distemperature thereof. It cleanses the blood exceedingly: and in spring, if you boil the tender plant, it will change your blood as the season changes, which is a very sure way to preserve health.

WOOLLY, OR COTTON THISTLE

DESCRIPTION this has many large leaves lying on the ground, somewhat cut in, and as it were crumpled, on the edges, of a green colour on the upperside, but covered over with a long hairy wool, or cottony down, set with sharp pricks; from the middle of whose heads of flowers come forth many purplish-crimson threads, sometimes white, although but seldom. The seed, that follows in these white downy heads, is somewhat large, long, and round, resembling the seed of our lady's thistle, but paler. The root is great, and thick, spreading much, yet usually dies after seed-time.

PLACE It grows on divers ditch banks, and in the corn-fields and highways, generally throughout England; and is often found growing in gardens.

TIME It flowers and bears seed about the end of summer, when other thistles flower and seed.

GOVERNMENT AND VIRTUES It is a plant of Mars. Galen says, that the roots and leaves hereof are good for such persons as have their bodies drawn together by some spasm or convulsion, or other infirmities, as the rickets in children; being a disease that hinders their growth, by binding their nerves, ligaments, and whole structures of their body.

THOROUGH-WAX, OR THOROUGH-LEAF

DESCRIPTION common thorough-wax sends forth one straight round stalk, and sometimes more, two feet high and better, whose lower leaves, being of a bluish-green colour, are smaller and narrower than those up higher, and stand close thereto, not compassing it, but, as they grow higher, they more and more encompass the stalk, until it wholly (as it were) pass through them, branching towards the top into many parts, where the leaves grow smaller again, every one standing singly. The flowers are very small and yellow, standing in tufts at the heads of the branches, where afterwards grow the seed, and blackish, many thick thrust together. The root is small, long, and woody, perishing every year after seed-time, and rising again plentifully of its own sowing.

PLACE It is found growing in many corn-fields and pasture-grounds in Great Britain.

TIME It flowers in July, and the seed is ripe in August.

GOVERNMENT AND VIRTUES Both this and the former are under the influence of Saturn. Thorough-wax is of singular good use for bruises and wounds, and ulcers and sores likewise, if the decoction of the herb with water or wine be drunk, and the places washed therewith, or the juice, or green herb bruised or boiled, either by itself or with other herbs, in oil or hog's grease, be made into an ointment to serve all the year. The decoction of the herb, or the powder of the dried herb, taken inwardly, and the same, or the green leaves bruised and applied outwardly, is singularly good to cure ruptures.

THYME

GOVERNMENT AND VIRTUES It is under the government of Venus. This herb is a notable strengthener of the lungs. It purges the body of phlegm, and is an excellent remedy for shortness of breath. An ointment made of it takes away hot swellings and warts, helps the sciatica, takes away pains and hardness of the spleen. It is excellent good for those that are troubled with the gout; it eases pains in the loins and hips. The herb taken any way inwardly comforts the stomach much, and expels wind.

WILD THYME, OR MOTHER OF THYME

PLACE It may be found in commons and other barren places throughout the nation.

GOVERNMENT AND VIRTUES This is likewise under the dominion of Venus, though under the sign Aries, and therefore chiefly appropriated to the head. If you make a vinegar of the herb, and anoint the head with it, it will soon ease the pain thereof. It is excellent good to be given either in a frenzy or lethargy, although they are two contrary diseases. It comforts and strengthens the head, stomach, reins, and womb; expels wind, and breaks the stone.

TOBACCO, ENGLISH, AND INDIAN

DESCRIPTION english tobacco rises up with a thick round stalk, about two feet high, whereon grow thick fat green leaves, not so large as the Indian, round-pointed, and not dented about the edges; at the top stand divers flowers in green husks, scarcely above the brims of the husk, round-pointed also, and of a greenish-yellow colour. Its seed is not very bright, but large, contained in great heads. The roots perish every winter, but rise generally of its own sowing.

Tobacco

Small tobacco

NAMES It is called in Latin *petum* and *nicotiana*.

PLACE AND TIME English tobacco grows much about Winscomb in Gloucestershire, as delighting in a fruitful soil; the other, which we smoke, grows best in Virginia, and is thence carried to some parts of Spain, and there made up and then brought to us, and named Spanish tobacco.

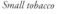

Short-leaved tobacco

GOVERNMENT AND VIRTUES It is a martial plant. It is found by good experience to be available to expectorate tough phlegm from the stomach, chest, and lungs; the juice thereof being made into a syrup, or the distilled water of the herb drunk; or the smoke taken by a pipe as is usual, but fasting. The seed hereof is very effectual to help the tooth-ache, and the ashes of the burnt herb to cleanse the gums and make the teeth white. The herb bruised, and applied to the place grieved with the king's-evil, helps it in nine or ten days effectually. The distilled water is often given with some sugar before the fit of an ague, to lessen it, and takes it away in three or four times using. The green herb, bruised and applied, cures any fresh wound or cut whatsoever: and the juice, put into sores, both cleanses and heals them.

TORMENTIL, OR SEPTFOIL

DESCRIPTION this has many reddish, slender, weak, branches, rising from the root, lying upon the ground, rather leaning than standing upright, with many short leaves that stand closer to the stalks than cinquefoil does (which this is very like) with the footstalk encompassing the branches in several places; but those that grow next to the ground are set upon long footstalks, each whereof are like the leaves of cinquefoil, but somewhat longer and smaller, and dented about the edges, many of them divided into five leaves only, but most of them into seven, whence it is also called septfoil; yet some may have six, and some eight, according to the fertility of the soil. At the tops of the branches stand small yellow flowers, consisting of five leaves, like those of cinquefoil, but smaller. The root is smaller than biltort, somewhat thick, but blacker without, and not so red within, yet sometimes a little crooked, having many blackish fibres.

PLACE It grows as well in woods and shadowy places as in the open country, about the borders of fields in many places of England, and almost in every broomfield in Essex.

TIME It flowers all the summer.

GOVERNMENT AND VIRTUES This is an herb of the Sun. Tormentil is most excellent to stay all kinds of fluxes of blood or humours in man or woman. The juice does wonderfully open obstructions of the liver and lungs, and thereby in short space helps the yellow-jaundice. The powder also, or decoction to be drunk, or to sit therein as a bath, is a fine remedy against abortion in women. Tormentil is no less effectual and powerful a remedy for outward wounds, sores, and hurts; and to put either the juice or powder of the root into such ointments, plasters, and such things as are to be applied to wounds and sores.

TREACLE-MUSTARD

DESCRIPTION it rises up with a hard round stalk about a foot high, parted into some branches, having divers soft-green leaves somewhat long and narrow

PLATE 26

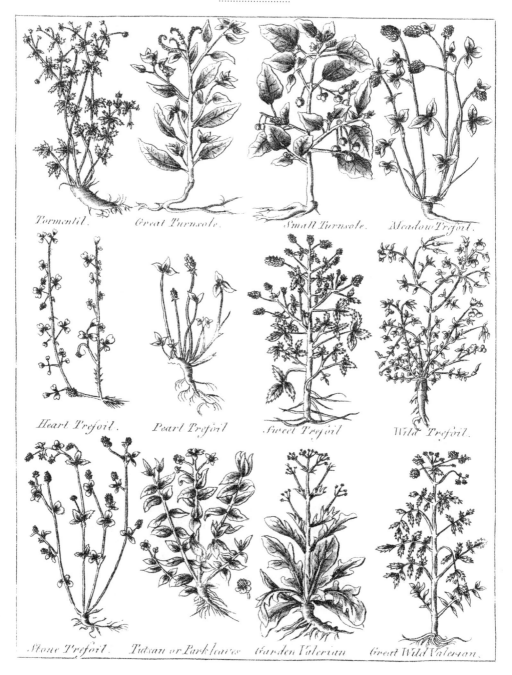

Tormentil.   Great Turnsole.   Small Turnsole.   Meadow Trefoil.

Heart Trefoil.   Pearl Trefoil   Sweet Trefoil   Wild Trefoil.

Stone Trefoil.   Tutsan or Parkleaves   Garden Valerian   Great Wild Valerian.

set thereon, waved, but not cut in on the edges, broadest towards the ends, and somewhat round-pointed; the flowers are white that grow at the tops of the branches, spike-fashion, one above another: after which come large round pouches parted in the middle with a furrow, having one blackish-brown seed on either side, somewhat sharp in taste, and smelling of garlic, especially in the fields where it is natural, but not so much in gardens: the roots are small and thready, perishing every year.

HEART-TREFOIL

Besides the ordinary sorts of trefoil, there are two more remarkable, and one of which may probably be called the heart trefoil, not only because the leaf is triangular like the heart of a man, but also because each leaf contains the perfection of a heart, and that in its proper colour, *viz.* a flesh-colour.

PLACE   It grows near Bow, and parts adjacent.

GOVERNMENT AND VIRTUES   It is under the dominion of the Sun; and, if it were used, would be found a strengthener of the heart and cherisher of the vital spirits, relieving the body against faintings and swoonings.

MEADOW-TREFOIL, OR HONEY-SUCKLES

Meadow-trefoil

GOVERNMENT AND VIRTUES   Mercury has dominion over the common sorts. Dodoneus says, the leaves and flowers are good to ease the griping pains of the guts, the herb being boiled and used in a clyster. If the herb be made into a poultice and applied to inflammations, it will ease them. The juice dropped into the eyes is a familiar medicine with many country people to take away the pin and web (as they call it) in the eyes; it also allays the heat and blood-shooting of them. It is held likewise to be good for wounds. The seed and flowers boiled in water, and after made into a poultice with some oil, and applied, help hard swellings and imposthumes.

Honey-suckle

PEARL-TREFOIL

It differs not from the common sort, save only in this one particular, that it has a white spot in the leaf like a pearl; it is particularly under the dominion of the Moon, and its icon shews that it is of singular virtue against the pearl, or pin and web, in the eye.

TURNSOL, OR HELIOTROPIUM

Great turnsol

Small turnsol

DESCRIPTION the greater turnsol rises up with one upright stalk about a foot high or more, dividing itself almost from the bottom into smaller branches of a hoary colour. At each joint of the stalk and branches grow two small broad leaves, somewhat white or hoary. At the top of the stalks and branches stand many small white flowers, consisting of four and sometimes five very small leaves, set in order one above another, upon a small crooked spike, which turns inwards, opening by degrees as the flowers blow open; after which in their places come forth small cornered seeds, four for the most part standing together. The root is small and thready, perishing every year; and the seed, shedding every year, raises it again the next spring.

PLACE It grows in gardens, and flowers and seeds with us in England, notwithstanding it is not natural to Great Britain, but to Italy, Spain, and France, where it grows plentifully.

GOVERNMENT AND VIRTUES It is an herb of the Sun. Dioscorides says, that a good handful of this, which is called the greater turnsol, boiled in water, and drunk, purges both choler and phlegm; and, boiled with cummin, and drunk, helps the stone in the reins, kidneys, or bladder, provokes urine and the menses, and causes an easy and speedy delivery in child-birth. The leaves bruised and applied to places pained with the gout, or that have been newly set, do give much ease. The seed and the juice of the leaves also being rubbed with a little salt upon warts will, by often using, take them away.

TUTSAN, OR **PARK-LEAVES**

DESCRIPTION it has brownish shining stalks, crested all the length thereof, rising to be two and sometimes three feet high, branching forth even from the bottom, having divers joints, and at each of them two fair large leaves, of a dark bluish-green colour on the upper-side, and of a yellowish-green underneath, turning reddish towards autumn, but abiding on the branches all the winter. At the tops of the stalks and branches stand large yellow flowers, and heads with seed, which being greenish at the first, and afterwards reddish, turn to be of a blackish-purple colour when they are thoroughly ripe, with small brownish seed in them, and then yield a reddish juice or liquor, of a reasonable good scent, somewhat resinous, and of an harsh and styptic taste, as the leaves also and the flowers be, although much less. The root is of a brownish colour, somewhat great, hard, and woody, spreading well in the ground.

PLACE It grows in many woods, groves, and woody-grounds, as parks and forests, and by hedge sides, in many places in Great Britain.

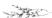

TIME It flowers later than St John's or St Peter's wort.

GOVERNMENT AND VIRTUES It is an herb of Saturn, and a great antivenerean. Tutsan purges choleric humours, as St Peter's wort is said to do; for therein it works the same effects, both to help the sciatica and gout, and to heal burnings by fire. It stays also the bleeding of wounds, if either the green herb be bruised or the powder of the dry be applied thereto. It has been accounted, and certainly is, a sovereign herb to heal any wound or sore either outwardly or inwardly, and therefore always used in drinks, lotions, balms, oils, ointments for any sort of green wound, or old ulcers and sores, in all which the continual experience of former ages has confirmed the use thereof to be admirably good, though it be not so much in use now as when physicians and surgeons were so wise as to use herbs more than they do at present.

GARDEN VALERIAN

DESCRIPTION this has a thick short greyish root, lying for the most part above ground, shooting forth on all sides other such-like small pieces or roots, which have all of them many long and great strings or fibres under them, in the ground, whereby it draws nourishment. From the heads of these roots spring up many green leaves, which at first are somewhat broad and long, without any division at all in them, or dented on the edges; but those that rise up after are more and more divided on each side, some to the middle-rib, made of many leaves together on a stalk, and those upon the stalk in like manner more divided, but smaller towards the top than below. The stalk rises to be a yard high or more, sometimes branched at the top, with many small whitish flowers, sometimes dashed over at the edges with a pale-purplish colour of a little scent; which passing away, there follows small brownish-white seed that is easily carried away with the wind.

PLACE It is generally kept with us in our gardens.

TIME It flowers in June and July, and continues flowering until the frost pull it down.

GOVERNMENT AND VIRTUES This is under the influence of Mercury. Pliny says, that the powder of the root, given in drink, or some of the decoction thereof taken, helps all stoppings and stranglings in any part of the body, whether they proceed of pains in the chest or sides, and takes them away. The root of valerian, boiled with liquorice, raisins, and anise-seed, is good for those that are short winded, and for those that are troubled with a cough, and helps to open the passages and to expectorate phlegm easily. The green herb with the root taken fresh, being bruised and applied to the head, stays rheum and thin distillations.

VERVAIN

Flat vervain

Low vervain

DESCRIPTION   the common vervain has somewhat long and broad leaves next the ground, gashed about the edges, and some only deeply dented, or cut all alike, of a blackish-green colour on the upper side, and somewhat grey underneath. The stalk is square, branched into several parts, rising about two feet high, especially if you reckon the long spike of flowers at the tops of them, which are set on all sides one above another, and sometimes two or three together, being small and gaping, of a purplish-blue colour, and white intermixed; after which come small round seed in small and somewhat long heads. The root is small and long, but of no use.

Upright vervain

PLACE   It grows generally throughout England, in divers places by the hedges, and way-sides, and other waste grounds.

TIME   It flowers about July, and the seed is ripe soon after.

GOVERNMENT AND VIRTUES   This also is an herb of Venus, and an excellent herb for the womb, to strengthen it, and remedy all the cold griefs of it, as plantain does the hot. Vervain is hot and dry, opening obstructions, cleansing and healing. It consolidates and heals also wounds both inward and outward, and stays bleedings; and, used with some honey, heals ulcers in the legs or other parts of the body, as also those ulcers that happen in the mouth.

VINE

VIRTUES   the leaves of the English vine, being boiled, make a good lotion for sore mouths; being boiled with barley-meal into a poultice, it cools inflammations of wounds. The ashes of the burnt branches will make teeth that are black as a coal to be as white as snow, if you do but every morning rub them with it. It is a tree of the Sun, very sympathetical with the body of man.

VIOLETS

Purple violet

TIME   They flower until the end of July, but are best in March and the beginning of April.

Yellow violet

GOVERNMENT AND VIRTUES   They are a fine pleasing plant of Venus, of a mild nature, no way harmful. All the violets are cold and moist while they are fresh and green, and are used to cool any heat or distemperature of the body either inwardly or outwardly. The powder of the purple leaves of the flowers

Strange violet

only, picked and dried, and drunk in water, is said to help the quinsey, and the falling sickness in children, especially in the beginning of the disease. The flowers of the white violets ripen and dissolve swellings.

VIPER'S BUGLOSS

DESCRIPTION this has many long rough leaves lying on the ground, from among which rises up divers hard round stalks, very rough as if they were thick set with prickles or hairs, whereon are set long, rough, hairy, or prickly, sad-green, leaves, somewhat narrow, the middle rib for the most part being white. The flowers stand at the top of the stalks, branched forth into many long spiked leaves of flowers, bowing or turning like the turnsol, all of them opening for the most part on the one side, which are long and hollow, turning up the brims a little, of a purplish-violet colour in them that are fully blown, but more reddish while they are in the bud, as also upon their decay and withering: but in some places of a paler purple colour, with a long pointel in the middle, feathered or parted at the top. After the flowers are fallen, the seeds, growing to be ripe, are blackish, cornered, and pointed somewhat like the head of a vine. The root is somewhat great, and blackish, and woolly, when it grows toward seed-time; and perishes in the winter.

There is another sort, little differing from the former, only in that it bears white flowers.

PLACE The first grows wild almost every where. That with white flowers about Lewes, in Sussex.

TIME They flower in summer, and their seed is ripe quickly after.

GOVERNMENT AND VIRTUES This is an herb of the Sun. The roots or seed are thought to be most effectual to comfort the heart, and expel sadness, or cause less melancholy; it tempers the blood, and allays hot fits of agues. The seed drunk in wine procures abundance of milk in women's breasts. The same also eases the pains in the loins, back, and kidneys.

Wall-flower

WALL-FLOWERS, OR WINTER GILLIFLOWERS

DESCRIPTION The common single wall-flowers, which grow wild abroad, have sundry small, long, narrow, and dark green, leaves, set without order upon small round whitish woody stalks, which bear at the tops divers single yellow flowers one above another, every one having four leaves a piece, and of a very sweet scent: after which come long pods containing reddish seed. The root is white, hard, and thready.

Winter gilliflower

PLACE It grows upon church walls, and other stone walls in divers places. The other sorts in gardens only.

TIME All the single kinds do flower in the end of autumn, and, if the winter be mild, especially in the months of February, March, and April, and until the heat of the spring do spend them; but the double kinds continue not flowering in that manner all the year long, although they flower very early sometimes, and in some places very late.

GOVERNMENT AND VIRTUES The Moon rules them. Galen, in his seventh book of simple medicines, says, that the yellow wall-flowers work more powerfully than any of the other kinds, and are therefore of more use in physic. They cleanse the blood and free the liver and reins from obstructions, stay inflammations and swellings, and are a singular remedy for the gout, and all aches and pains in the joints and sinews. A conserve made of the flowers is used for a remedy both for the apoplexy and palsy.

WALNUT-TREE

TIME It blossoms early, before the leaves come forth; and the fruit is ripe in September.

GOVERNMENT AND VIRTUES This is a plant of the Sun; let the fruit of it be gathered accordingly, which you shall find to be of most virtue whilst they are green, before they have shells. The bark of the tree binds and dries very much, and the leaves are much of the same temperature; but the leaves, when they are older, are heating and drying in the second degree, and harder of digestion than when they are fresh.

The juice of the outer green husks, boiled up with honey, is an excellent gargle for sore mouths, the heat and inflammations in the throat and stomach. The kernels, when they grow old, are more oily, and therefore not so fit to be eaten, but are then used to heal the wounds of the sinews, gangrenes, and carbuncles. The said kernels, being burned, are then very astringent, and will then stay lasks and women's menses, being taken in red wine; and stay the falling of the hair. The green husks will do the like, being used in the same manner. The kernels, beaten with rue and wine, being applied, help the quinsey. A piece of the green husk, put into a hollow tooth, eases the pain. The young green nuts, taken before they be half ripe, and preserved with sugar, are of good use for those that have weak stomachs, or defluxions thereon.

PLATE 27

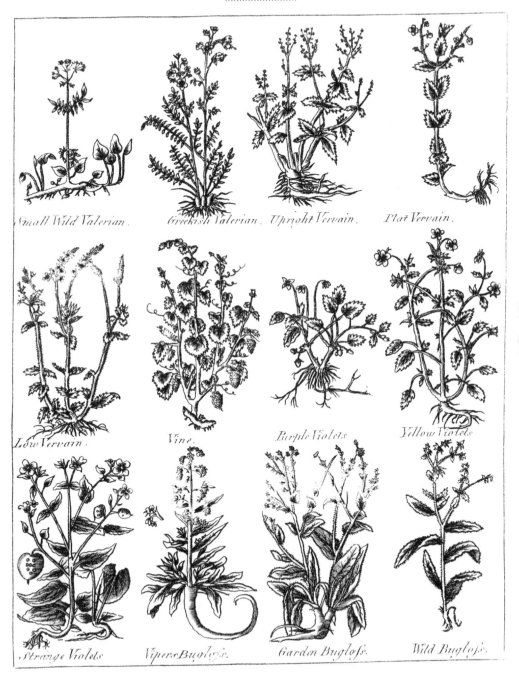

Small Wild Valerian.   Greekish Valerian.   Upright Vervain.   Flat Vervain.

Low Vervain.   Vine.   Purple Violets.   Yellow Violets.

Strange Violets.   Vipers Buglofs.   Garden Buglofs.   Wild Buglofs.

PLATE 28

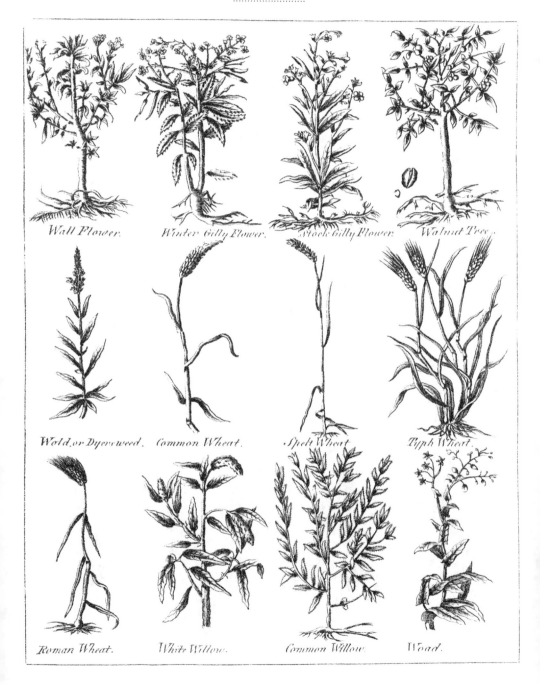

Wall Flower.   Winter Gilly Flower.   Stock Gilly Flower.   Walnut Tree.

Wold, or Dyersweed.   Common Wheat.   Spelt Wheat   Typh Wheat.

Roman Wheat.   White Willow.   Common Willow.   Woad.

Common wheat

Roman wheat

Spelt wheat

Typh wheat

WHEAT

GOVERNMENT AND VIRTUES It is under Venus. Pliny says, that the corns of wheat roasted upon an iron pan, and eaten, are a present remedy for those that are chilled with cold. The oil, pressed from wheat between two thick plates of iron or copper heated, heals all tetters and ringworms, being used warm. The flour of wheat, mixed with the juice of henbane, stays the flux of humours to the joints, being laid thereon. The said meal boiled in vinegar helps the shrinking of the sinews, says Pliny. The decoction of the bran of wheat or barley is of good use to bathe those places that are bursten by a rupture, and the said bran boiled in good vinegar, and applied to swollen breasts, helps them, and stays all inflammations. The leaves of wheat-meal, applied with salt, take away hardness of the skin, warts, and hard knots in the flesh.

Common willow

White willow

WILLOW-TREE

GOVERNMENT AND VIRTUES   the Moon owns it. The leaves, bark, and seed, are used to staunch bleeding at nose and mouth. It helps also to stay thin, hot, sharp, salt, distillations from the head upon the lungs, causing a consumption. The leaves bruised with some pepper, and drunk in wine, much help the wind cholic. The leaves bruised, and boiled in wine and drunk, stay the heat of lust. Galen says, the flowers have an admirable faculty in drying up humours, being a medicine without any sharpness or corrosion. The bark works the same effects, if used in the same manner; and the tree has always bark upon it, though not always flowers. The burnt ashes of the bark, being mixed with vinegar, takes away warts, corns, and superfluous flesh. The decoction of the leaves or bark in wine, takes away scurf, or dandruff, by washing the place with it. It is a fine cool tree, the boughs of which are very convenient to be placed in the chamber of one sick of a fever.

Woad

Wild woad

WOAD

DESCRIPTION   it has divers large leaves, long, and somewhat broad, like those of the greater plantain, but larger, thicker, of a greenish colour, and somewhat blue; from among which leaves rises up a lusty stalk, three or four feet high, with divers leaves set thereon; the higher the stalk rises, the smaller are the leaves: at the top it spreads into divers branches, at the end of which appear very pretty little yellow flowers, which, after they pass away, come husks, long, and somewhat flat; in form they resemble a tongue; in colour, they are black, and hang downwards. The seed contained within these husks, if it be a little chewed, gives an azure colour. The root is white and long.

PLACE It is sowed in fields for the benefit of it, where it is cut three times a year.

TIME It flowers in June, but it is long after before the seed is ripe.

Garden woad

GOVERNMENT AND VIRTUES It is a cold and dry plant of Saturn. The herb is so drying and binding, that it is not fit to be given inwardly. An ointment made thereof staunches bleeding. A plaister made thereof, and applied to the region of the spleen, takes away the hardness and pains thereof. The ointment is excellent good in such ulcers as abound with moisture, and takes away corroding and fretting humours. It cools inflammations, and stays defluxions of blood to any part of the body.

WOLD, WELD, OR DYER'S WEED

DESCRIPTION the common kind grows bushing with many leaves, long, narrow, and flat upon the ground, of a dark bluish-green colour, somewhat like unto woad, but nothing so large; a little crumpled, and as it were round-pointed, which do so abide the first year; and, the next spring, from among them rise divers round stalks two or three feet high, beset with many such-like leaves thereon, but smaller, and shooting forth some small branches, which with the stalks carry many small yellow flowers in a long spiked head at the tops of them, where afterwards comes the seed, which is small and black, inclosed in heads that are divided at the tops into four part. The root is long, white, and thick, abiding the winter. The whole herb changes to be yellow after it has been in flower a while.

PLACE It grows every where by the way-sides, in moist grounds as well as dry, in fields and lanes. In Sussex and Kent they call it green-weed.

TIME It flowers about June.

GOVERNMENT AND VIRTUES Mathiolus says, that the root hereof cuts tough phlegm, digests raw phlegm, thins gross humours, dissolves hard tumours, and opens obstructions. The people in some parts of England bruise the herb, and lay it to cuts or wounds in the hands or legs.

WOLF-BANE

DESCRIPTION It has a root shining within like alabaster. There are many kinds, all extremely pernicious and poisonous; for, if a man or beast be wounded with arrow, knife, sword, or any other instrument, dipped in the juice of this herb, they die incurable within half an hour. The reason this herb goes by the name of wolf-bane was this: men in former ages hunting for wolves used to poison pieces of raw flesh with the juice of this herb and lay them as baits, on which the wolves died presently.

WOODBINE, OR HONEY-SUCKLE

TIME They flower in June, and the fruit is ripe in August.

GOVERNMENT AND VIRTUES It is an herb of Mercury, and appropriated to the lungs. It is fitting a conserve, made of the flowers of it, were kept in every house; I know no better cure for an asthma.

WORMWOOD

PLACE It grows familiarly in England by the sea-side.

Sea-wormwood

DESCRIPTION It starts up out of the earth with many round woody hoary stalks from one root; its height is four feet, or three at the least. The leaves are long, narrow, white, hoary, like southernwood, only broader and longer, in taste rather salty than bitter, because it grows so near the salt water: at the joints with the leaves, toward the tops, it bears little yellow flowers. The root lies deep, and is woody.

Common wormwood

PLACE It grows upon the tops of the mountains; but is usually nursed up in gardens for the use of the apothecaries in London.

TIME All wormwoods usually flower in August, a little sooner or later.

GOVERNMENT AND VIRTUES Wormwood is an herb of Mars. It is hot and dry in the first degree. Moths are under the dominion of Mars; his herb, wormwood, being laid amongst clothes, will hinder moths from hurting them. Wormwood is good for an ague.

YARROW

Called also nose-bleed, mil-foil, and thousand-leaf.

DESCRIPTION It has many long leaves spread upon the ground, finely cut and divided into many small parts. Its flowers are white, upon divers green stalks which rise from among the leaves.

PLACE It is frequent in all pastures.

TIME It flowers not until the latter end of August.

GOVERNMENT AND VIRTUES It is under the influence of Venus. An ointment of it cures wounds, and is most fit for such as have inflammations. The ointment of it is not only good for green wounds, but also for ulcers and fistulas. It stays the shedding of hair, the head being bathed with the decoction of it. Inwardly taken, it helps the retentive faculty of the stomach, and such as cannot hold their water. The leaves, chewed, ease the tooth-ache.

YUCCA, OR JUCCA

DESCRIPTION This Indian plant has a thick tuberous root, spreading in time into many tuberous heads, whence shoot forth many long, hard, and hollow, leaves, very sharp-pointed, compassing one another at the bottom, of a greyish-green colour, abiding continually, or seldom falling away, with sundry hard threads running in them, and, being withered, become pliant to bind things. From the midst thereof springs forth a strong round stalk, divided into sundry branches, whereon stand divers somewhat large white flowers, hanging downwards, consisting of six leaves with divers veins, of a weak reddish or bluish colour, spread on the back of three outer leaves, from the middle to the bottom, not reaching to the edge of any leaf; which abide not long, but quickly fall away.

PLACE AND TIME It grows in divers places of the West Indies, as in Virginia and New England, and flowers about the latter end of July.

VIRTUES There has no property hereof conducible to physical use as yet been heard of, but some of its vices. The natives in Virginia use, for bread, the roots hereof. The raw juice is dangerous, if not deadly. It is very probable that the Indians used to poison the heads of their darts with this juice, which they usually keep by them for that purpose.

PLATE 29

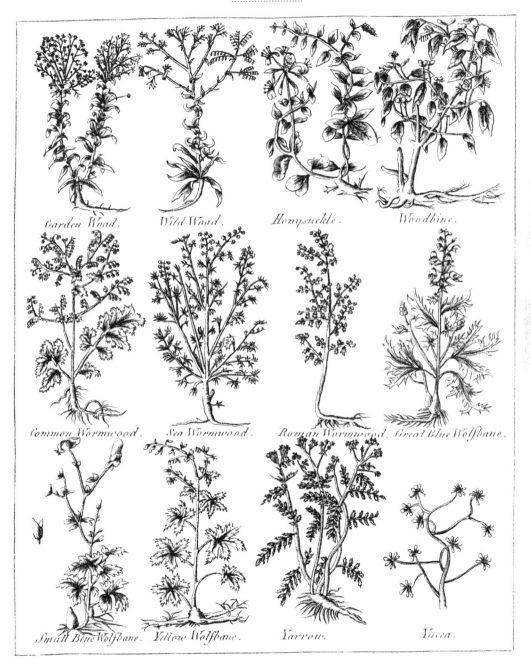

Garden Woad.   Wild Woad.   Honysuckle.   Woodbine.

Common Wormwood.   Sea Wormwood.   Roman Wormwood.   Great Blue Wolfbane.

Small Blue Wolfbane.   Yellow Wolfbane.   Yarrow.   Yucca.

OF THE GATHERING, DRYING, AND PRESERVING OF PLANTS, HERBS, AND FLOWERS

THE LEAVES OF HERBS OR TREES

Choose only such as are green and full of juice, pick them carefully, and cast away such as are declining, for they will putrify the rest.

Note in what place they most delight to grow, and gather them there; for betony that grows in the shadow is far better than that which grows in the Sun, because it delights in the shadow: so also such herbs as delight to grow near the water should be gathered near the water, though you may find some of them on dry ground.

The leaves of such herbs as run up to seed are not so good when they are in flower as before (some few excepted, the leaves of which are seldom or never used): in such cases, if through ignorance they were not known, or through negligence forgotten, you had better take the top and the flower than the leaf.

Dry them well in the Sun, and not in the shade; for, if the Sun draw away the virtues of herbs, it must needs do the like by hay; which the experience of every country farmer will explode as a vulgar error.

Let the planet that governs the herb be angular, and the stronger the better. In herbs of Saturn, let Saturn be in the ascendant; in herbs of Mars, let Mars be in the mid-heaven, for in those houses they delight: let the Moon apply to them by good aspect, and let her not be in the houses of their enemies; if you cannot well stay till she apply to them, let her be with a fixed star of their nature.

Having well dried them, put them up in brown-paper bags, and press them not too hard together, and keep them in a dry place near the fire. As for the duration of dried herbs, a just time cannot be given, for, first, such as grow upon dry grounds will keep better than such as grow on moist; secondly, such herbs as are full of juice will not keep so long as such as are drier; thirdly, such herbs as are well dried will keep longer than such as are ill dried. Yet by this you may know when they are corrupted, *viz.* by their loss of colour, or smell, or both; and, if they be corrupted, reason will tell you that they must needs corrupt the bodies of those people that take them. Remember to gather all the leaves in the hour of that planet that governs them.

OF FLOWERS

The flower, which is the beauty of the plant, and of none of the least use in physic, grows yearly, and it is to be gathered when it is in its prime.

As for the time of gathering them, let the planetary hour, and the plant they come of, be observed, as above directed; as for the time of day, let it be when the Sun shines upon them, that they may be dry; for, if you gather either flowers or herbs when they are wet or dewy, they will not keep. Dry them well in the Sun, and keep them in papers near the fire. So long as they retain their colour and smell they are good; either of them being gone, so is their virtue also.

OF SEEDS

The seed is that part of the plant which is endued with faculty to bring forth its like, and it contains potentially the whole plant itself.

As for place, let them be gathered from the places where they delight to grow. Let them be fully ripe when they are gathered, and forget not the celestial harmony before-mentioned, for I have found by experience that their virtues are twice as great at such times as others: there is an appointed time for every thing under the Sun. When you have gathered them, dry them a little in the Sun before you lay them up. You need not be so careful of keeping them so near the fire as the other before mentioned, because they are fuller of spirit, and therefore not subject to corrupt. As for the time of their duration, it is palpable they will keep a great many years; yet, they are best the first year, and this I make appear by a good argument, they will grow soonest the first year they be set, therefore then are they in their prime, and it is an easy matter to renew them yearly.

OF ROOTS

Of roots, choose such as are neither rotten nor worm-eaten, but proper in their taste, colour, and smell; such as exceed neither in softness nor hardness.

Give me leave here to deny the vulgar opinion, that the sap falls down into the root in the autumn, and rises again in the spring, as men go to bed at night, and rise again in the morning; which idle tale of untruth is so grounded in the heads not only of the vulgar, but also of the learned, that men cannot drive it out by reason: If the sap fall into the root in the fall of the leaf, and lie there all the winter, then must the root grow only in the winter, as experience witnesses: but the root grows not at all in winter, as the same experience teaches, but only in the summer; for example: If you set an apple kernel in the spring, it will grow to a pretty bigness in that summer, and be no bigger next spring: the truth is, when the Sun declines from the tropic of Cancer, the sap begins to congeal both in root and branch; when he touches the tropic of Capricorn, and ascends to upward, it begins to get thin again by degrees, as it congealed.

The drier time you gather your roots in, the better they are: for they have the less excrementitious moisture in them. Such roots as are soft should be dried in the Sun, or else hang them in the chimney corner upon a string: as for such as are hard, you may dry them any where. Such roots as are large will keep longer than such as are small: yet most of them will keep a year. Such roots as are soft should be always kept near the fire; and take this general rule for it, if in winter you find any of your roots, herbs, or flowers, begin to grow moist, as many times they will (for it is best to look to them once a month) dry them by a very gentle fire; or, if you can with convenience keep them near the fire, you may save this trouble.

OF BARKS

Barks which physicians use in medicines are of three sorts: of fruits, of roots, of boughs.

The barks of fruits are to be taken when the fruits are full ripe, as oranges, lemons, &c. The barks of trees are best gathered in the spring, if it be of great trees, as oaks, or the like; because then they come easiest off, and so you may dry them if you please: but your best way is to gather all barks only for present use.

As for the bark of roots, it is thus to be gotten: take the roots of such herbs as have pith in them, as parsley, fennel, &c. slit them in the middle, and when you have taken out the pith (which you may easily and quickly do) that which remains is called the bark, and is only to be used.

OF JUICES

Juices are to be pressed out of herbs when they are young and tender, and also of some stalks and tender tops of herbs and plants, and also of some flowers.

Having gathered the herb you would preserve the juice of, when it is very dry, bruise it well in a stone mortar with a wooden pestle; then, having put it into a canvas bag, press it hard in a press, then take the juice and clarify it.

When you have clarified it, and it is cold, put it into a glass, and put so much oil on it as will cover it the thickness of two fingers; the oil will swim at top, and so keep the air from coming to putrify it; or, instead of oil, when you have clarified the juice as before, boil it over the fire till (when cold) it be the thickness of honey: then tie it down close, and keep it for use.

Whatever you gather of plants, herbs, fruits, flowers, roots, barks, seeds, &c. for medicinal purposes, either for distillation, syrups, juleps, decoctions, oils, electuaries, conserves, preserves, ointments, and the like, must be gathered when they are in the greatest vigour and fullest perfection; for in that state only are they fit to be applied for the restoration and preservation of our health; and, when they are applied, let it be done under the sympathetic influence of planets participating in the same nature; the benefits of which are so amply demonstrated in my *Display of the Occult Sciences*.

INDEX

Printed in the United States
by Baker & Taylor Publisher Services